A Manual of
Paediatric Dentistry

Train up a child in the way he should go: and when he is old, he will not depart from it.

Proverbs xxii 6

For Churchill Livingstone:

Publisher: Mike Parkinson
Project Manager: Ninette Premdas
Copy Editor: Alison Gale
Project Controller: Nancy Arnott

A Manual of Paediatric Dentistry

FOURTH EDITION

R.J. Andlaw
Unversity of Bristol Dental School

W.P. Rock
University of Birmingham Dental School

With illustration by
G.C. van Beek BDS

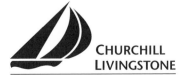

CHURCHILL
LIVINGSTONE

NEW YORK EDINBURGH LONDON MADRID MELBOURNE SAN FRANCISCO
TOKYO 1996

CHURCHILL LIVINGSTONE
Medical Division of Pearson Professional Limited

Distributed in the United States of America by Churchill
Livingstone Inc., 650 Avenue of the Americas, New York,
N.Y. 10011, and by associated companies, branches and
representatives throughout the world.

First published as *A Manual of paedodontics* 1982
Second edition 1987
Third edition 1992
Fourth edition 1996

ISBN 0 443 053723

British Library Cataloguing in Publication Data
A catalogue record for this book is available from the British
Library.

Library of Congress Cataloging in Publication Data
A catalog record for this book is available from the Library of
Congress.

Medical knowledge is constantly changing. As new
information becomes available, changes in treatment,
procedures, equipment and the use of drugs become
necessary. The authors and the publishers have, as far as it is
possible, taken care to ensure that the information given in
this text is accurate and up to date. However, readers are
strongly advised to confirm that the information, especially
with regard to drug usage, complies with current legislation
and standards of practice.

The
publisher's
policy is to use
**paper manufactured
from sustainable forests**

Printed in Singapore.

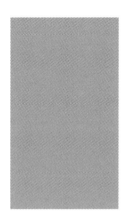

Preface to the Fourth Edition

Since this book was first published in 1982, new editions have been produced at about 5-year intervals. For this fourth edition the process of revision and updating has continued, but without extending the objectives beyond those set for the first edition. The emphasis, therefore, remains firmly on the practical aspects of paediatric dentistry. Nearly every chapter has been subjected to some revision, and a short chapter on dental erosion has been added.

The most obvious change is in the title, in which *paediatric dentistry* has been substituted for *paedodontics*. We considered making this change for the previous edition, because *paediatric dentistry* has become established in the UK as the official title of our specialty, but we were persuaded that it was more undesirable to change the name of an established book than to run the risk of sounding old-fashioned. We now feel the balance has tipped in the other direction and that the change is justified. Keeping the cost of the book within the reach of undergraduate students has always been an important consideration, and we have decided against introducing clinical photographs in addition to, or instead of, some of the line drawings. We feel the drawings adequately complement the text; some new drawings have been added, and others modified.

A questionnaire was sent to colleagues in all the UK dental schools to obtain feedback and ideas for improving the book. We are grateful to those who responded, and also to Linda Shaw for advice regarding erosion, to Iain Mackie for helpful comments, and to Glyn Duggan for general assistance.

Bristol, 1996   R.J.A.
                                                                 W.P.R.

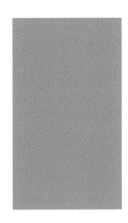

Preface to the First Edition

This book has been written primarily for under-graduate dental students but we hope it will also be of interest and value to practising dentists. Our aim has been to write a practical manual, not a comprehensive textbook. Thus, treatment aspects have been considered in detail but other aspects such as aetiology, clinical features and histopathology, have been excluded or considered only briefly. We have included most of the common forms of treatment in paedo-dontics, but there are some omissions; for example, we have not described the extraction of teeth or other surgical procedures.

We would greatly value constructive criticisms from our colleagues, which would be most helpful in preparing further editions. The book is strongly influenced by current ideas and practices in the United Kingdom and, inevitably, it is orientated towards the British reader; for this we beg the indulgence of our overseas readers.

The tabular format chosen for describing many of the clinical techniques is a modification of that used by Dr Milton Houpt in *Tas Analyses of Procedures in Paedodontics* (U.W. Public Health Service, 1975). To avoid disrupting the continuity of the tables, illu-strations are placed at the end of each table. We hope students will find this format instructive and easy to follow.

We wish to record our gratitude to the following colleagues who read sections of the drafts and made helpful suggestions: Tom Dowell, Glyn Duggan, Don Glenwright, Hugh Edmondson, Stephen Kneebone and Roger Smith. We also thank Mrs Elaine Collings, who typed the manuscript, and all those at Churchill Livingstone who helped in the publication of this book.

Bristol, 1982
R.J.A.
W.P.R.

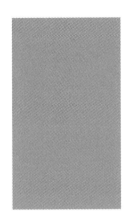

Contents

The child patient

Part 1

1 The first appointment

The practice of paediatric dentistry, as indeed of all branches of dentistry, should be governed by a simple but fundamental philosophy: treat the patient not the tooth. Implicit in this philosophy is a commitment to consider the child's feelings, to gain the child's confidence and cooperation, to perform treatment in a kind, sympathetic manner, and to be concerned not only with providing the treatment currently required but also with promoting the child's future dental health by stimulating positive attitudes and behaviour regarding dental care.

The child's first dental visit should be used to establish a sound basis for achieving these aims. The visit should be organized in such a way that it becomes an enjoyable experience for the child. It should be regarded primarily as a mutual assessment session during which the dentist assesses the child, and the child assesses the dentist and the surgery environment. It is recognised that sometimes, for example when the child attends in acute pain, the ideal procedure may have to be modified, but the fundamental aims of the first session should never be abandoned.

A child's first dental appointment may not be made until the child is about $2\frac{1}{2}$ to 3 years old, when the primary dentition is fully erupted. Parents should, however, receive information regarding the prevention of dental disease during ante- and post-natal care, and those who visit a dentist should also receive such information. It is important to give parents advice about diet, oral hygiene, and the use of fluorides. These topics are discussed in Chapters 3 and 4. In addition, parents should be encouraged to introduce their child to the dentist at an early age in order to encourage the child to accept the dentist and the dental environment without fear. The infant may be examined as described and illustrated on page 7, comfortably cradled in a parent's arms.

1.1 PREPARATION FOR THE CHILD'S FIRST VISIT

Parents usually try in some way to prepare their child for the dental visit. Some parents, through their own fears or ignorance, do more harm than good in this attempt. It is therefore sensible to advise parents on how to prepare their child, and a letter that has been prepared for this purpose is presented on page 4.

The aims of the first session with a child patient are:

1. To establish good communication with the child and parent.
2. To obtain important background information (i.e. the patient's social, dental and medical history).
3. To examine the child, and to obtain radiographs if required.
4. To introduce the child to a simple treatment procedure.
5. To explain treatment aims to the child and parent.

Dear parents

I enclose an appointment card for your child. I hope the date and time will be convenient—please contact me if you cannot attend.

Most people (adults included) are rather nervous at the prospect of visiting a dentist for the first time. I hope the following notes will be helpful.

Preparation for the visit

Parents sometimes try to prepare their children for the visit by saying that the dentist 'will not hurt', or by bribing them to be good with the promise of a toy (or even a sweet!). I suggest that it is better to be as casual as possible. Simply inform your child, either on the morning of the appointment or on the day before, that you will be taking him/her to visit me and that I will count his/her teeth and help to look after them. Avoid conversation in the home that might include unfavourable references to dentistry.

What will be done?

My aim will be to make the visit enjoyable, to set a good foundation for gaining your child's trust and confidence. I will first ask you and your child a few questions to obtain essential background information, for example, about general health, any past dental experience etc. I will then examine your child's mouth and, if necessary, take X-ray pictures— you will be welcome to remain with your child during these procedures if you wish. Finally I will outline what I can do to help, not only in dealing with any problems that may be present but also in preventing dental disease.

If your child has toothache or any other dental problem I will attend to it, but ideally I will not carry out treatment during the first visit.

Further visits

Any treatment that may be required can usually be started at the second visit, but will only be started if the child's confidence and cooperation have been obtained. Some children require several introductory visits before treatment can proceed.

Parents usually remain in the waiting room, but you will be welcome to come into the surgery if your child needs your support.

I look forward to meeting you soon, and I hope your child will enjoy coming to see me.

1.2 COMMUNICATION WITH CHILD AND PARENT

Most patients have some anxiety about visiting a dentist for the first time, and it should therefore be an important objective for the dentist and staff to allay this anxiety. The receptionist should greet the child in a friendly and cheerful manner, and the waiting room should contain evidence that children are welcome (e.g. children's posters, periodicals, books and toys). Thus, the whole environment of reception and waiting areas should communicate a warm sense of friendship and welcome.

On meeting the child and parent, the dentist should establish friendly communication with them while at the same time obtaining the information that constitutes the parent's history. Ideally, this meeting should not take place in the surgery, but in another room (Swallow et al 1975); if in the surgery, it is preferable to offer the child a chair other than the dental chair. This approach allows the dentist time to assess and, if necessary, to allay the child's anxiety before placing the child in a more stressful situation.

It is desirable to meet the parent with the child mainly to obtain a full history, important details of which may not be provided by the child. Moreover, very young or apprehensive children usually need the psychological support of a parent in the surgery, at least at their first visit. On subsequent visits, the dentist must decide whether to separate child and parent by asking the parent to remain in the waiting room. Some dentists invariably insist on working with the child alone; others are more flexible and base their decisions on the age and behaviour of the child, and on the character of the parent. However, it is always important to gain the parent's interest and cooperation, so that effective home care is encouraged. There is some evidence that most children, especially the very young, are more cooperative when a parent is present, and that parents generally prefer to be present for all or some of their child's treatment (Fenlon et al 1993).

Some dentists find communicating with children easy, others find it difficult. An essential ingredient in successful communication is to show interest in the child, and this can readily be achieved by asking simple questions about the home, school and favourite leisure activities. The dentist should also communicate visually by appearing relaxed, friendly and cheerful, and should use opportunities that may arise to communicate physically, for example by shaking hands or patting the child on the shoulder, or by stroking a girl's 'beautiful hair' or tickling a young child; there are many opportunities depending on the child's age and sex. Especially with the very young child, and with the mentally handicapped, this visual and physical communication is most important.

1.3 HISTORY

The information that constitutes the patient's history is divided into three parts: the social, dental and medical histories. History-taking provides essential information on which treatment planning is based. A suggested outline for history-taking is given on pages 5 and 6.

It is important to appreciate that details of the social, dental and medical histories are accurate only at the time they are recorded; they can change considerably within a short period of time. For example, the birth of another child or a change of address can affect the parent's ability to take the child to the dental surgery; the child's attitudes may change for better or worse during a course of treatment; and medical status can change significantly. Therefore the details recorded at the first meeting with a child patient cannot be assumed to be accurate and relevant at a review visit 4–6 months later. It is important to keep the history up to date by further questioning at review visits.

An outline for history-taking

	Information	Rationale	Notes
Social history	Name (including any abbreviated name or nickname) Address School	A child should be addressed by the name he/she prefers.	
	Brothers and sisters Pets Favourite activity at home, at school	Simple questioning about home and school is the most natural way of communicating with a child. In addition, the answers provide an insight into the child's interests and home environment. Recording these details provides the dentist with topics of conversation at subsequent meetings.	The type of response to questioning immediately gives some indication of the child's character and state of mind. The child may respond in an easy, friendly manner, indicating a happy and relaxed state of mind, or may refuse to respond at all, indicating shyness, anxiety or defiance.
	Mother's occupation— any difficulties in bringing the child for further appointments?	Most commonly it is the mother who accompanies the child. Any difficulty in attending would have to be considered in treatment planning, especially if a long course of treatment is required.	
	Father's occupation	Classifying the family by social class, based on the father's occupation, allows some prediction to be made of family attitudes towards dentistry (Beal 1996).	Often, the father's occupation emerges while establishing the mother's occupation. Sometimes, however, it may seem inappropriate to question on this point, in which case the information may be obtained at a subsequent meeting, perhaps after asking the child "what do you want to be when you grow up?"
Dental history	C/o—*Complaining of:* Is the patient attending because of a specific complaint? If not, what is the reason for attendance e.g. routine check-up, or referred following dental inspection at school?	It is essential to establish the reason for the patient's attendance.	
	HPC—*History of present complaint:* If complaint is toothache, obtain the following information: location of pain when did it start? is it intermittent or continuous? if intermittent, how long does it last? is it brought by hot, cold or sweet stimuli, or when eating?	The symptoms of toothache give an indication of the probable pathology of pulp, e.g. intermittent pain of short duration brought on by hot, cold or sweet—pulp hyperaemia; spontaneous pain, severe, keeps child awake—acute pulpitis, abscess.	Unfortunately, the symptoms described by a child or parent may be vague and of little diagnostic value.

An outline for history-taking *(contd)*

	Information	Rationale	Notes
	does pain keep child awake at night? is pain relieved by analgesics? *PDH—Past dental history:*		
	Has dental care been regular or irregular in the past?	The regularity of past dental care gives an indication of the parent's attitudes to dental health.	
	Has previous dental treatment been given elsewhere? If so, why has the parent changed dentist?	If previous treatment upset the child, the reasons need to be pursued in such a way as to show the child that the dentist is interested and sympathetic, and that every effort will be made to overcome the problem.	
	Has the child had any experience of dental treatment? If so, what treatment e.g. 'fillings' extractions local analgesia general anaesthesia?		When asking a child about previous experience of local analgesia, it is better to ask "was your tooth made to go to sleep?" than "did you have an injection?" or "did you have a needle?", which would be considered threatening by many children. Similarly, when asking about general anaesthesia, "did you go to sleep?" is better than "did you have gas?"
	Attitudes of the child to any of the above treatments (with a young child, the parent's opinion is relevant)	Any unfavourable attitudes to specific items of treatment must be taken into account in treatment planning. To pursue any form of treatment ignorant of the child's attitudes to that treatment reflects a lack of consideration for the child's feelings which is incompatible with the principles of good patient management	The child's attitudes to previous treatment may be assessed by the response to simple questions like "did you find it easy?", "was it OK?"
	Attitudes of the parent to dental treatment	Parent's attitudes and expectations regarding dental treatment differ greatly; a treatment plan beyond their expectations should not be started without first explaining and justifying its value.	It may be anticipated that some parents would not appreciate the value of, for example, conservative treatment of primary teeth, or of preventive treatment.
Medical history	*Heart* congenital heart disease rheumatic fever, chorea *Blood* anaemia, thalassaemia sickle cell trait/anaemia bleeding disorder *Respiratory tract* infections asthma *Endocrine* diabetes *Gastrointestinal* *Liver* jaundice hepatitis *Kidney* *Bone and joint* *Central nervous system* epilepsy mental or physical handicap *Recent or current medication* *Allergies* *Previous operations or serious illnesses* *Family history of serious illness*	The health risks that medical conditions present have been considered in detail by Moore & Hobson (1989, 1990).	It is important to adopt a systematic approach to obtaining a medical history. The current recommendations for the prevention of infective endocarditis have been reviewed by Longman & Martin (1993).

1.4 EXAMINATION

1.4.1   Clinical examination

Extra-oral examination

Any obvious extra-oral abnormalities noted during history-taking should be examined more closely. An outline of points to note is given in Table 1.1.

Intra-oral examination

It is hoped that any anxiety that the child may have felt on arrival will have been reduced or eliminated during history-taking. The child should then be happy to sit on the dental chair.

A good approach is to ask "how many teeth do you have?" and to suggest "let's count your teeth"; this is probably less threatening to a child than to say "I want to look at your teeth". It is highly desirable that the child should respond favourably to this approach, but there is always a chance, especially with young children, that they will become anxious and uncooperative when asked to leave their parent's side and sit on the dental chair. Therefore the preferred approach with a young child (less than about 5 years old), even when the child appears happy and relaxed during history-taking, is to ask the parent to sit on the chair and lay

the child across his/her lap; the child's head is supported by the parent's right arm (Fig. 1.1). This arrangement allows the child to retain the sense of security provided by the parent, and the child's reclined position is excellent for oral examination and for simple introductory treatment procedures; in contrast, a child placed for the first time on a dental chair may feel ill-at-ease, especially in the reclined position.

If the child was confident enough during the first visit to sit on the chair alone, the level of confidence would be even higher at the second visit and transfer to the chair could easily be made; but the position in the parent's lap is so satisfactory that there need be no urgency to make this transfer.

The initial examination need only be superficial, the most important objective being to gain the child's confidence and allay anxiety. It is reasonable, therefore, not to wear surgical gloves at this stage because the unnatural appearance they give the dentist's hands might create anxiety, and because the dentist's fingers need not extend into the child's mouth for this initial

Table 1.1 An outline for clinical examination

Extra-oral
General appearance—size and weight
Gait
Skin, complexion
Eyes, lips
Facial symmetry
Lymph glands

Intra-oral
Soft tissues
   cheeks
   lips
   tongue
   tonsils
   hard and soft palate
   gingiva
Teeth
   oral cleanliness
   teeth present
   position of teeth—crowding, spacing, drifting
   occlusion
      permanent first molars and canines
      incisors—overjet, overbite
   mobility—exfoliating primary tooth, abscess,
         periodontitis
   colour—non-vital tooth, intrinsic staining, caries
   structure—hypoplasia, hypomineralisation, caries

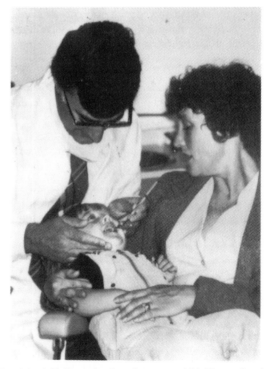

Fig. 1.1   Initial examination of a young child. The mother is seated on the dental chair. Her right arm provides a rest for the child's head and her left hand is available to restrain undesirable movements if necessary. It is not essential to wear surgical gloves at this stage (see text).

examination. Gloves should, of course, be worn for more detailed examination involving palpation of soft tissues and for treatment, after the child's confidence has been gained.

During the initial examination the teeth may be counted aloud to provide interest and distraction. If a probe is used to aid diagnosis it may be described as "a pointer, to help me count your teeth", but its sharp end should be kept out of the child's field of vision and it should be used very gently to avoid causing discomfort.

The approach outlined above clearly is not practicable with an older child who is too large to lie on a parent's lap. If such a child remains uncooperative after the history-taking period and is unwilling to sit on the dental chair, it may be preferable to postpone oral examination and to plan a series of introductory visits, as outlined on page 15. Although this situation does not frequently arise, it is not uncommon with mentally handicapped children. Clearly, if the child was brought because of a specific problem requiring urgent treatment, some means must be found of examining the child (under general anaesthesia if absolutely necessary), but if the reason for attendance was a routine 'check-up', postponement of the oral examination until the child's cooperation has been gained is often the most reasonable decision and the most successful in the long term.

1.4.2 Radiographic examination

Sometimes the clinical examination provides all the necessary information about the patient, in which case radiographs are not required. More commonly, however, radiographs are required for one of the following reasons:

1. To diagnose dental caries in tooth surfaces not accessible to clinical examination.
2. To detect abnormalities in the developing dentition.
3. To investigate specific problems, for example the condition of periapical tissues associated with non-vital or traumatized teeth.

Dental caries

Bite-wing radiographs are essential for the diagnosis of approximal surface caries. Several studies have shown that at least half the approximal lesions in primary molars of children aged 3–7 years would not be detected without radiographs (Kidd & Pitts 1990). Approximal lesions may progress to form large cavities, which may even involve the pulp, before they are detectable clinically.

If bite-wing radiographs cannot be obtained because the child is uncooperative, rotated lateral oblique radiographs (see below) may provide satisfactory views of approximal lesions.

With the increasing use of fissure sealants in recent years, bite-wing radiographs have become important for the diagnosis of occlusal caries that might occur if sealants are defective (although early occlusal caries is not easily diagnosed on radiographs).

Abnormalities in the developing dentition

An important aim in dentistry for children is to monitor the developing dentition and, if possible, to prevent or alleviate undesirable effects that might be caused by an abnormality in the dentition. Early detection of abnormalities is important, so that appropriate action can be taken at the most favourable stage of dental development, before any undesirable changes have occurred. Early detection of abnormalities requires a full radiographic survey.

Although it may be of interest to know of the existence of an abnormality during the primary dentition stage, it is of little practical importance at this time. It is normally preferable to wait until the early mixed dentition stage before obtaining the necessary radiographs.

A full radiographic examination of child patients at about 8 years old should be routine practice, and may be achieved by one of the following combinations of radiographs:

1. a. Panoramic radiograph—to show the complete dentition.
   b. Maxillary anterior occlusal—to show the maxillary anterior region more clearly.
   Panoramic radiography is a convenient method of obtaining a picture of the whole dentition on one film, but the equipment is expensive and therefore is not available in every dental practice.
   The anterior region of both jaws is the least well defined on panoramic radiographs, and supernumerary teeth lying out of the line of the arch may not be detected. In the early mixed dentition, it is important to detect the presence of supernumerary teeth and other abnormalities, and therefore it is essential to take a maxillary anterior occlusal radiograph in addition to the panoramic radiograph.
2. a. Right and left rotated lateral oblique radiographs—to show maxillary and mandibular teeth distal to the canines.
   b. Maxillary anterior occlusal—to show the maxillary anterior region.

c. Mandibular anterior occlusal—to show the mandibular anterior region. Abnormalities in this region are rare, and this view may be excluded unless there is a definite reason to include it.

Right and left rotated lateral oblique views can be projected on to one 13 × 18 cm film, which is then called a bimolar radiograph (Bowdler Henry 1955). No special equipment is required (except a film cassette) and the technique is therefore useful when facilities for panoramic radiography are not available.

3. a. Periapical radiographs—to show posterior teeth.
   b. Maxillary anterior occlusal and, possibly, mandibular anterior occlusal.

Usually, four periapical films are required (one for each posterior segment), but eight films may be required for older children. Because of this, and because intra-oral techniques require greater cooperation from the child than do extra-oral techniques, this approach is less convenient.

Specific problems

If the general radiographic survey is done by extra-oral radiography, selected periapical views may be required to show the periapical condition of, for example, a tooth with suspected pulp exposure, or of a tooth that has been traumatized or received root canal treatment.

If an unerupted tooth or odontome is found in the radiographic survey, it will be necessary to determine whether it is placed labial or palatal to the roots of erupted teeth; this information is commonly required in the case of an unerupted supernumerary or canine tooth. The labio-palatal position may be determined by applying the principle of parallax to two periapical radiographs taken of the same area but at different angles; alternatively, a maxillary anterior occlusal and an off-centre periapical radiograph may be used.

A standard occlusal radiograph of the mandible may be useful in locating the bucco-lingual position of an unerupted mandibular tooth.

Techniques

Brief details of recommended techniques are outlined on page 10.

It is important to note that the rotated lateral oblique (bimolar) radiograph should show teeth distal to the canine in both the maxilla and the mandible (Fig. 1.2). To obtain this view, it is essential to rotate the head by placing the tip of the patient's nose as well as the cheek in contact with the cassette; this rotation lifts the mandible on the side of the X-ray tube

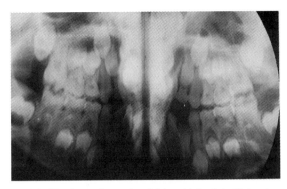

Fig. 1.2 Bimolar radiograph—right and left rotated lateral obliques on one 13 × 18 cm film.

upwards, so that it does not become superimposed over the opposite canine and premolar region. It is convenient and economical to use one 18 × 13 cm film for views of both sides of the mouth; this is done by using a lead rubber or metal sheet to cover each half of the cassette in turn.

An alternative method of taking bimolar radiographs is to place the cassette on a flat surface and to position the child's head over it. A simple apparatus is available (Qualident Head Positioner, Orthomax Ltd) which makes this method particularly easy to use (Fig. 1.3); it incorporates a board on which to place the cassette, a device for positioning the child's head correctly, and a lead rubber sheet that can be moved to cover each half of the cassette in turn.

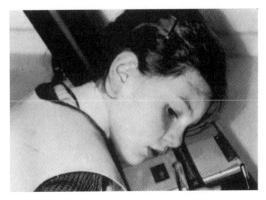

Fig. 1.3 Using a head positioner to take a bimolar radiograph.

Radiographic techniques

	Bite-wing	Maxillary anterior occlusal	Rotated lateral oblique (bimolar)	Periapical
Head position	The imaginary line joining alar of nose to tragus of ear should be horizontal.	Alar–tragus line horizontal.	Sit the child sideways on the chair (armrest lowered).	Alar–tragus line horizontal.
Film size	For young child (e.g. under 5 years) —2.2 × 3.5 cm. For older child—3.1 × 4.1 cm. Place the film in a bite-wing film holder —several types are available—or attach an adhesive tab.	'occlusal' film in 5.7 × 7.6 cm.	13 × 18 cm film in cassette with intensifying screens.	For young child—2.2 × 3.5 cm. For older child—3.1 × 4.1 cm.
Film position	Close to the lingual surfaces of maxillary and mandibular teeth, anterior border in line with the canines. Nearly vertical. The anterior corners of the film may be bent lingually if they cause discomfort.	Held between maxillary and mandibular anterior teeth. Longer dimension across the mouth, anterior border projecting a few mm beyond the incisal edges.	Rest the cassette on the chair's head-rest at an angle of about 45°. Position the child's head so that the nose and cheek touch the surface of the cassette and the lower border of the mandible lies parallel to its bottom edge. Ask the child to support the cassette with a hand. (For alternative method see text.)	For incisors and canines, insert the film with its length running from the incisal edges of the teeth to the palate (or floor of the mouth), with its anterior border projecting a few mm beyond the incisal edges. For molars, place the film with its length running antero–posteriorly. Ask the child to support the film with a thumb or finger.
Direction of tube	Perpendicular to the tube.	Between the tip and bridge of nose, at an angle of about +65°.	Just behind the angle of the mandible and just below the ear, aiming at the opposite premolar region at an angle of about +10°.	Perpendicular to a plane bisecting the angle formed by the long axis of the tooth and the plane of the film.

	maxillary teeth	mandibular teeth
prim. incisor	+45°	−10°
perm. incisor	+55°	−20°
prim. canine	+40°	−10°
perm. canine	+50°	−20°
molars	+20°	−5°

The exposure times are dependent on the type of X-ray machine and film used.
A protective lead-plastic apron should always be used.

Guidelines for radiography of child patients

	New patient	Recall patient
For caries *(high caries rate)* *(low caries rate)*	Bite-wings	 Bite-wings, if previous bite-wings taken > 1year ago Bite-wings, if previous bite-wings taken > 2 years ago
For developmental abnormalities	Radiographs usually not indicated below age 8. Age 8 upwards, panoramic or bimolar + maxillary anterior occlusal (+ mandibular anterior occlusal?)	Radiographs usually not indicated, unless to monitor an abnormality detected previously, or to assess dental development following interceptive treatment, or to plan active orthodontic treatment
For periodontal disease or other specific problem	Periapicals of areas where periodontal disease (other than gingivitis) is noted clinically.	Further periapicals may be indicated to assess progress or arrest of lesion

Guidelines for radiography of child patients

A summary of recommendations for dental radiography of child patients is presented above. This summary is based on recommendations of the American Dental Association (1989) but differs from them in some respects.

1.5 DIAGNOSIS

Information gathered from the history and from the clinical and radiographic examinations usually allows a diagnosis to be made. Sometimes, further diagnostic aids are required, for example pulp vitality tests for a traumatized tooth, or study models for orthodontic assessment. The diagnosis is a statement of any disease affecting the patient's oral health, or of any abnormality affecting dental development.

The diagnosis defines the problem for which treatment must be planned.

1.6 INTRODUCTORY TREATMENT

After examining the child, a simple operative procedure should be introduced. Ideally, when the child has not presented with pain or any other complaint, the treatment should be a simple 'polish' using a brush or rubber cup in a slow-speed handpiece. The objectives are to introduce the child to the sensation of the dentist working in the mouth and to show that this is a pleasant experience; this is especially important when the child is attending for the first time. The Tell-Show-Do method (Ch. 2) is very effective. With a young child, brushing may be limited to a few incisors and take only a minute or two, the prime objective being to introduce the child happily to dentistry; whether plaque is removed or not is unimportant, and prophylaxis paste need not be used. With an older child, a full-mouth prophylaxis may be completed, and this treatment may conveniently be extended to the application of topical fluoride. Ideally, operative treatment involving injections or cavity preparation is not started during the first visit; even a child with previous experience of dentistry elsewhere has, by this stage in the visit, been introduced to enough new situations.

Unfortunately, children are often first taken to a dentist when in pain and the ideal form of introduction described above may not be possible. However, the important aim of influencing the child's long-term attitudes to dentistry should not be abandoned in the concern to treat pain. Certainly, immediate intervention is essential on some occasions but if intermittent pain has been tolerated for some time it may be preferable to recommend an analgesic and to arrange another appointment, thus delaying operative treatment until the child's confidence has been obtained.

1.7 CONCLUDING THE SESSION

Before dismissing the child, the dentist should give the parent a brief explanation of the treatment that is required. If restorations are necessary, this should be pointed out, but also it should be emphasized that attention to reparative treatment alone is of little long-term benefit, and that prevention of further dental disease must also be an important aim. Perhaps it is enough at the first visit to make this one fundamental point about preventive treatment rather than to discuss in detail the methods that will be used. However, since oral hygiene instruction forms a part of the preventive plan, parents may be asked to bring the child's toothbrush when they next attend.

Finally, some indication should be given to the parent of the probable length of the course of treatment; parents may become disillusioned if they expect to bring their child for two or three visits and later find that many more visits are needed. Especially if the child is uncooperative and several introductory visits are envisaged during which little or no operative treatment will be performed, the plan of action should be clearly explained to the parent (see page 16).

1.8 SUMMARY OF THE FIRST APPOINTMENT

The recommended procedure for a child's first visit may be summarised as follows:

1. Take the history
   a. social
   b. dental
   c. medical
2. Examine the child
   a. extra-orally
   b. intra-orally
3. Take radiographs if required
   a. to show dental caries—bite-wings
   b. to show the developing dentition (in patients over age 8 years)
      — panoramic + maxillary anterior occlusal
   or— rotated lateral obliques (bimolar)
      + maxillary anterior occlusal
   c. to investigate specific problems
      — periapicals

4. Perform a simple operative procedure
   a. prophylaxis: incisors only (in young child) or full mouth, including removal of calculus if required
   b. perform simple palliative treatment if necessary
   c. possibly topical fluoride treatment or other non-traumatic procedure
5. Explain aims of treatment to parent
   a. emphasize the need for preventive as well as operative treatment
   b. request that the child's toothbrush be brought at the next visit
   c. give an estimate of the number of visits that will be required to complete treatment

1.9 TREATMENT PLANNING

Good treatment planning is at the very heart of good dentistry for children. Essential to good planning is a firm commitment to benefit the whole child, not merely the dentition, and to influence the child's attitudes to dentistry in addition to performing any necessary treatment. A course of treatment that is successful in completing operative treatment but that fails to establish or strengthen positive attitudes may be of only short-term benefit to the child; if negative attitudes are introduced more harm than good may be done. The essence of good dentistry for children is to plan and pursue treatment in such a way that the child benefits in the broadest sense, in the long term as well as in the short term.

To achieve these aims it is necessary to know more than just the state of the child's dentition. Much of the necessary information is provided by the patient's social, dental and medical histories, and their

An outline for treatment planning

	Points to consider	Relevance in treatment planning
Behaviour management	The attitudes of the child and the parent to dental health, assessed by the regularity of past dental care, oral hygiene, etc.	The approach necessary to interest a family in dental health and to motivate them to practise preventive measures will inevitably be greatly influenced by their initial attitudes.
	Parents' attitudes to dental treatment.	Some parents do not value preventive or restorative dentistry, particularly for primary teeth. It would be necessary to change these attitudes before an ideal treatment plan could be made for their child.
	Child's attitudes to previous dental treatment; in particular, fears of specific items of treatment.	The selection of the most appropriate method of behaviour management must be based on a knowledge of the individual child's attitude to treatment.
Preventive treatment *General*	Caries experience. Medical history, especially cardiac conditions, bleeding disorders, debilitating disease with poor resistance to infection, mental or physical handicap.	All types of preventive treatment are especially important for children with high caries experience and for those particularly at risk from oral disease.

An outline for treatment planning *(contd)*

	Points to consider	Relevance in treatment planning
Oral hygiene instruction	Standard of oral hygiene, and state of gingival tissues.	If oral hygiene is poor and gingival inflammation is present, intensive oral hygiene instruction is required; if oral hygiene and gingival condition are good, re-emphasis and encouragement only may be required.
	Child's age.	When the child is younger than about 6 years of age, or mentally or physically handicapped, the parent should be instructed in brushing the child's teeth.
Diet counselling	Caries experience.	Diet counselling is always important but is especially so if the child's caries experience is high.
Fluoride		
— tablets (or drops)	Parental interest.	Since parents must administer or supervise the use of the tablets, their interest is essential.
	Child's age.	Fluoride tablets are most strongly indicated for infants and young children; once started they may be continued to age 12–13 years.
— mouthrinsing	Parental interest.	As above.
	Child's age.	Mouthrinsing is only feasible for children from about the age of 6–7 years, because younger children cannot manage the recommended procedure, which involves retaining solution in the mouth for 1–2 minutes.
— topical application	Is the child receiving systemic fluoride or using a mouthrinse regularly at home?	Topical fluoride application may not be justified for children receiving systemic fluoride or using a mouthrinse regularly, but is justified for children with high caries rates or for those who are medically-at-risk, or mentally or physically handicapped.
Fissure sealing	Child's age. Caries experience. Morphology of pits and fissures.	Sealing of caries-free pits and fissures is particularly justified for newly erupted permanent first molars that have deep pits and fissures, especially for children with high caries experience (as assessed from the condition of the primary dentition), and for those who are medically-at-risk, or mentally or physically handicapped.
Operative treatment		
General	Medical history.	Precautions are necessary for some forms of dental treatment of children who have certain types of medical condition (e.g. congenital heart disease, blood disorders).
Restorations	Depth of caries.	The depth of caries will influence the type of material chosen to restore the tooth. If it is predicted that one or more primary teeth have pulp exposures, a decision must be made either to conserve by pulp treatment or to extract.
	Extent of caries.	Teeth with extensive lesions may be better restored with stainless steel crowns than with amalgam or other restorative material.
	Use of local analgesia.	Ideally, restorative dentistry is performed under local analgesia. However, if the child's attitudes are unfavourable, a decision must be made either: a) to attempt to change the child's attitude b) to introduce some form of sedation c) to pursue treatment without local analgesia (usually only possible if caries is minimal).
	Order of restoring teeth.	If local analgesia is to be used, a maxillary premolar or primary molar should be chosen if possible for the first restoration, as it is easiest to give a painless injection in this region.
Extractions	Are one or more teeth unsaveable, or have teeth already been extracted?	If extraction of a primary molar is necessary, the need for a 'balancing' extraction or space maintenance must be considered. If a permanent first molar must be extracted, extraction of one or more of the other permanent first molars may be desirable.
	Use of local analgesia or general anaesthesia.	A decision must be made to extract teeth under local analgesia (with or without sedation), or under general anaesthesia. The child's attitudes should be considered.
Orthodontic treatment	Crowding or spacing of: a. erupted teeth b. unerupted teeth, i.e. deficiency or excess of space in the arch for their eruption.	If there is crowding, extractions may be required immediately or be planned for the future. In cases of doubt, an orthodontist's opinion should be sought.
	Developmental abnormalities.	Some abnormalities may be treated early.
	Established malocclusion.	Orthodontic treatment may be indicated.

influence on treatment planning has been noted on pages 5 and 6. Every child is different, and the most appropriate treatment plan for each individual patient can only be made on the basis of relevant background information. With this information, possible problems can be anticipated and treatment planned in such a way as to overcome or avoid them; without it, treatment can only proceed blindly, with the possibility of encountering unexpected problems. Thus, an adequate history, together with a detailed examination and an accurate diagnosis, are essential requirements for good treatment planning.

An outline of points to consider in treatment planning is presented on pages 12–13.

Having decided which forms of preventive and operative treatment are most appropriate for the patient, it is necessary to plan the order in which the treatment is to be carried out, because this can have a crucial bearing on the success of the course of treatment. General guidance is given below, based on the principles of behaviour shaping that are considered in Chapter 2. The final plan should be flexible and open to modification as treatment progresses.

1.10 THE UNCOOPERATIVE CHILD

Careful management of all procedures during the first session with a child patient usually succeeds not only in allaying any initial anxiety but also in obtaining cooperation for oral examination, radiography and a

Order of treatment: general guidance

	Procedure	Rationale
1st visit	Introduce the child to operative treatment—'polish' a few teeth or full prophylaxis.	This is a simple, painless introductory procedure.
	Take radiographs.	If radiographs are required it is logical to obtain them at the first visit, not only because they complement the clinical examination and contribute to the diagnosis but also because the procedures are not traumatic and therefore provide a suitable introduction to treatment.
2nd visit	Assess toothbrushing technique — observe the child brushing — determine Oral Debris Index. Start oral hygiene instruction.	Activities involved in oral hygiene instruction, if carried out imaginatively, not only stimulate the child's (and parents') interest in dental health but also help to establish good rapport, an essential pre-requisite for gaining the child's cooperation for other treatment.
	Topical fluoride or fissure sealant or preventive resin restoration.	These are painless procedures. Local analgesia is not required for a preventive resin restoration.
	Provide a diet record leaflet and explain its purpose to the parent and/or child.	Having introduced oral hygiene instruction at the beginning of this visit, it is convenient at the end to introduce another important aspect of prevention.
3rd visit	Collect diet record leaflet.	It is preferable simply to collect the diet leaflet at this visit rather than to attempt instant assessment and counselling.
	Continue oral hygiene instruction.	Giving praise, encouragement and further instruction at each visit helps to motivate and maintain interest.
	Amalgam restoration in maxillary molar—infiltration local analgesia.	An infiltration in the maxillary molar region is the simplest injection to administer painlessly and therefore should always be chosen if possible when introducing a child to local analgesia.
4th visit	Continue oral hygiene instruction. At this and subsequent visits, introduce progressively more complex restorations, delaying treatment of mandibular teeth if possible until the child happily accepts maxillary infiltrations.	
	Diet counselling.	Inferior dental alveolar nerve block injection is often considered unpleasant despite the greatest care being taken in its administration. The diet record collected at the previous visit will have been studied and advice prepared.

simple introductory operative procedure. Unfortunately not all patients respond in a positive manner: little or no communication can be established with some patients and they remain uncooperative. This presents a problem that the dentist must be able to handle confidently because uncertain, indecisive behaviour will compound the problem.

The child's attitudes usually become evident during history-taking. Crying at this early stage clearly is an unfavourable sign, but the dentist should be alert to other signs of potentially uncooperative behaviour, for example, lack of response to simple questions, or clinging tightly to the parent. The dentist must not show any sign of being disturbed, even by the loudest protests. Conversation with the parent should continue as normally as possible, from time to time directing a friendly comment or question to the child in the hope of eliciting a favourable response, but not showing concern if there is none. It is hoped that the child, observing the relaxed and friendly relationship between dentist and parent, will be encouraged also to relax.

It is, of course, not abnormal for a young child to cry or show other signs of anxiety when confronted by a stranger in unfamiliar surroundings, but it is not unusual for such a child, supported by a parent, to adapt quickly and accept the new situation. Thus, many children who initially appear uncooperative may, after only a few minutes of history-taking, cooperate for an oral examination. If, however, the child remains uncooperative, an important decision must be made: either to postpone the examination or to proceed despite possible protests. The latter course of action is only possible with young children who are small enough to be placed on a parent's lap (as described on page 7), and with the parent's consent and cooperation; frequently the sense of security provided by the parent is sufficient to enable the child to accept the examination without protest. If, however, the child does protest the parent is well placed gently to restrain any undesirable arm movements, and the dentist similarly can restrain head movements while examining the mouth. Again, it is important for the dentist to appear unconcerned and undisturbed by any protests, and counting the teeth aloud, whilst ignoring the disruptive behaviour, helps to achieve this. An examination carried out under such conditions should be kept as brief as possible and may not be very detailed, but important objectives are to demonstrate to the child that an oral examination is not a painful or unpleasant procedure and that the dentist is not diverted by disruptive behaviour (behaviour that perhaps is successful when applied to parents or other adults). This approach may seem rather severe, but it is important to appreciate that it is only considered appropriate when carrying out a completely atraumatic procedure; it cannot be condoned as a means of performing an operative procedure. This simple show of authority may succeed in establishing a basis for cooperation, because by ignoring undesirable behaviour and not allowing it to be rewarded by avoidance of the examination, that behaviour is less likely to be repeated at subsequent visits; conversely if the behaviour is rewarded it is more likely to be repeated. Immediately after the examination the child is allowed to sit up and friendly conversation is continued without any reference to the child's behaviour.

Postponing oral examination of an uncooperative child may sometimes be justified, for example when the parents are confident of the child's oral health but simply wish to introduce the child to the dental surgery; however, if the child interprets the dentist's inaction as being the result of the disruptive behaviour the chances are increased that the same behaviour will be repeated at subsequent visits. Postponement may be necessary with older children who cannot be placed and gently restrained on a parent's lap; if an examination is essential because of suspicions of a dental problem that might require urgent treatment, sedation or general anaesthesia may be required.

Having either examined or decided to postpone examination of an uncooperative child, a plan for further action is required (Hill & O'Mullane 1976). A suggested outline for such a plan is given on page 16 (the plan assumes that the child does not need urgent treatment).

Plan of action for an uncooperative patient

Procedure	Rationale
Discuss the problem with the parents — operative treatment is not possible without cooperation (unless sedation of general anaesthesia is used) — need to give the child time to acclimatize — need to control existing disease and prevent further disease.	It is in the long-term interest of the child to be helped to accept normal treatment, without resorting to sedation or general anaesthesia. Since operative treatment cannot be performed immediately it is all the more important to control existing disease and prevent further disease.
Advise three-four introductory visits — to gain the child's confidence and cooperation — to give advice on all possible preventive measures.	During three to four visits a behaviour shaping plan can be pursued (Ch. 2), and comprehensive advice and help can be given regarding oral hygiene and diet (Ch. 3) and, if appropriate, home use of fluoride (Ch. 4). Even if the child does not become cooperative enough for operative treatment to begin, the series of visits will benefit the child if the parents respond favourably to the advice.
Inform the parents that, after the introductory visits, a decision will be made: *either* to proceed with normal treatment	It is important to perceive the way ahead following the introductory visit—a protracted series of visits, if unrewarded by significant success in gaining the child's cooperation, can be disheartening for the parent and dentist.
or to postpone treatment	Operative treatment may be postponed if the child still cannot cooperate and treatment is not urgently required. An appointment is made to see the patient again in 2–3 months.
or to extract selected teeth	If treatment cannot be postponed further, extraction of one or more teeth may be the treatment of choice. General anaesthesia may be used if suitable facilities are available. The use of general anaesthesia for restorative treatment is generally considered justifiable only for special categories of patient (e.g. the mentally, physically or medically handicapped patient).
or to carry out treatment under some form of sedation.	Treatment under sedation may be feasible with some patients —unfortunately not usually with very young uncooperative patients (Ch. 2).
Obtain the parent's agreement to this plan	It is important that the parent responsible for bringing the child understands and agrees with the aims of the plan, to ensure that appointments are kept and to avoid possible misunderstandings.

REFERENCES

American Dental Association 1989 Council on Dental Materials, Instruments and Equipment. Recommendations on radiographic practices: an update 1988. Journal of the American Dental Association 118: 115–117

Beal J 1989 Social factors and preventive dentistry. In: Murray J J (ed) The prevention of oral disease, 3rd edn. Oxford University Press, Oxford, ch 16

Bowdler Henry C 1955 A maxillostat. British Dental Journal 19: 80–83

Fenlon W L, Dobbs A R, Curzon M E J 1993 Parental presence during treatment of the child patient: a study with British parents. British Dental Journal 174: 23–28

Hill F J, O'Mullane D M 1976 Preventive programme for the dental management of frightened children. Journal of Dentistry for Children 43: 30–36

Kidd E A M, Pitts N D 1990 A reappraisal of the value of the bitewing radiograph in the diagnosis of posterior approximal caries. British Dental Journal 169: 195–200

Longman L P, Martin M V 1993 Prevention of infective endocarditis—paedodontic considerations. International Journal of Paediatric Dentistry 3: 63–70

Moore R S, Hobson P 1989 A classification of medically handicapping conditions and the health risks they present in the dental care of children. Part I—Cardiovascular, haematological and respiratory disorders. Journal of Paediatric Dentistry 5: 73–83

Moore R S, Hobson P 1990 A classification of medically handicapping conditions and the health risks they present in the dental care of children. Part II—Neoplastic, renal, endocrine, metabolic, hepatic, musculoskeletal, neuromuscular, central nervous system and skin disorders. Journal of Paediatric Dentistry 6: 1–14

Swallow J N, Jones J M, Morgan M F 1975 The effect of environment on a child's reaction to dentistry. Journal of Dentistry for Children 42: 290–292

RECOMMENDED READING

Holloway P J, Swallow J N 1982 Child dental health, 3rd edn. Wright, Bristol, ch 3

Myerscough P R 1989 Talking with patients—a basic clinical skill. Oxford University Press, Oxford

Wright G Z 1975 Behavior management in dentistry for children. Saunders, Philadelphia, chs 3, 4

Wright G Z, Starkey P E, Gardner D E 1987 Child management in dentistry. IOP Publishing, Bristol, ch 8

2 Techniques of behaviour management

To obtain the cooperation of a child patient the dentist must not only establish good rapport with the child but also use effective techniques of behaviour management. Clearly, some knowledge of normal child development is essential, but this subject is outside the scope of this book; the reader is referred to the texts listed at the end of this chapter.

Managing a child patient may be considered simply a matter of applying common sense, based on previous experiences with children but not on any formal knowledge of child psychology. Unfortunately, the application of common sense is not necessarily common practice. Therefore it is instructive to consider techniques that have proved successful in psychology and which can be applied in dentistry. Many dentists use these techniques intuitively, but when they are defined and described their basic principles can be applied consciously and, therefore, more effectively.

2.1 BEHAVIOUR SHAPING

Psychologists use the term 'behaviour shaping' to refer to the process of influencing behaviour towards a desired ideal. An essential part of behaviour shaping is to define a series of steps on the path to the desired behaviour, and then to progress step by step to the goal. In relation to dentistry, it may be stated that ideal behaviour is shown by a patient who maintains excellent oral hygiene, exercises sensible diet control, and is relaxed and cooperative during operative treatment. It would be unrealistic to expect all patients to show this type of behaviour at their first visit to the dentist, but it would be wrong to accept as unchangeable the behaviour of those who do not show it, or simply to hope that it will improve in time. The proper course of action is to plan treatment in such a way that the child's behaviour is gradually improved to the desired standard. Only by so doing can the fundamental aims in dentistry for children be fulfilled: to influence positive attitudes and behaviour in addition to carrying out any necessary treatment.

Behaviour shaping is based on a planned introduction of treatment procedures, so that the child is gradually trained to accept treatment in a relaxed and cooperative manner. Steps that may be defined for the introduction of restorative treatment to an average school-aged child are:

1. Examination and prophylaxis.
2. Fissure sealant or topical fluoride application.
3. Minimal occlusal restoration in a primary tooth without local analgesia.
4. Infiltration analgesia and restoration.
5. Inferior dental nerve block and restoration.

The time spent on each step will depend on the child's behaviour. Thus, some children might require several short sessions at the early steps before being taken further, while others could be taken to step 5 within one or two sessions. Indeed, some children could be taken to step 5 at their first visit, but this would not be considered good practice; even if the child accepts the treatment, such an approach rejects the principles of behaviour shaping and is less likely to succeed.

For very frightened young children, the following steps may be planned:

1. To carry out a brief oral examination; child lying across parent's lap (page 7).
2. To use a prophylaxis brush or rubber cup gently, first by hand and then in a slow-speed handpiece; child lying across parent's lap.
3. Child to demonstrate toothbrushing with own toothbrush.
4. Parent, and then dentist, to brush the child's teeth with the toothbrush.
5. Child to sit on the dental chair; use of prophylaxis brush in slow-speed handpiece.
6. Proceed as with normal child.

Again, the number of steps included in each session, or the number of sessions devoted to each step, will depend on how the child responds. The gradual approach implicit in behaviour shaping may initially delay the progress of treatment, but when the child's full cooperation is obtained this delay is more than compensated, so that time spent initially can be regarded as a sound investment.

2.2 TELL—SHOW—DO (TSD)

The essentials of TSD are to *tell* the child about the treatment to be carried out, to *show* at least some part of how it will be done, and then to *do* it. The technique is used routinely in introducing a child to prophylaxis, which is always chosen as the first operative procedure. Thus, the child is told that the teeth are to be brushed, shown the 'special' brush and how it revolves in the handpiece, and then the teeth are brushed. To the TSD sequence should be added 'praise', because good behaviour during this initial treatment, and indeed during any subsequent treatment, should immediately be reinforced (see below).

The transition from a brush to a bur is easily made; the bur may be introduced as a 'special cleaner' that cleans 'the places that the brush cannot reach'.

Some compromise is necessary in applying this method to the administration of local analgesia. Most dentists consider that the needle should not be shown, because most children (and adults too) are apprehensive about needles. Therefore the child is told that his/her tooth will be 'made to go to sleep', and shown

the surface analgesic on cotton wool; the injection follows without further demonstration (Ch. 6).

For whatever treatment TSD is being employed, it is important to ensure a smooth continuity through the T—S—D stages. The explanations should not be detailed and protracted, as this would tend to confuse the child and perhaps arouse anxiety; they should be given simply and casually. Similarly, the demonstration should be given briefly and in a matter-of-fact manner, so that the actual treatment follows without undue delay.

2.3 REINFORCEMENT

Reinforcement may be defined as the strengthening of a pattern of behaviour, which increases the probability of that behaviour being displayed in the future. Psychologists who adhere to the social-learning theories of child development believe that a child's behaviour is a reflection of responses to the rewards and punishments of the environment, and that a very important form of reward (and therefore a strong motivating factor for behaviour change) is the approval obtained first from parents and later from peers. Therefore, good behaviour by children in the dental situation, whether it be in brushing their teeth efficiently or in cooperating well in operative procedures, should be rewarded by a show of approval from the dentist. This approval is expected to reinforce the good behaviour, thus increasing the probability of it being repeated in subsequent treatment, because it becomes a normal pattern of behaviour for the child in that situation.

The dentist's approval should be shown frequently during treatment, whenever the child responds positively to directions (Rosenberg 1974). Usually this approval is given verbally, but smiles and nods are also appropriate. The wording is not important and dentists have their own favourite phrases ranging, for example, from a simple "that's good", through "well done, that's terrific" to "you are one of my best patients". The important point is that the child's good behaviour should be reinforced frequently.

The reward should be closely linked to the action. For example, if a child is asked to open his mouth wide and he responds well, he should receive an immediate sign of approval. Approval given only at the end of a session, for example "we've finished now, you've been a very good boy" is not by itself effective because it will not be clear to the child what precise behaviour brought such approval. Much worse, however, is to ignore the child's good cooperation during treatment; not only does this waste an excellent opportunity of strengthening that behaviour but may, by acting as a form of punishment, reduce the probability of that behaviour being repeated.

Another form of reward is a present. Many suitable items are available, such as colouring sheets, balloons and 'stickers', but even a cotton wool roll or a prophylaxis brush may be prized by a young child. A present should only be given at the end of a session as a sign of approval of good behaviour; it should not be offered as a bribe in the hope of encouraging good behaviour, and should certainly not be given if the child has not been cooperative.

It is important to avoid reinforcement of poor behaviour. If a child is obstructive and the planned treatment cannot be completed, abrupt termination of treatment and return to the parent for consolation is very likely to reinforce that poor behaviour. It would be preferable to appear undisturbed and to pretend that treatment has been completed (for example by placing a temporary dressing). The dentist should not ridicule the child for poor behaviour, or show anger. The forms of punishment that can be used are limited to showing disappointment and disapproval, and withholding any kind of reward.

2.4 DESENSITIZATION

Desensitization is one of the techniques used most frequently by psychologists in the treatment of fears. Classically, the technique involves three stages: first, training the patient to relax; second, constructing a hierarchy of fear-producing stimuli related to the patient's principal fear; and third, introducing each stimulus in the hierarchy in turn to the relaxed patient, starting with the stimulus that causes least fear and progressing to the next only when the patient no longer fears that stimulus (Wolpe & Lazarus 1966). It is important to note that the patient must be helped to relax before fear is overcome; simply repeating the stimulus many times increases rather than decreases fear. Relaxation and fear are incompatible; if relaxation is achieved, fear is abolished. The technique has been used to overcome many types of fear, for example, of heights, of crowded places, or of isolation, as well as fear of dentistry (Gale & Ayer 1969).

To apply the technique in its classical form, a series of preliminary sessions is required to teach the patient how to relax. Although some dentists (especially those familiar with hypnosis) may be prepared to do this, and others may refer the patient to a psychologist, the basic concepts may be applied in dentistry without the preliminary sessions. It is important to know the basis of the child's fear, which may be a general fear of dentists, doctors, hospitals or clinics, or a more specific fear of 'the needle', 'the drill' or other aspects of dental treatment. When this information is known, a hierarchy of fear-producing stimuli can be constructed and worked through. If, for example, the child is frightened of the dental environment in general, desensitization might include the successive introduction of the child to the following stimuli:

1. Reception and waiting rooms.
2. Dentist and nurse.
3. Dental surgery.
4. Dental chair.
5. Oral examination.
6. Prophylaxis.

If, on the other hand, the child fears 'the drill', the selected stimuli might be:

1. Brushing the child's teeth with a prophylaxis brush held by hand.
2. Brushing with a prophylaxis brush in a slow-speed handpiece.
3. Using a fine finishing bur in a slow-speed handpiece, revolving in the mouth but not in contact with teeth.
4. Applying the finishing bur gently to a restoration or tooth surface.

At each stage of a hierarchy the Tell—Show—Do procedure is followed, the child's fears are allayed by the kind, friendly and reassuring manner of the dentist, and positive behaviour shown by the child is strongly reinforced. When the child appears relaxed and contented, progress is made to the next stage. Some children's fears are quickly overcome in this way, allowing rapid progress through the hierarchy. On the other hand, others are more resistant, and this no doubt discourages many dentists from using the method.

Desensitization from fear of 'the needle' is more difficult, especially with young children, who cannot be expected to react favourably to the sight of a needle or, even less, to its introduction into their mouth. If this fear persists despite careful behaviour shaping during introductory visits, some form of sedation may be considered (p. 20).

2.5 MODELLING

Modelling is another technique used by psychologists in the treatment of fears; for example, children frightened of dogs have been helped to overcome their fears by watching other children playing happily with dogs, the happy children being the models which the frightened children later imitated.

This simple technique may be applied to a variety of dental treatment situations but perhaps its most frequent application is in the introduction of an anxious child to oral examination in the dental chair. A parent or, preferably, another child is asked to act as the model, submitting to an examination and prophylaxis; the relaxed, cooperative behaviour of the model will, it is hoped, later be imitated by the anxious child. Tell—Show—Do and reinforcement should be used to supplement the modelling procedure. Together with desensitization, this is an effective approach to the problem of introducing simple treatment to a frightened child (Adelson & Goldfried 1970).

2.6 HAND-OVER-MOUTH

The 'hand-over-mouth' technique is generally regarded as being rather an extreme measure in dealing with an uncooperative child. It is rarely used in the UK but has had its adherents in the USA (Levitas 1974).

The technique involves restraining the protesting child gently but firmly in the dental chair, placing a hand (or towel) over the child's mouth to subdue the protests and, speaking quietly but clearly into the child's ear, explaining that the hand will be removed as soon as the crying stops (Craig 1971). When this happens, the hand is removed immediately and the child is praised. If protests start again, the procedure is repeated.

This technique has always been controversial and cannot be popular with any dentist who cares for children and whose aim is to influence positive attitudes in addition to carrying out treatment. Its only possible justification might be in dealing with a spoilt child who has learned to manipulate over-indulgent parents with temper tantrums, or with a defiant child who has found that silent but firm defiance always succeeds. Such children are not frightened; they simply do not wish to cooperate and know how to avoid doing so. Their behaviour usually soon becomes evident during their first visit and is confirmed by the manner of their refusal to be examined. If such a child is picked up and placed on the chair or on a parent's lap, strong protests may be expected, but the dentist may proceed as described in Chapter 1. Sometimes this simple show of authority by the dentist succeeds in establishing some basis for cooperation in the future. However, if the child behaves in a similar manner at the next visit, a decision has to be made about further action. It is in these cases that the hand-over-mouth technique may be justified, because unless the child learns that the dentist is not impressed or deterred by tantrums or defiance, no treatment is possible (except by recourse to general anaesthesia). The technique should never be used with frightened children, for whom desensitization and other methods are appropriate. Correct assessment of the reasons for a child's uncooperative behaviour is therefore essential.

2.7 SEDATION

The great majority of children introduced to dentistry by the methods described above become relaxed and cooperative patients who readily accept most operative procedures. Unfortunately a minority remain, or become, uncooperative. The most common reason for lack of cooperation is fear, often of a specific procedure such as the injection or 'the drill'. If fear persists despite carefully conducted introductory sessions, some form of sedation may be helpful. In general, it may be said that sedation will be most effective with children who are genuinely frightened but who understand the need for treatment and who wish to be helped; children whose lack of cooperation has no rational basis and who simply do not wish to cooperate are less likely to respond favourably to any form of sedation.

It should be emphasized that by sedation is meant the allaying of anxiety. Although reducing anxiety tends to raise the patient's pain threshold, sedation does not produce analgesia. Therefore, the use of local analgesia in normally required, but this usually presents no problems when the patient is sedated. However, sedation with nitrous oxide (p. 21) produces some analgesia in addition to sedation, and local analgesia is then not always required.

It must also be emphasized that the sedated patient is conscious and in command of all normal protective reflexes, including the cough reflex. Therefore, sedation may be administered by the dentist who performs the dental treatment, in sharp contrast to anaesthesia, which must not be administered by the person responsible for the dental treatment.

Sedation may be administered by the following routes:

1. Inhalational.
2. Oral.
3. Intramuscular.
4. Intravenous.
5. Rectal.

The inhalational method is the most widely used in the UK, but where the necessary equipment and facilities are not available other methods may be considered.

2.7.1 Inhalational route

The technique of sedation by inhalation of nitrous oxide and oxygen has become well established. It was pioneered principally by Langa (1976) who named the technique Relative Analgesia. This term was introduced by Guedel (1937) who, having described the stages of inhalation anaesthesia, divided the first stage (analgesia) into 'relative analgesia' and 'total analgesia'. Although nitrous oxide has analgesic properties, the principal aim of the technique is to sedate the patient, and for this reason the term 'inhalational sedation' is preferred. The sedated patient communicates freely with the dentist and is relaxed, fear having been reduced or eliminated. The pain threshold is raised, often to a point that allows simple conservative dentistry to be performed without added local analgesia. Local analgesia is, nevertheless, normally required, but the injection is usually accepted by patients who previously were afraid and would not accept it. Inhalational sedation and local analgesia have also been used successfully for dental extractions in children who would otherwise have been treated under general anaesthesia (Crawford 1990).

The levels of nitrous oxide analgesia have been described by Roberts and Rosenbaum (1991) as follows:

Plane 1: Moderate sedation and   5–25% N_2O
analgesia

Plane 2: Dissociation sedation and   20–55% N_2O
analgesia

Plane 3: Total analgesia   50–70% N_2O

Moderate analgesia is characterized by relaxation and mild analgesia; the patient may feel 'tingling' sensations in the toes, fingers or other parts of the body. At the lower levels of dissociation analgesia (about 30% nitrous oxide), analgesia is more marked; the patient still reacts to pain but feels detached from and little concerned by it. The patient may report mild sensations of drowsiness, of detachment from the immediate environment, or of euphoria similar to that associated with alcoholic intoxication; these sensations are generally, but not always, regarded as pleasant. At higher levels of dissociation analgesia, these sensations become more marked and unpleasant, making such levels incompatible with relaxation. Thus, the desired level of sedation is within the zone of moderate analgesia or in the lower levels of dissociation analgesia, generally achieved by inhalation of between 15% and 35% nitrous oxide. The concentration cannot be specified more precisely because patients vary considerably in their responses; the concentration administered is based on close observation of the patient. However, satisfactory results have been reported using a fixed concentration of 25% nitrous oxide, achieved by using Entonox (50% nitrous oxide + 50% oxygen) diluted with an equal volume of air (Edmunds & Rosen 1977).

Technique

Before employing inhalational sedation for the first time it is important to understand the principles of the technique, which have been fully discussed by Langa (1976), Bennett (1978) and Roberts (1991).

Specially designed continuous-flow machines are recommended for administering nitrous oxide and oxygen; they have several safety features, and are more convenient and economical to use than anaesthesia machines. The machines used in the UK are the Quantiflex 'RA' and 'MDM' machines. The 'RA' has separate controls to regulate the flow rates of nitrous oxide and oxygen; the more modern 'MDM' has one control to regulate the gas mixture (that is, the proportions of nitrous oxide and oxygen) and another to regulate the total flow rate.

It is important to use a lightweight nosepiece. Three sizes are available, the smaller two being suitable for most children. The nosepiece has an expiratory valve and an air inlet. The expiratory valve is open and cannot be adjusted (although in older nosepieces it can be closed). The air inlet can be opened and closed. In the techniques recommended below for using both the 'RA' and 'MDM' machines, the air inlet is closed when nitrous oxide is introduced. Langa (1976) kept the air inlet one-quarter open, but this method is not generally used; allowing entry of air makes it necessary to use more nitrous oxide to achieve the required concentration, which is an unnecessary waste of gas.

When using the standard type of nosepiece, expired gases pass through the expiratory valve into the surgery atmosphere, and it is therefore important to have adequate ventilation in the room. It is preferable, however, and highly desirable, to use a 'scavenging' system, which channels expired gases through the expiratory valve into a length of flexible tubing, the end of which is passed out of a window or through a hole in an outside wall. A vacuum unit incorporated in the system increases its efficiency, and the use of a high-volume dental aspirator also helps to reduce ambient nitrous oxide levels (Henry & Borganelli 1995).

Full cylinders of nitrous oxide and oxygen must be connected to the machine in addition to the cylinders in use. Before using the machine, the pressures in the cylinders in use must be checked to confirm that they are not empty.

Before administering inhalational sedation, it is important to ensure that 'a second appropriate person' (for example a suitably-trained dental nurse) is present and that resuscitation equipment is readily available (General Dental Council 1993).

Success with nitrous oxide sedation is dependent on establishing close communication with, and gaining the cooperation of, the patient. Therefore, the method is most suitable for the patient who is frightened of dentistry but who wishes to receive treatment. Very young or mentally handicapped children present special problems, but sedation can sometimes be successful if their attention and interest can be gained. For these, or for particularly nervous patients, an orally-administered sedative may be helpful in overcoming the initial fear of the inhalation method itself.

An important advantage of inhalational sedation over other forms is that patients recover rapidly and can be dismissed within 5 minutes of the termination of treatment, with no limitations on the activities they may undertake during the rest of the day. In addition, most (but not all) children prefer the nosepiece to an intravenous injection.

No special instructions need be given to a parent bringing a child for nitrous oxide sedation, but to reduce the slight possibility of vomiting, the parent may be advised to give the child no more than a light meal 2 or 3 hours before the dental appointment. Contraindications are few, but include upper respiratory infections (e.g. the common cold) and pulmonary disease. Clearly, nasal obstruction due to any cause, if it prevents easy breathing through the nose, makes the method difficult or impossible to use. If the patient is under psychiatric care, it is prudent to consult with the psychiatrist before proceeding with this or with any other form of sedation.

Technique: inhalational sedation

Procedure	Method	Rationale	Notes
Introductory session			
1. Prepare the patient	Explain the technique in terms that the child can understand: e.g. "happy air", "magic wind", "helps you to feel good, relaxed, happy". Emphasize that the child will not go to sleep. Mention that many children have tried it, as well as the dentist and nurse; all think "it's great".	Good psychological preparation is essential. The child's attention, interest and cooperation must be obtained before the technique can be introduced.	It cannot be emphasized too strongly that the success of the technique is greatly dependent on the dentist's participation in relaxing the patient. It is strongly recommended that the dentist should experience inhalational sedation, so that the sensations can be described accurately to the patients.
	Reassure the child that no dental treatment will be done at this session.	Removing the threat of treatment increases the chances of the child accepting the procedure.	Sometimes treatment is essential and ideal introduction is not possible.
2. Fill the reservoir bag with O_2. Open the air inlet on the nosepiece	Allow the bag to fill slowly, or fill quickly by using the 'O_2 flush' control.		If using an old type of nosepiece, the expiratory valve should be fully open.
		An open air inlet ensures that the patient can breathe freely.	Patients may initially feel a slight sense of suffocation if the nosepiece is introduced with the air inlet closed, even if oxygen flow is adequate.
3. Introduce the nosepiece	Position the nosepiece gently on the nose and ask the child to "make it comfortable". Adjust the position and the tension of the tubes behind the chair in such a way that the nosepiece is held securely but not tightly on the patient's nose.	It is essential to ensure that the child does not feel restricted by the nosepiece.	
	Give praise and suggestions of pleasant, relaxing sensations, while the child breathes O_2 and air.	It is important to have the child comfortably relaxed even before the N_2O is introduced.	

Technique: inhalational sedation *(contd)*

Procedure	Method	Rationale	Notes
4. Set O$_2$ flow rate to about 4 litres/min. Close the air inlet	Observe the reservoir bag to check that the flow rate is adequate; increase if necessary. Give the child encouragement, reassurance and praise as appropriate.	A volume of 4 litres/min of gas is usually adequate for comfortable breathing by children (adults require 6–8 litres/min). The flow rate should be sufficient to prevent the reservoir bag from emptying.	
5. Introduce N$_2$O	Introduce N$_2$O only if the child is cooperating.	If the child is not cooperating, further psychological preparation is advisable before proceeding.	
	'RA' machine — Keep O$_2$ flow at 4 litres/min. Introduce N$_2$O at 0.5 litres/min. 'MDM' machine — Set gas mixture control to about 90% O$_2$ (i.e. 10% N$_2$O); the total flow rate remains constant.		4 litres/min O$_2$ + 0.5 litres/min N$_2$O = 11% N$_2$O. This does not take into account leakage around the nosepiece, or mouthbreathing.
6. Inform and make suggestions about sensations to be expected	Sit near the child and speak quietly and calmly with a soothing voice. *Suggest* that the "happy air" has a "nice" smell. *Suggest* that a slight tingle m*a*y be felt in the toes, fingers or other parts; suggest that it is a "funny feeling". *Suggest* that the whole body *may* feel very light, or very heavy; *suggest* that it is a "lovely feeling", like "floating in the clouds" or "lying comfortably in bed".	Since patients' responses differ, it is wise to use the word 'may' rather than 'will', and to suggest alternative sensations.	Verbal communication is essential, but it is also helpful to maintain physical communication by placing a hand on the child's shoulder from time to time.
	From time to time, ask the patient to describe the sensations. Reinforce all the pleasant sensations described.	Asking the child what is felt is better than to ask how it feels; the latter suggests the possibility of an unpleasant feeling.	
7. Increase the proportion of N$_2$O if desired	If the expected sensations are not reported within about 2 minutes, or to deepen the level of sedation, increase the concentration of N$_2$O. 'RA' machine — increase N$_2$O by 0.5 litres/min and, if desired after 1–2 min, by another 0.5 litres/min to total 1.5 litres/min. 'MDM' machine — set gas mixture to 80% O$_2$ and, if desired after 1–2 min, to 70% O$_2$.	It is important: a. to increase the concentration of N$_2$O gradually, b. to allow at least 1 minute for the new concentration to have its effect, c. to check on the effect by observing and by questioning the patient.	1.5 litres/min N$_2$O + 4 litres/min O$_2$, with no air dilution, produces N$_2$O concentration of 30%.
8. Terminate the session	When the patient has enjoyed the experience for 1–2 minutes, the session may be terminated. Before doing so, suggest that at subsequent visits the feeling of happiness and relaxation will be even greater and that dental treatment will be easy to accept. Reduce N$_2$O to zero and give 100% O$_2$ for at least 2 minutes.	As N$_2$O is rapidly eliminated through the lungs, the relative concentration of O$_2$ in the lung alveoli might fall to a hypoxic level if O$_2$ is not administered.	The patient may be shown that mouthbreathing lightens the level of sedation. Knowledge that they have this control gives some patients added confidence.

Technique: inhalational sedation *(contd)*

Procedure	Method	Rationale	Notes
Subsequent sessions			
1. Prepare the patient	Remind the child of the pleasant sensations experienced at the last visit.		
2, 3, 4	As at introductory session.		
5. Introduce N_2O	Introduce 10% N_2O, and increase by 10% increments at 1–2 minute intervals until reaching the level found satisfactory at the introductory session.		
6. Inform and make suggestions about sensations	Inform the child that the sensations will begin to be noted in about 1 minute. Repeat the suggestions made at the last visit.	Continued close communication with the child is essential.	
7. Proceed with dental treatment	When the patient is comfortably sedated, start dental treatment. Reinforce feelings of comfort and relaxation, and suggest that in this happy state treatment will be easy to accept. Local analgesia may not be required for conservative dentistry. If local analgesia is required, introduce with care if this is known to have caused anxiety previously. Inform the child, in a casual manner, that it will be given, and suggest that it is nothing to worry about. Regularly reinforce good behaviour with praise. When treatment is completed, reduce N_2O to zero and give 100% O_2 for at least 2 minutes.	The pain threshold may be sufficiently elevated in the sedated patient to obviate the need for local analgesia. The dentist should not use sedation to break faith with the child by carrying out treatment without consent.	If the degree of sedation is not adequate, further increments of about 5% N_2O may be added. Beyond about 40% N_2O, symptoms of dissociation may be unpleasant.

2.7.2 Oral route

Many drugs and combinations of drugs have been administered orally to sedate anxious children, including chloral hydrate, meperidine, promethazine, and diazepam (Houpt 1993).

Diazepam has probably been used most frequently, either in a single dose (1 hour before the dental appointment) or in three doses (on the evening before the appointment, on rising on the day of the appointment, and 1 hour before the appointment). Although diazepam has been shown to be effective in helping adult patients to accept dental treatment (Baird & Curson 1970), studies with children have given conflicting results. Auil et al (1983) administered a single dose of 0.5 mg diazepam to 4- to 8-year-old children in the waiting room 1 hour before treatment and found it to be ineffective. Lindsay & Yates (1985) also reported no effect with slightly older children (aged 4–13 years), using either a single dose of 0.2 mg/kg given in the waiting room 1 hour before treatment, or a series of three doses (2 mg the evening before treatment, and 0.2 mg/kg on rising on the day of treatment and again 1 hour before treatment in the afternoon). On the other hand, Yanase et al (1996) found a single dose of 0.3 mg/kg, given to 1- to 8-year-olds by their parents at home 1 hour before the appointment, to be effective; they suggested that administration of the drug by parents at home is preferable because a 1-hour wait in the dentist's waiting room probably increases fear and tension in a child, thus reducing the sedative effect of the drug.

Temazepam, a minor metabolite of diazepam, has also been studied; given to preschool children in a dose of 0.3 mg/kg it was found to be as effective as a combination of chloral hydrate and hydroxyzine (Tsinidou et al 1992).

Before prescribing a sedative, the dentist should gain the trust and confidence of the child. The sedative must be portrayed as something that will help to produce relaxation and therefore to overcome fear. It is important that patients do not feel threatened by imagining that the sedative will force them into submission; rather they should feel that it is being used to help them. Unfortunately this approach based on trust and understanding is impracticable with very young, uncooperative children.

If it is decided to ask a parent to administer the drug at home, it is preferable for the child not to attend school before the dental visit, because the drug may cause drowsiness.

Although it is simple and convenient to administer a drug orally, the effects are less predictable than when it is given by other routes, because of many factors that influence absorption. Therefore the use of an orally-administered sedative should not necessarily be abandoned if the desired effects are not obtained at the first attempt; the dose may be increased until the appropriate dose for the individual patient is reached.

2.7.3 Intramuscular route

The advantage of administering a drug intramuscularly rather than orally is that its action is more rapid and its effect more predictable. A disadvantage, however, is that a nervous, uncooperative child inevitably finds the intramuscular injection an unpleasant procedure.

Various types of drugs have been used (Musselman & McClure 1975). An effective combination is promethazine hydrochloride (Phenergan) and pethidine. Promethazine is an antihistamine that has sedative and anti-emetic properties. Pethidine is a potent analgesic but has little sedative effect. In combination they provide sedation and analgesia, and the anti-emetic action of promethazine counteracts the nausea that may be produced by pethidine. The doses for intramuscular injection are pethidine 1.5 mg/kg and promethazine 0.75 mg/kg. The injection may be given in the upper lateral quadrant of the buttock, the anterior aspect of the upper thigh or the lateral aspect of the upper arm (Musselman & McClure 1975, Bennett 1978). The method has been widely used in the USA, particularly to produce deep sedation in very uncooperative young patients who generally cannot be adequately sedated by oral, intravenous or inhalational methods. In the UK such patients are usually treated under general anaesthesia.

2.7.4 Intravenous route

The principal advantages of the intravenous route over the oral and intramuscular routes are that the injected drug has a very rapid effect and that the dose can be given in increments until the desired level of sedation is achieved.

Intravenously administered sedation for dental patients was introduced by Jorgensen & Leffingwell (1961), who used a mixture of pentobarbitone, pethidine and hyoscine. Later, diazepam became the drug of choice for intravenous sedation. Diazepam produces effective sedation, muscle relaxation and amnesia but it has the disadvantages that it is only slowly eliminated from the body, and its injection into a vein is often painful. The more recently introduced midazolam (Hypnovel) has similar sedative, relaxant and amnesic properties to those of diazepam but it is more quickly eliminated from the body and does not cause pain on injection (McGimpsey et al 1983).

Patients selected for intravenous sedation must be cooperative despite their anxieties, because they must be prepared to accept an intravenous injection. Their cooperation generally is based on trust and confidence in the dentist, and on their desire to receive treatment. For these and, perhaps, other reasons, the technique of intravenous sedation has been found to be more successful with adults than with children. However, some children can be successfully treated in this way (Healy & Hamilton 1971).

To administer a drug intravenously requires a mastery of the technique of venepuncture; the technique is well described by Rosenbaum (1991). Midazolam is injected into a vein in the dorsum of the hand. The dose required to produce satisfactory sedation is about 0.1 mg/kg body weight; this is injected slowly, over a period of 1–2 minutes, during which time the child is spoken to in a relaxing and reassuring manner. Sedation is deepest immediately following the injection and for the next 10 minutes; during this period the injection of local analgesic is given and treatment is commenced. There is complete or partial amnesia from the time of the intravenous injection; thus, the patient may remember the intravenous but not the intraoral injection, even if the latter caused discomfort. The depth of sedation becomes progressively lighter and the patient usually appears normal about 1 hour after injection. However, the drug may continue to have an effect for several hours; the patient should be required to rest for about 1 hour before leaving the surgery, and then to rest at home for the rest of the day. The need for a period of postoperative recovery, and the subsequent restriction of activities, are the main disadvantages of this technique.

The General Dental Council (1993) has stipulated that, when employing intravenous or inhalation sedation techniques, 'a second appropriate person' must be present throughout the treatment session. This person might be a suitably trained dental surgery assistant who is capable of monitoring the condition of the patient and of assisting the dentist in case of emergency. It is also essential to have appropriate facilities for resuscitation readily available.

2.7.5 Rectal route

The rectal route for the administration of drugs is frequently used in medical practice but rarely in dentistry. However, it is employed successfully in Sweden for the dental treatment of young, anxious patients (Lundgren et al 1978), using a preparation containing 5 mg or 10 mg diazepam in 2.5 ml solution. The same preparation has been used in the UK for sedating young children requiring treatment of maxillofacial injuries (Lowey & Halfpenny 1993); its administration was not considered by the parents or the children to be traumatic. Rectally administered diazepam has also proved effective for sedating young children prior to restorative treatment, using a dosage of 0.6 mg diazepam/kg body weight (Flaitz et al 1985), and rectally administered midazolam (0.25 or 0.35 mg/kg body weight) has been used successfully in children undergoing the extraction of teeth (Roelofse et al 1990).

2.8 HYPNOSIS

Hypnosis has been defined as 'a particular state of mind which is usually induced in one person by another . . . a state of mind in which suggestions are not only more readily accepted than in the waking state but are also acted upon more powerfully than would be possible under normal conditions' (Hartland 1971).

Hypnosis has long been a controversial and misunderstood subject, shrouded by an aura of mysticism which has been encouraged by public entertainers. However, much progress has been made during the last 40–50 years in the scientific investigation of hypnosis, and it now holds an accepted place in medical and dental practice (Waxman 1989, Gibson & Heap 1991, Shaw & Niven 1996).

It is estimated that 90% of individuals can be induced into a light hypnotic trance, which is characterized by relaxation and reduction of anxiety; 70% of these individuals can be deepened to a medium trance, in which some analgesia may be produced; and a further 20% of these can reach a deep trance in which considerable analgesia is possible. Hypnosis can only be induced in individuals who wish to cooperate. Although this might suggest that children are often unsuitable subjects, the reverse is the case. The apparent paradox is explained by the fact that children generally are more amenable to persuasion and suggestion than adults, and more accustomed to accepting instructions without question. It is, however, essential to gain their confidence and to hold their attention, and this may not be possible with very young, frightened or timid children.

Hypnosis is used most commonly in dentistry as a method of helping the anxious patient to relax. A light trance is usually sufficient to achieve this objective; the relaxed patient can then accept treatment procedures which previously were unacceptable. Some patients may be taken to deeper levels, at which sufficient analgesia of teeth or oral tissues may be produced to perform treatment without the need for injection of a local analgesic. Hypnosis may also be useful in helping patients who 'gag' when anything is placed in their mouth; in encouraging children to wear orthodontic appliances; and in introducing children to inhalational sedation or to general anaesthesia.

No doubt many dentists relax their patients by using a calm, kind, understanding approach, without the aid of hypnosis, and the depth of relaxation they achieve may be similar to that of a light hypnotic trance. However, techniques that have been established for the induction of hypnosis are more precise and more likely to be effective with most anxious patients. Various techniques have been described by Lampshire (1975), Smith (1977) and Waxman (1989).

Before proceeding to induce hypnosis, the dentist must prepare the patient by explaining what is to be done. Although adults require careful preparation to correct misconceptions and to remove suspicions and fears of hypnosis, children require only minimal preparation. The word 'hypnosis' need not be used with children. Young children may be told that they will have a special kind of sleep, when their eyes will be closed as if they were asleep but that it will be different because they will hear everything that the dentist says and will be able to talk without waking up. Older children need only be informed that the purpose is to help them to relax so that their worries about dental treatment may be overcome. Parents may be informed that this form of deep relaxation is called 'hypnosis', but it is not essential to offer this information. It is clear that both the child and the parent must have trust in the dentist.

As with inhalational sedation, the ideal approach is to devote the first session to the introduction of hypnosis, having informed the patient that no dental treatment will be performed; removing anxiety about impending treatment increases the chances of success. With the reassurance of a pleasant experience, together with the use of post-hypnotic suggestion, hypnosis is induced more easily and more rapidly at subsequent meetings.

REFERENCES

Adelson R, Goldfried M R 1970 Modelling and the fearful child patient. Journal of Dentistry for Children 37: 476–489

Auil B, Cornejo G, Gallardo F 1983 Flunitrazepam and diazepam compared as sedatives in children. Journal of Dentistry for Children 50: 442–444

Baird E S, Curson I 1970 Orally-administered diazepam in conservative dentistry. British Dental Journal 128: 25–27

Bennett C R 1978 Conscious sedation in dental practice, 2nd edn. Mosby, St Louis

Craig W 1971 Hand over mouth technique. Journal of Dentistry for Children 38: 387–389

Crawford A N 1990 The use of nitrous oxide-oxygen inhalational sedation with local anaesthesia as an alternative to general anaesthesia for dental extractions in children. British Dental Journal 168: 395–398

Edmunds D H, Rosen M 1977 Sedation for conservative dentistry: further studies on inhalation sedation with 25 per cent nitrous oxide. Journal of Dentistry 5: 245–251

Flaitz C M, Nowak A J 1985 Evaluation of the sedative effect of rectally administered diazepam for the young dental patient. Pediatric Dentistry 7: 292–296

Gale E N, Ayer W A 1969 Treatment of dental phobias. Journal of the American Dental Association 78: 1304–1307

General Dental Council 1993 Professional conduct and fitness to practise, p 7

Gibson H B, Heap M 1991 Hypnosis in therapy. Lawrence Erlbaum Associates, London, chs 11, 12

Guedel A E 1937 Inhalational anaesthesia. Macmillan, New York

Hartland J 1971 Medical and dental hypnosis and its clinical applications, 2nd edn. Baillière Tindall, London

Healy T E J, Hamilton M C 1971 Intravenous diazepam in the apprehensive child. British Dental Journal 130: 25–27

Henry R J, Borganelli G 1995 High-volume aspiration as a supplemental scavenging method for reducing ambient nitrous oxide levels in the operatory: a laboratory study. International Journal of Paediatric Dentistry 5: 157–161

Houpt M 1993 Project USAP – the use of sedative agents in pediatric dentistry: 1991 update. Pediatric Dentistry 15: 36–40

Jorgensen N B, Leffingwell F 1961 Premedication in dentistry. Dental Clinics of North America (July) 299–308

Lampshire E L 1975 Hypnosis in dentistry for children. In: Wright G Z (ed) Behaviour management in dentistry for children. Saunders, Philadelphia, ch 6

Langa H 1976 Relative analgesia in dental practice, 2nd edn. Saunders, Philadelphia

Levitas T C 1974 Home: hand over mouth exercise. Journal of Dentistry for Children 41: 178–182

Lindsay S J E, Yates J A 1985 The effectiveness of oral diazepam in anxious child dental patients. British Dental Journal 159: 149–153

Lowey M N, Halfpenny W 1993 Observations on the use of rectally administered diazepam for sedating children before treatment of maxillofacial injuries: report of nine cases. International Journal of Paediatric Dentistry 3: 89–93

Lundgren S, Ekman A, Blomback U 1978 Rectal administration of diazepam in solution. A clinical study on sedation in paediatric dentistry. Swedish Dental Journal 2: 161–166

McGimpsey J G, Kawar P, Gamble J A S, Browne E S, Dundee J W 1983 Midazolam in dentistry. British Dental Journal 155: 47–50

Musselman R J, McClure D B 1975 Pharmacotherapeutic approaches to behaviour management. In: Wright G Z (ed) Behaviour management in dentistry for children. Saunders, Philadelphia, ch 8

Roberts G J 1991 Relative analgesia: inhalation sedation with oxygen and nitrous oxide. In: Roberts G J, Rosenbaum N L A colour atlas of dental analgesia and sedation. Wolfe, London, ch 5

Roelofse J A, Vander Bijl P, Stegmann D H 1990 Preanaesthetic medication with rectal midazolam in children undergoing dental extractions. Journal of Oral and Maxillofacial Surgery 48: 791–796

Rosenbaum N L 1991 The techniques of intravenous sedation. In: Roberts G J, Rosenbaum N L A colour atlas of dental analgesia and sedation. Wolfe, London, ch 12

Rosenberg H M 1974 Behaviour modification for the child dental patient. Journal of Dentistry for Children 41: 111–114

Shaw A J, Niven N 1996 Theoretical concepts and practical applications of hypnosis in the treatment of children and adolescents with dental fear and anxiety. British Dental Journal 180: 11–16

Smith S R 1977 A primer of hypnosis. British Society of Medical and Dental Hypnosis, London

Tsinidou K G, Curzon M E J, Sapsford D J 1992 A study to compare the effectiveness of temazepam and a chloral hydrate/hydroxyzine combination in sedating paediatric dental patients. International Journal of Paediatric Dentistry 2: 163–169

Waxman D 1989 Hartland's medical and dental hypnosis, 3rd edn. Baillière Tindall, London

Wolpe J, Lazarus A A 1966 Behaviour therapy techniques: a guide to the treatment of neuroses. Pergamon, Oxford

Yanase H, Braham R L, Fukuta O, Kurosu K 1996 A study of the sedative effect of home-administered oral diazepam for the dental treatment of children. International Journal of Paediatric Dentistry 6: 13–18

RECOMMENDED READING

Behaviour Management

Bennett A E 1976 Communication between doctors and patients. Oxford University Press, Oxford

Christen A G 1977 Piagetan psychology: some principles helpful in treating the child dental patient. Journal of Dentistry for Children 44: 48-52

Ingersoll B D 1982 Behavioral aspects in dentistry. Appleton-Century-Crofts, New York

Kent G, Blinkhorn A S 1991 The psychology of dental care, 2nd edn. Wright, Bristol

Kreinces G H 1975 Ginott psychology applied to pedodontics. Journal of Dentistry for Children 42: 119–122

Malamed S F 1995 Sedation – a guide to patient management, 3rd edn. Mosby-Year Book

Ripa L W, Barenie J T 1979 Management of dental behaviour in children. PSG, Littleton, M A

Wright G Z 1975 Behavior management in dentistry for children. Saunders, Philadelphia, ch 5

Wright G Z, Starkey P E, Gardner D E 1987 Child management in dentistry. IOP Publishing, Bristol, chs 9, 18

Psychological Development

Alpern G 1975 Child development: basic concepts and clinical considerations. In: Wright G Z (ed) Behaviour management in dentistry for children. Saunders, Philadelphia, ch 2

Blain S M 1982 Behaviour. In: Barber T K, Luke L S (eds) Pediatric dentistry. Wright, Bristol, ch 4

Butler N R, Golding J 1986 From birth to five. A study of the health and behaviour of Britain's 5-year-olds. Pergamon Press, Oxford

Kenna M D, Smith B A 1985 Psychologic growth and development. In: Braham R L, Morris M E (eds) Textbook of pediatric dentistry, 2nd edn. Williams & Wilkins, Baltimore, ch 3

Gesell A L 1954 The first five years of life. Methuen, London

Gesell A L, Ilg F J 1946 The child from five to ten. Hamilton, London

Holloway P J, Swallow J N 1982 Child dental health, 3rd edn. Wright, Bristol, ch 2

Lowrey G H 1973 Growth and development of children, 6th edn. Year Book Medical Publishers, Chicago

Sarles R M 1981 Psychologic growth and development. In: Forrester D J (ed) Pediatric dental medicine. Lea & Febiger, Philadelphia, ch 3

Sheridan M D 1975 From birth to five years, 3rd edn. NFER-Nelson, Windsor

Treatment of dental caries—preventive methods

Part 2

3 Dental health education

It is generally accepted that dental caries is initiated by acids produced during the bacterial degradation of dietary carbohydrate in the dental plaque. It follows that two important methods of preventing dental caries must be to control dietary carbohydrate and to remove dental plaque from the teeth. It should be an important aim of all dentists to educate their patients about these methods and, indeed, of the dental profession to educate the public at large. To be effective, methods used in dental health education should be planned and carried out skilfully. The aim must be not only to instruct, but also to persuade; success depends greatly on the sincerity and interest shown by each member of the dental team.

3.1 THE INDIVIDUAL

3.1.1 Toothbrushing instruction

Although about 75% of children in the UK claim to brush their teeth at least twice a day, the majority have plaque on their teeth (O'Brien 1994); this indicates that toothbrushing generally is done ineffectively. In teaching children how to brush their teeth, the aim must be to instruct and to encourage them to remove all debris and plaque from all accessible tooth surfaces.

A suggested method is outlined below.

Technique: toothbrushing instruction

Procedure	Method	Rationale	Notes
1. Assessment		An assessment of the patient's oral cleanliness provides a baseline against which the effects of instruction can be evaluated. An objective assessment is preferred to a simple statement of 'good', 'fair' or 'poor'. The surfaces that are examined are those on which debris readily accumulates unless toothbrushing is carried out effectively.	The method outlined is based on the Oral Debris Index described by Greene & Vermillion (1964). Examining only six tooth surfaces is a quick and simple procedure. The plaque index of Silness and Loe (1964), in which all surfaces of six teeth are examined, is more comprehensive but also more time-consuming. The simpler procedure adequately fulfils the purpose of providing baseline information for oral hygiene instruction.
a. Assess oral cleanliness	Examine in turn the following tooth surfaces: buccal buccal | buccal 6 1 6 ————————— 6 1 6 lingual | buccal | lingual (buccal 11, 16, 26, 31; lingual 36, 46)		

31

Technique: toothbrushing instruction (*contd*)

Procedure	Method	Rationale	Notes

Rest a probe against the tooth surface in the distal embrasure, with its tip at the gingival margin. Draw the probe mesially, keeping it in contact with the tooth surface (Fig. 3.1). Observe the distribution of debris, and score as follows:

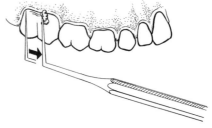

Fig. 3.1

0—no debris.
1—debris within gingival $\frac{1}{3}$ only.
2—debris beyond gingival $\frac{1}{3}$ but within gingival $\frac{2}{3}$.
3—debris beyond gingival $\frac{2}{3}$ (i.e covering most of surface).

Method: Record results, e.g.

$$\begin{array}{c|c} 1 \quad\;\; 1 & 2 \\ \hline 2 \quad\;\; 2 & 2 \end{array}$$

Rationale: Recording the results in this way indicates where the emphasis in instruction need to be given:

e.g. $\begin{array}{c|c} 0 \quad\;\; 0 & 0 \\ \hline 2 \quad\;\; 0 & 2 \end{array}$ instruction required only in cleaning lingual surface of mandibular molars;

e.g. $\begin{array}{c|c} 2 \quad\;\; 0 & 0 \\ \hline 2 \quad\;\; 0 & 0 \end{array}$ instruction required only in cleaning right side of mouth;

e.g. $\begin{array}{c|c} 2 \quad\;\; 1 & 2 \\ \hline 2 \quad\;\; 1 & 2 \end{array}$ general instruction required.

Notes: If the specific tooth is not present in the mouth, use the tooth just mesial or distal to it—regions of the mouth are more important than specific teeth. Debris scores noted on the patient's record card can be of value in motivating the patient, by showing how toothbrushing has improved at subsequent visits.

---

b. Assess tooth-brushing technique

Method: Observe the child using a toothbrush.
Note: 1. Whether all surfaces of teeth are brushed.
2. Whether teeth are brushed in any particular order.
3. Whether any specific technique is used.

Rationale: Instruction should be tailored to the needs of the patient. Observing the patient's technique indicates whether full instruction is required or whether attention need be given only to specific aspects.

Notes: It has been recommended (p. 11) that, at the first visit, the parents should be asked to bring the child's toothbrush on their next visit. Not only will the child brush more comfortably with this brush but the adequacy of the brush can be assessed. Brushes should be available for those who forget to bring their own.

---

2. Start instruction

a. Explain the reasons for tooth-brushing

Method: According to the child's age and intelligence, give a brief explanation of the cause of gingivitis and dental caries. Indicate the role of 'germs', plaque and foods. Use models, posters, extracted teeth or other visual aids to illustrate gingivitis and the progress of caries.

Rationale: It is essential to stimulate the child's interest.

Notes: Ideally, a parent should be present to listen and observe; a good parent will remind the child at home of the dentist's instructions.

Technique: toothbrushing instruction (*contd*)

Procedure	Method	Rationale	Notes
b. Demonstrate on models and in the child's mouth	(Assuming that the child's toothbrushing efficiency is poor, as assessed by the state of oral cleanliness and the observed toothbrushing technique.) On a model, demonstrate that 'back' teeth have 3 'sides'—cheek, tongue and biting surfaces—and that 'front' teeth have 2 'sides' (Fig. 3.2a). Explain that all these 'sides' need to be brushed. So as not to miss any, a system is needed—suggest a starting point and an order for brushing all the teeth (Fig. 3.2b). Now demonstrate the method in the child's mouth, with the child observing in a mirror. Then ask the child to do the same on the model and then in the mouth.	It is important to give the child a mental picture of what must be brushed, and to emphasize the need for a systematic approach.	If the child's toothbrushing efficiency is good, praise and encouragement should be given. It is reasonable to exclude mention of approximal surfaces at this stage.

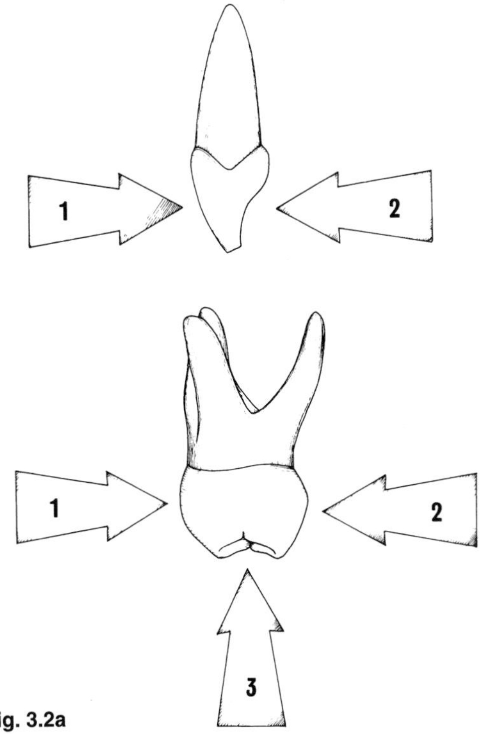

Fig. 3.2a

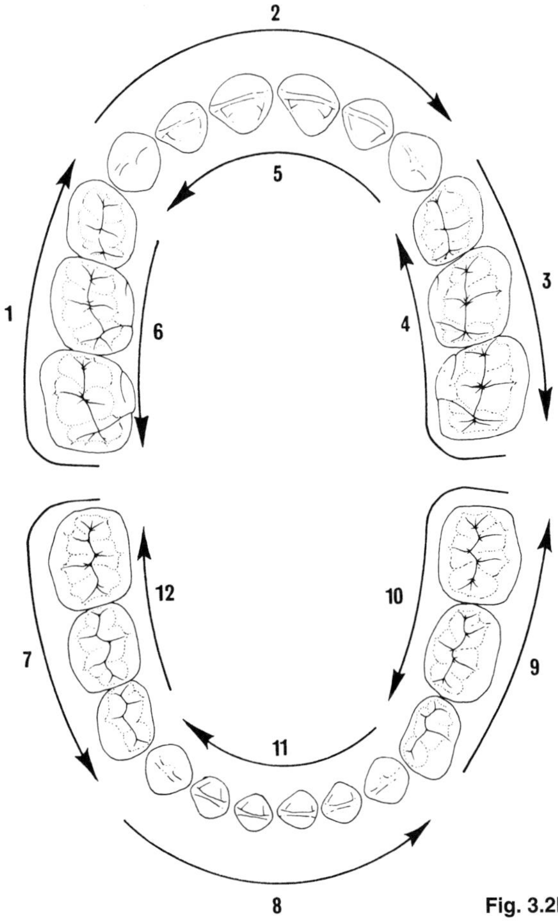

Fig. 3.2b

c. Give advice to the child and/ or parent:	With a child younger than 5–6 years of age, show the parent how to hold the child (see page 35) and ask him/ her to demonstrate the brushing technique.	Young children cannot be expected to brush efficiently.	Although young children should be encouraged to brush their own teeth, parents should also be encouraged to assume responsibility.

Technique: toothbrushing instruction (*contd*)

Procedure	Method	Rationale	Notes
(i) toothbrush	Recommend a high-quality brush (as supplied by specialist companies)—these have soft, fine filaments (about 0.018 mm diameter). Recommend a brush with a handle small enough for the child to handle comfortably and with a brush head not more than 2 cm long.	Soft, fine-filament brushes are more likely to penetrate interdentally and into the gingival crevices without causing gingival damage. Parents tend to provide their child with a brush that is too large.	The tips of the filaments of the best brushes are rounded and smooth (Silverstone & Featherstone 1988).
(ii) toothpaste	Recommend a fluoride-containing toothpaste.	Fluoride-containing toothpastes are effective in reducing caries incidence. 'Brush after breakfast and before going to bed' has long been an accepted dental health message.	Most toothpastes on the market in the UK now contain fluoride. Although brushing at least twice a day should be recommended, it is more important to remove plaque thoroughly once a day than to brush inefficiently more frequently.
(iii) frequency	Recommend that teeth are brushed very thoroughly last thing at night before going to bed and after breakfast.		
(iv) duration	Advise the child to take 2 or 3 minutes for brushing.	Thorough toothbrushing cannot be accomplished very hurriedly.	A systematic and efficient technique is more important than the duration of brushing.

3. Next visit

a. Evaluate progress

Determine oral debris scores, and compare with scores recorded at the previous visit. Then observe the child brushing or (with young children) the parent brushing the child's teeth. Note any improvements and praise the child and/or parent. Encourage rather than criticize.

Efficient toothbrushing is not easy. Rapid improvement should not be expected—the child should be given time to improve gradually.

Ideally, the child will have brough his/her own toothbrush (if requested to do so at their previous visit).

b. Introduce a self-assessment method

With a cotton pledget, apply disclosing solution to all surfaces of the teeth (Fig. 3.2c). Alternatively ask the child to chew a disclosing tablet. Demonstrate the disclosed plaque, then ask the child to brush it off and to check efficiency.

Use of disclosing solution is of doubtful value with a young child who cannot understand its significance (but the parent may find it instructive).

c. Give more detailed instruction on technique

If the child uses a recognizable technique, develop that technique to a greater level of efficiency. If a haphazard technique is used, introduce either a *gentle* scrubbing action, or the Bass technique, or any other.

If the child and/or parent shows sufficient interest, recommend the occasional use of a disclosing tablet at home.

There is no evidence that any particular technique is more effective than others. Especially with children, who may become discouraged by a difficult exercise, it is more important to emphasize the need to reach all tooth surfaces than to insist on a particular technique.

Fig. 3.2c

4. Subsequent visits

Evaluate progress and emphasize previous instruction

Assess oral cleanliness and toothbrushing technique as before. Instruct as necessary to maintain standards or to improve in specific aspects. Reinforce good performance by praising and giving an appropriate reward (e.g. a 'sticker').

Good behaviour, if reinforced, is more likely to be continued.

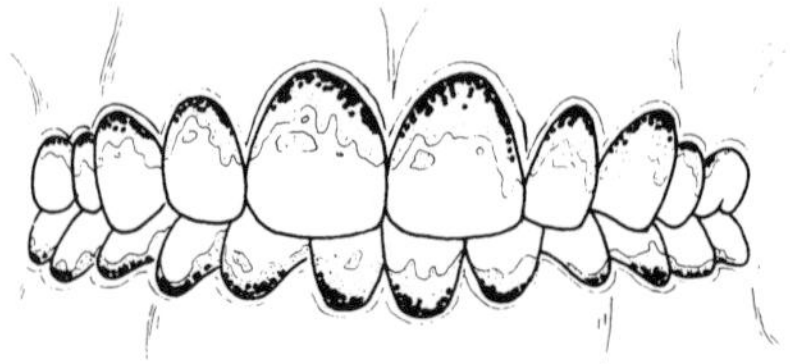

It is not easy to master an effective technique of toothbrushing, and some children do not have the manual dexterity to succeed. This is especially the case with young children below the age of 5–6 years, and with the mentally or physically handicapped. To help such patients, the dentist must involve a parent (or guardian), who must be encouraged to accept responsibility. Young and mentally or physically handicapped children should be encouraged to brush their own teeth, but also to allow parents to help. Instruction concerning technique should then be directed at the parent. Electric toothbrushes may be useful for such patients.

If not instructed, parents usually stand or sit face-to-face with their child when brushing the child's teeth. A much better approach is as illustrated in Figure 3.3; this provides good support for the child's head and gives the parent much greater control. The parent should be instructed to use the fingers of the left hand to retract cheeks and lips as required, to improve access for the toothbrush; most parents will

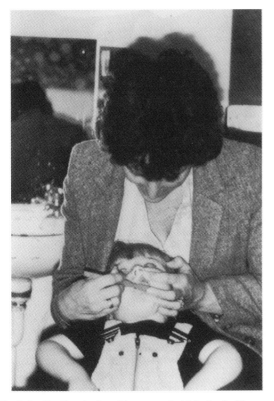

Fig. 3.3 Position for brushing a small child's teeth. The parent either stands or sits, depending on the child's height. The child's head is tilted backwards and rests on the parent's chest or abdomen.

not do this unless instructed, using their left hands only to support the child's head. Parents should be advised to start brushing their child's teeth as soon as the first tooth erupts, so that toothbrushing becomes accepted as part of the normal bathroom routine.

Several toothbrushing techniques have been proposed; these are summarized in Table 3.1 and illustrated in Figure 3.4. There is no evidence that one technique is superior to others in removing dental plaque, although it might be expected that the Scrub method would not penetrate the gingival sulcus or interdental areas as readily as others. All except the Scrub method require some manual dexterity. To insist on a method that the child finds difficult risks discouraging the child from brushing at all. It is usually wiser to start with the Scrub technique and to introduce one of the other techniques only after some progress has been made in developing the child's interest and cooperation. The Bass technique is generally favoured and, if the parent brushes the child's teeth, this method may be recommended; the child may learn to imitate the technique.

The relationship between toothbrushing and gingivitis is easy to demonstrate; every dentist has noted marginal gingivitis associated with plaque deposits, and resolution of the gingivitis when efficient toothbrushing is instituted. This relationship was confirmed long ago in clinical studies with adults and with children (Koch & Lindhe 1965). However, the relationship between toothbrushing and dental caries is less easy to demonstrate. With individual patients, the introduction of efficient toothbrushing may be seen to be followed by the arrest of, for example, early cervical lesions, but various types of studies with groups of children have shown only a weak relationship between oral hygiene and dental caries (Andlaw 1978, Sutcliffe 1996). It is probable that toothbrushing must be done very effectively to have an effect in preventing dental caries; in addition, its effect is limited by the fact that toothbrush bristles cannot penetrate deep pits or fissures, or interdental spaces. Therefore, although oral hygiene instruction should be aimed at achieving an excellent standard of oral cleanliness, patients and their parents should not be led to believe that this is all that is required to prevent dental caries; other factors, especially dietary factors, are also involved (p. 38).

3.1.2 Dental floss and tape

'Flossing' with dental floss or tape removes plaque from approximal tooth surfaces that are inaccessible to the toothbrush. Ideally, therefore, flossing should accompany toothbrushing as part of normal oral hygiene practice. However, flossing is a difficult

Table 3.1 Summary of toothbrushing techniques

| Method | Starting position | | Movements* |
	Tips of bristles	Direction of bristles	
Scrub	On gingival margin	Horizontal.	Scrub in antero–posterior direction, keeping brush horizontal.
Roll	On gingival margin	Pointing apically, parallel to the long axis of the teeth.	Roll brush occlusally, maintaining contact with gingiva, then with the tooth surface.
Bass	On gingival margin	Pointing apically, about 45° to the long axis of the teeth.	Vibrate the brush, not changing the position of the bristles.
Stillman	On gingival margin	Pointing apically, about 45° to the long axis of the teeth.	Apply pressure to blanch the gingiva, then remove. Repeat several times. Slightly rotate the brush occlusally during the procedure.
Modified Stillman	On gingival margin	Pointing apically, about 45° to the long axis of the teeth.	Apply pressure as in Stillman method, but at the same time vibrate the brush and gradually move it occlusally.
Fones	On gingival margin	Horizontal.	With the teeth in occlusion, move the brush in a rotary motion against the maxillary and mandibular tooth surfaces and gingival margins.
Charters	Level with occlusal surfaces of teeth	Pointing occlusally, about 45° to the long axis of the teeth.	Vibrate the brush while moving it apically to the gingival margin.

* For occlusal surfaces, a vigorous scrubbing action is recommended, except by Charters, who recommends small rotary movements to encourage the bristles to penetrate pits and fissures.

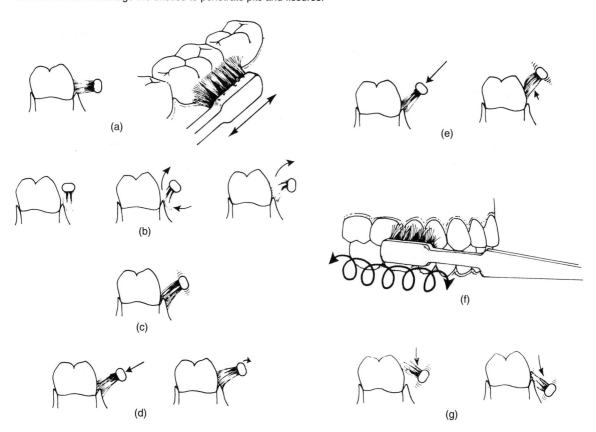

Fig. 3.4   Toothbrushing techniques: (a) Scrub (b) Roll (c) Bass (d) Stillman (e) Modified Stillman (f) Fones (g) Charters.

procedure, requiring considerable practice before it is mastered. Most children need constant encouragement to maintain an adequate standard of toothbrushing, and it would be unreasonable to expect all children to perform an additional procedure. Therefore, flossing should only be introduced to children who use a toothbrush easily, efficiently and with some enthusiasm. They may be shown how to floss on anterior teeth first, later extending to posterior teeth. Alternatively, a motivated parent who flosses may be encouraged to floss the child's teeth. It is important for the dentist or hygienist to supervise the procedure periodically, because a poor flossing technique can do more harm than good.

The following advice may be given to the child and parent:

1. Use unwaxed floss or tape. Wax left on the tooth surface may inhibit the uptake of fluoride from toothpaste or from topical treatment.
2. Cut off a length of about 30–40 cm and lightly wrap the ends round the middle fingers (Fig. 3.5a, b).
3. The tips of the fingers or thumbs controlling the floss should not be more than about 2 cm apart, to give maximum control (Fig. 3.5c, d).
4. Pass the floss gently through the contact points by moving the floss bucco-lingually until it slides through slowly. Avoid forcing it through roughly, which would traumatize the interdental papilla.
5. Move the floss gently occluso-gingivally and bucco-lingually against each approximal surface; the floss should be allowed to spread just below the gingival margin (Fig. 3.5e, f).

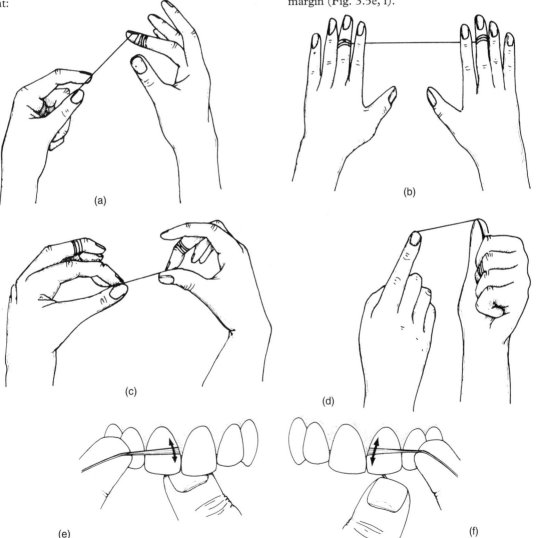

Fig. 3.5   Flossing technique.

6. After flossing all the teeth, rinse the mouth vigorously to remove the plaque and debris dislodged from the interdental spaces.

The effect of flossing on dental caries has been investigated in only one study, which showed that caries incidence was reduced in approximal surfaces of primary molars that were flossed daily for 20 months by research assistants (Wright et al 1977).

3.1.3 Diet counselling

A good, balanced diet is essential for optimal general health; this is important for the mother and fetus during pregnancy and for the growing child. However, there is no evidence that nutritional deficiencies during the period of tooth development affect the teeth or oral soft tissues in such a way as to make them later more susceptible to disease. Other than the possible supplementation of the diet with fluoride (Ch. 4) there are no specific recommendations that need be given concerning the nutritional value of the diet and its relationship to oral health.

The most important factor in the relationship of diet and dental health is the frequency of eating foods containing refined carbohydrate. After eating a carbohydrate-containing food, acid is produced in the dental plaque (Stephan 1940). When acid depresses plaque pH below about pH 5.5, enamel demineralization may occur, and this is generally accepted as being the first stage in the initiation of dental caries. The relationship between the frequency of eating carbohydrate-containing foods and the incidence of dental caries has been demonstrated in a variety of studies (Andlaw 1977, Rugg-Gunn 1989). Thus, the most important aim in diet counselling in relation to dental health is to encourage the patient to control the frequency of eating carbohydrate-containing foods.

Although oral bacteria can break down many carbohydrates to acid, sucrose is particularly implicated in dental caries (Rugg-Gunn & Edgar 1984). Unfortunately, sucrose is a constituent of the majority of snack foods.

The problems of diet counselling are formidable. Many people have acquired at an early age the habit of frequent eating of sweets and snack foods, and consider this to be normal and acceptable behaviour. For an individual patient to change these habits requires a fundamental change in attitude; for the dentist (or ancillary) to achieve this presents a considerable challenge. To have any chance of success, the methods used in diet counselling should be planned not only to give information but also to persuade the child and parent to act on this information. At least for the younger children, parental involvement is essential.

It is easy to explain the reasons for controlling the frequency of eating: the child and parent may be given a brief explanation (perhaps with visual aids) of the production of acid on teeth, including the interaction of 'germs' and food in the plaque. Although such an exercise at least fulfils the dentist's responsibility to impart information, it usually has limited impact and therefore may not motivate patients to improve their diet habits. No known method is certain to have the desired effect, but the use of a diet record form, on which the parent is asked to record the child's diet for a number of days, is recommended. The advantages of this method are that the parent (and child if old enough) becomes actively involved in recording the diet, and that the advice subsequently given is more personal, being based on the child's own diet.

Various diet record forms have been designed, varying considerably in their complexity. A simple form is illustrated on page 39.

It is most important to be tactful in introducing a diet record form to parents. It should be presented as a means of helping them; this is printed on the form but should be emphasized. If introduced in this way, most parents are pleased to cooperate, but a careless approach can antagonize them by giving the impression that their care of the child is to be criticized.

When the completed diet form is returned by the patient, there are two principal ways of proceeding. The simpler but perhaps the less effective way is for the dentist to peruse the form in the presence of the child and parent, and to comment and advise on the good or bad points that emerge from it. The other, more effective, approach is to receive the form, expressing thanks for their interest and help in completing it, and to inform them that the diet will be analysed in time for their next visit. At the next visit, the results of the analysis, accompanied by written recommendations, are presented on a Diet Analysis and Recommendations form, an example of which is illustrated on page 39. The advantages of this approach are that a more objective assessment of the diet is given, and that the care and interest of the dentist or hygienist are more clearly demonstrated to the parent; both of these are strong motivational factors.

Several methods of analysing diet records have been proposed. A very simple method is outlined below. More detailed methods have been described by Holloway et al (1969), Nizel and Papas (1989), and Nikiforuk (1985). The simplest type of analysis is adequate if the aim is specifically to recommend control of the frequency of eating. If the aim were to give broader nutritional advice, a more detailed analysis would be required.

Diet Record Form

Dental decay is caused by acids which are formed by bacteria (germs) acting on food particles on the tooth surface.

FOOD + BACTERIA → ACIDS → DECAY

The information requested below will enable us to estimate the severity of the attack on the teeth, and will help us to advise you on how this attack may be reduced.

Please record all foods and drinks taken each day for *THREE DAYS* including 'extras' eaten between meals.

Include one weekend day, if possible.

Estimate the approximate amounts of the foods eaten as follows:

vegetables, puddings, sugar, cereals .... teaspoons or tablespoons
bread, cheese .... slices
drinks .... tumblers or cups
meat, fish .... size of portions
fruits, sweets, biscuits, chocolates .... type and number

NAME: date of birth:

1st Day – Date ....
                            Food or drink   Quantity
Breakfast

Between breakfast and lunch

Lunch

Between lunch and tea

Tea

After tea

(The reverse side of the form provides space for recording the diet on the second and third days.)

Simple method of analysing the diet

'Exposures of teeth to acid attack' are scored as follows:

Meals	*Score*
Average meal containing carbohydrate	2
Meal followed by toothbrushing	1

Between meals

Non-cariogenic item (e.g. cheese, carrot, nuts)	0
Item eaten within 5 minutes (e.g. a sweet or biscuit or small bar of chocolate)	1
Item eaten over longer period (e.g. packet of sweets)	2

Diet Analysis and Recommendations

Day	Exposures of teeth to acid attack	
	Recorded diet	Recommended diet
1 Meals	6	3
Between meals	3	0
2 Meals	6	3
Between meals	4	0
3 Meals	6	3
Between meals	2	0
Total number of acid attacks:	27	9

Note: If the recommendations are followed, the acid attack on (child's name)'s teeth can be reduced by two thirds.

Recommendations:

This method of analysing the diet is arbitrary and unscientific, but it produces scores for the recorded diet and for a recommended modified diet that are intelligible to the parents. These scores are entered on the Diet Analysis and Recommendations form, as in the example shown above. The contribution of between-meal snacks is clearly highlighted, as is the reduction that can be achieved in the total number of exposures of teeth to attack if the recommendations were followed. It is hoped that the size of the reduction will impress parents as something worth striving to achieve.

In giving recommendations, the following guidelines are suggested:

1. First, praise good points in the diet. The aim must be to encourage rather than to criticize.
2. Emphasize the danger of between-meal snacks, and comment on the between-meal items in the child's diet.
3. Recommend substitution of non-cariogenic between-meal foods for cariogenic items.
   Based on research evidence, only meat and meat-based products, bread and butter, cheese, carrots and other vegetables, potato crisps and nuts can be classified as non-cariogenic (Rugg-Gunn et al 1978). In the past, apples would have been included in this list, but this is not strictly justified because it has been shown that they cause a pH drop in dental

plaque. Nevertheless, apples and other fruits are generally recommended (see below).

4. Emphasize the desirability of eating good, nutritious meals, which reduce the demand for between-meal snacks.

5. Point out that a low-sugar, low-fat, moderate-protein diet is recommended not only for dental health but also for optimum general health.

6. Sweets are a special problem. Advise that they should be consumed at the end of a meal rather than between meals, or restricted to weekends. To advise complete elimination of sweets is not realistic in most cases.

'Toothfriendly sweets', which are now being promoted in the UK (British Society of Paediateric Dentistry 1995) may offer an alternative. To qualify as 'toothfriendly' a product must contain, instead of sugar, an approved non-sugar sweetener or sugar substitute. Toothfriendly sweets have been available in Switzerland since 1982 and have been introduced in several other countries, notably in Finland. Most research has been done with xylitol, a sugar substitute, but all non-sugar sweeteners and sugar substitutes are considered to be non-cariogenic (Imfeld 1993).

Sugarless chewing gum can be recommended as an alternative to sweets between meals, or to be used immediately after a meal, because saliva flow is increased and plaque acid neutralized (Edgar & Geddes 1990, Manning & Edgar 1993). However, many parents regard gum-chewing as an unpleasant habit and are reluctant to give gum to their children. It should not, of course, be recommended for a child wearing an orthodontic appliance.

In the UK, the Committee on Medical Aspects of Food Policy (COMA) has classified dietary sugars as 'intrinsic' (those 'naturally integrated into the cell structure of the food') and 'extrinsic' (those 'free in the food or added to it') (Department of Health 1989). Although acid is produced in plaque from both intrinsic and extrinsic sugars (Hussein et al 1996), foods containing only intrinsic sugars, for example fresh fruit and vegetables, are recommended because they are the types of foods more likely to be eaten infrequently, at mealtimes, whereas most foods containing extrinsic sugars are snack foods normally consumed between meals. Milk contains extrinsic sugars but is considered a special case because it contains lactose, which is less acidogenic than other sugars. COMA recommended reduction in the amount and frequency of consumption of 'non-milk extrinsic sugars' in the diet.

Ideally, diet counselling should be given to mothers immediately after the birth of a child: it is easier to establish good habits than to change bad habits later.

In particular, mothers should be warned against allowing infants to drink on demand from a feeding bottle or reservoir-type pacifier, especially at night (unless the drink is water). Particularly popular are proprietary fruit drinks, which not only have a high sugar content but also are highly acidic. Rampant, 'nursing bottle', caries (page 104) may result from prolonged exposure of teeth to such drinks (Ripa 1988). Parents should be advised to encourage their infant to drink from a cup rather than from a bottle from as early an age as possible and to restrict sugar-containing drinks to mealtimes.

Rampant caries can, more rarely, be caused by frequent and prolonged exposure of teeth to cow's or human milk (Dilley et al 1980, Curzon & Drummond 1987); this has been termed 'nursing' caries (Ripa 1988). Acid is produced in dental plaque after drinking cow's or human milk, but human milk, being higher in lactose and lower in calcium and phosphate, causes a greater pH drop and more enamel dissolution in vitro (Rugg-Gunn et al 1985). Although breast-feeding is generally strongly encouraged for a variety of reasons, mothers who wish to feed their baby on demand throughout the day and night should be warned of the risk. Likewise, those who bottle-feed should be advised against making the bottle constantly available to the baby.

Parents should be encouraged to start brushing their baby's teeth as soon as the incisors erupt, at about 6 months, and at this time the use of fluoride drops may be considered (p. 47).

3.2 THE COMMUNITY

Dental health education has been pursued within communities in various ways, which are briefly discussed below. Any efforts that are made in community dental health education depend largely on the manpower and financial resources of the community and on the priority given to such activities in relation to other commitments of the dental service.

To be understood, the dental health message must be kept simple, and the Health Education Authority (1996) has recommended that it should be based on the following four statements:

1. Diet: reduce the consumption and especially the frequency of sugar-containing food and drink.

2. Toothbrushing: clean the teeth thoroughly twice every day with a fluoride toothpaste.

3. Fluoridation: request your local water company to supply water with the optimal fluoride level.

4. Dental attendance: have an oral examination every year.

3.2.1 Dental health campaigns

Dental health campaigns have been mounted from time to time with varying degrees of ingenuity but always with great enthusiasm. Some campaigns have been directed at specific groups (e.g. schoolchildren), others at a whole community. These campaigns always succeed in stimulating interest, but their effects on the dental health of the community are uncertain; any reported improvements have been of short duration.

3.2.2 Dental health education in schools

Dental health education is most commonly directed at schoolchildren; primary schoolchildren, in particular, have long been a favourite target group. Short-term improvements have been reported in dental health knowledge and in oral cleanliness (Howat et al 1984, Hodge et al 1985), but these improvements are generally not maintained (Rayner & Cohen 1971). Regular reinforcement, no doubt, is important and greater benefits might be obtained if parents could be involved. Unfortunately this is usually not practicable.

In recent years there has been a change of approach to dental health education in schools. The emphasis has turned towards developing programmes that can be integrated into normal school work and be used by schoolteachers. Several programmes have been developed and tested in the UK: in primary schools (McIntyre 1984, Towner 1984), in secondary schools (Craft et al 1981, Arnold & Doyle 1984) and in pre-school groups (Croucher et al 1985). In general, these studies have shown that programmes can be devised that are well received by teachers and children, that knowledge of dental health can be increased, and that some improvement in dental health behaviour (reflected by improved oral cleanliness and gingival health) can be obtained. Follow-up in some secondary schools several months after a programme ended showed that some of the improvements were maintained (Craft et al 1981) but the evidence regarding long-term benefits is inconclusive (Arnold & Doyle 1984).

REFERENCES

Andlaw R J 1977 Diet and dental caries: a review. Journal of Human Nutrition 31: 45–52

Andlaw R J 1978 Oral hygiene and dental caries: a review. International Dental Journal 28: 1–6

Arnold C, Doyle A J 1984 Evaluation of the dental health education programme 'Natural Nashers'. Community Dental Health 1: 141–147

British Society of Paediatric Dentistry 1995 A policy document on toothfriendly sweets. International Journal of Paediatric Dentistry 5: 195–197

Craft M, Croucher R E, Dickinson J 1981 Preventive dental health in adolescents: short and long term pupil response to trials of an integrated curriculum package. Community Dentistry and Oral Epidemiology 9: 199–206

Croucher R E, Rodgers A I, Franklin A J, Craft M H 1985 Results and issues arising from an evaluation of community dental health education: the case of the 'Good Teeth' programme. Community Dental Health 2: 89–97

Curzon M E J, Drummond B K 1987 Case report-rampant caries in an infant related to prolonged on-demand breast feeding and a lactovegetarian diet. Journal of Paediatric Dentistry 3: 25–28

Department of Health 1989 Dietary sugars and human disease. Report on health and social aspects 37. Her Majesty's Stationery Office, London

Dilley G J, Dilley D H, Machen J B 1980 Prolonged nursing habit: a profile of patients and their families. Journal of Dentistry for Children 47: 102–108

Edgar W M, Geddes D A M 1990 Chewing gum and dental health—a review. British Dental Journal 168: 173–177

Greene J C, Vermillion J R 1964 The simplified oral hygiene index. Journal of the American Dental Association 68: 7–13

Health Education Authority 1996 The scientific basis of dental health education: a policy document, 4th edn.

Hodge H, Buchanan M, Jones J, O'Donnell P 1985 The evaluation of the infant dental health education programme developed in Sefton. Community Dental Health 2: 175–185

Holloway P H, Booth E M, Wragg K A 1969 Dietary counselling in the control of dental caries. British Dental Journal 126: 161–165

Howat A P, Craft M, Croucher R, Rock W P, Foster T D 1984 Dental health education: a school visits programme for dental students. Community Dental Health 2: 23–32

Hussein I, Pollard M A, Curzon M E J 1996 A comparison of the effects of some extrinsic and intrinsic sugars on dental plaque pH. International Journal of Paediatric Dentistry 5: 000–000

Imfeld T 1993 Efficacy of sweeteners and sugar substitutes in caries prevention. Caries Research 27 (Supplement 1): 50–55

Koch G, Lindhe J 1965 The effect of supervised oral hygiene on the gingiva of children: the effect of toothbrushing. Odontologisk Revy 16: 327–335

McIntyre J, Wight C, Blinkhorn A S 1984 A reassessment of Lothian Health Board's dental health education programme for primary schools. Community Dental Health 2: 99–108

Manning R H, Edgar W M 1993 pH changes in plaque after eating snacks and meals, and their modification by chewing sugared or sugar-free gum. British Dental Journal 174: 241–244

Nikiforuk G 1985 Understanding dental caries 2: Prevention—basic and clinical aspects. Karger, Basel, ch 8

Nizel A E, Papas A S 1989 Nutrition in clinical dentistry, 3rd edn. Saunders, Philadelphia, p 262

O'Brien M 1994 Children's dental health in the United Kingdom 1993. Her Majesty's Stationery Office, London pp 61 & 64

Rayner J F, Cohen L K 1971 School dental health education. In: Richards N D, Cohen I K (eds) Social sciences and dentistry: a clinical bibliography. Sigthoff, The Hague, p 286

Ripa L W 1988 Nursing caries: a comprehensive review. Pediatric Dentistry 10: 268–282

Rugg-Gunn A J 1989 Diet and dental caries. In: Murray J J (ed) The prevention of dental disease. Oxford University Press, Oxford, ch 2

Rugg-Gunn A J, Edgar W M 1984 Sugar and dental health: a review of the evidence. Community Dental Health 1: 85–92

Rugg-Gunn A J, Edgar W M, Jenkins G N 1978 The effect of eating some British snacks upon the pH of human dental plaque. British Dental Journal 145: 95–100

Rugg-Gunn A J, Roberts G J, Wright W G 1985 Effect of human milk on plaque pH in situ and enamel dissolution in vitro compared with bovine milk, lactose and sucrose. Caries Research 19: 327–331

Silness J, Löe H 1964 Periodontal disease in pregnancy II. Correlation between oral hygiene and periodontal condition. Acta Odontologica Scandinavica 22: 121–135

Silverstone L M, Featherstone M J 1988 A scanning electron microscope study of the end-rounding of bristles in eight toothbrush types. Quintessence International 19: 3–23

Stephan R M 1940 Changes in the hydrogen ion concentration on tooth surfaces and in carious lesions. Journal of the American Dental Association 27: 718–723

Sutcliffe P 1996 Oral cleanliness and dental caries. In: Murray J J (ed) The prevention of oral disease, 3rd edn. Oxford University Press, Oxford, ch 4

Towner E M L 1984 The 'Gleam Team' programme: development and evaluation of a dental health education package for infant schools. Community Dental Health 1: 181–191

Wright G Z, Banting D W, Feasby G H 1977 The effect of interdental flossing on the incidence of proximal caries in children. Journal of Dental Research 56: 574–578

RECOMMENDED READING

Murray J J (ed) 1996 The prevention of oral disease, 3rd edn. Oxford University Press, Oxford

Catalogue of dental health education resources for England, Wales & Northern Ireland 1995 Eden Bianchi Press, 2 Ashwood Avenue, West Didsbury, M2O 8ZB, UK

DeBiase C B 1991 Dental health education: theory and practice. Lea & Febiger, Philadelphia

Schou L, Blinkhorn A S 1993 Oral health promotion. Oxford University Press, Oxford

4 Fluorides

4.1 METHODS OF USING FLUORIDE FOR THE CHILD PATIENT

4.1.1 Methods administered by dental personnel

Topical application of solution or gel

The idea of applying fluoride solution to teeth closely followed the demonstration in the USA of the caries-preventive effect of fluoride when present in public water supplies. The first topical fluoride technique that was shown to be effective involved the use of neutral 2% sodium fluoride solution (Knutson 1948). A disadvantage of this technique was that a series of four applications at about weekly intervals was required. The search for more effective agents led to the introduction of 8% stannous fluoride solution (Gish et al 1962). However, stannous fluoride has certain disadvantages: it is unstable in solution (which makes it necessary to prepare a fresh solution for each treatment), and it produces a brown stain in hypomineralized or demineralized enamel (for example, in early carious lesions and at the margins of restorations); this stain is unsightly if it occurs in anterior teeth. Acidulated phosphate-fluoride (APF) is now generally used for topical applications. The composition of APF is 2% sodium fluoride and 0.3% hydrofluoric acid in 0.1 M orthophosphoric acid; the pH is about 3.3.

The development of APF was reviewed by Brudevold & DePaola (1966), who pointed out that the presence of phosphate enhances fluoride uptake into enamel while preventing precipitation of calcium fluoride and dissolution of enamel, both of which were considered to be undesirable reactions that would occur in the absence of phosphate. However, it is now known that calcium fluoride is formed within the enamel and, by dissolving slowly, releases fluoride ions; although some fluoride is lost from the enamel, some remains and promotes the formation of fluorapatite (Mellberg & Ripa 1983).

APF is stable when stored in plastic or polythene containers. Its taste is less disagreeable than that of stannous fluoride, and is improved by the addition of flavouring agents. It does not stain enamel.

APF is available as either solution or gel and may be applied to the teeth either directly with a cotton applicator (direct technique) or indirectly in a tray (indirect technique). In addition, varnishes are available which are applied directly to the teeth.

It was only with the advent of APF gels that the indirect method became popular, since gels are particularly easy to use in a tray. This method is quicker than the direct method and therefore is usually preferred. However, the direct method is often better with a young, nervous child who may not tolerate a tray; direct application of solution, gel or varnish is a simple procedure that is useful in introducing the child to dental treatment. In addition, when treating a mixed dentition in which primary molars are missing, it may be preferable to apply directly to permanent incisors and permanent first molars only.

Technique: topical fluoride application

A. Direct technique: solution, gel or varnish

Procedure	Method	Rationale	Notes
1. Ask the child to brush his/her teeth	Supervise the child brushing (and flossing if normally done).	Food debris must be removed before fluoride application, Even if oral hygiene is satisfactory, observing the child brushing at this stage provides an opportunity to reinforce good technique.	In the past, a full prophylaxis was considered to be an integral part of the topical fluoride technique. However, sufficient evidence exists to show that it is not necessary (Ripa 1984).
2. Isolate teeth	Use saliva ejector, cotton wool rolls and/or absorbent pads to isolate the teeth to be treated. Isolate either one quadrant of teeth or a $\frac{1}{2}$ mouth (maxillary and mandibular teeth on one side) or a $\frac{1}{3}$ mouth (maxillary and mandibular primary and/or permanent molars on one side, or maxillary and mandibular incisors and canines).	Isolation allows the teeth to be dried and prevents dilution of the applied fluoride by saliva. The number of teeth that can be comfortably isolated depends on the patient. In general, quadrant isolation is most appropriate for young children: $\frac{1}{2}$ mouth for teenagers: $\frac{1}{3}$ mouth for mixed dentition-age children.	
3. Dry the isolated teeth	Dry the isolated teeth with compressed air.	Saliva on the tooth surface would dilute solution or gel.	
4. Apply solution, gel or varnish	With a small brush or cotton wool pledget held in tweezers, apply solution or gel to all tooth surfaces, working it especially into the interdental spaces from buccal and lingual sides. Keep cotton wool rolls away from the teeth. Keep the teeth covered with solution or gel for 4 minutes.	Solution or gel would be absorbed by cotton wool rolls. A 4-minute application has become accepted as standard practice.	It is not known whether a shorter application of solution or gel would be equally effective, or a longer application more effective.
	If using varnish, apply a thin layer specifically to approximal surfaces and any surfaces showing enamel demineralization; then allow contact with saliva or drip water on to the varnish.	It is not necessary to wait for varnish to set; it does so when wet.	Unless lingual and buccal surfaces show signs of demineralization they need not be treated, thus sparing the patient the mild discomfort caused by varnish on those surfaces.
5. (After 4 minutes) Remove solution or gel from accessible tooth surfaces (leave varnish)	With cotton wool roll or gauze, wipe solution or gel from accessible tooth surfaces but do not attempt to remove it from approximal surfaces.	The amount of solution or gel placed on the teeth is small, but it is undesirable for the child to ingest an unnecessary dose of fluoride. Moreover, the taste is often considered to be unpleasant.	
	Instruct the child to expectorate thoroughly but not to rinse.	It is desirable to eliminate excess fluoride.	

Isolate another quadrant or $\frac{1}{3}$ mouth, or the other $\frac{1}{2}$ mouth, and repeat the treatment.
At the end of treatment, advise the patient not to eat or drink for $\frac{1}{2}$ hour, to prolong contact of fluoride with approximal surfaces of the teeth; this results in greater fluoride uptake into enamel (Stookey et al 1986).

Technique: topical fluoride application *(contd)*
B. Indirect (tray) technique: gel

Procedure	Method	Rationale	Notes
1. Ask the child to brush his/her teeth	See procedure 1, direct technique.		
2. Select and prepare a tray	Select a tray and check that it is the correct size by trying it in the child's mouth. Place only enough gel to cover the base of the tray (2–3 ml).	Enough gel should be used to coat the teeth, but over-filling would result in it being squeezed out of the tray, which is not only unpleasant for the patient but may also be toxic (p. 46).	Various types of tray are available. A disposable tray with an absorbent sponge lining is recommended (Fig. 4.1).
3. Dry the teeth	Isolate the maxillary or mandibular arch by retracting the cheeks, and dry with compressed air. Do not place a saliva ejector at this stage, or cotton wool rolls.	A saliva ejector or cotton wool rolls would obstruct placement of the tray.	It has to be accepted that drying of lingual surfaces of mandibular teeth may be incomplete.
4. Insert the tray(s)	Sit the patient nearly upright.	If the patient is reclined, any excess solution or gel extruding from the tray would flow into the throat.	Usually, each arch is treated separately (the two parts of the tray can be separated by cutting the plastic connectors), but both arches can be treated at the same time by folding the tray so that the two parts are back-to-back.
	Keeping the cheeks away from the dry teeth, insert the tray. Apply finger pressure on the tray. Insert a saliva ejector.	Pressure squeezes gel into the interdental spaces. Suction is desirable to remove any excess gel extruding from the tray, and to avoid possible dilution of the gel by saliva.	
5. (After 4 minutes) Remove the tray and remove excess gel	Remove the tray(s) from the mouth. Before allowing the patient to swallow, remove excess gel from accessible surfaces by wiping with a cotton wool roll or gauze, or by using suction apparatus. Do not attempt to remove remaining gel from interdental spaces. Instruct the patient to expectorate thoroughly but not to rinse.	Many children find the taste of the gel unpleasant; a considerable excess of gel usually remains after removal of the tray.	

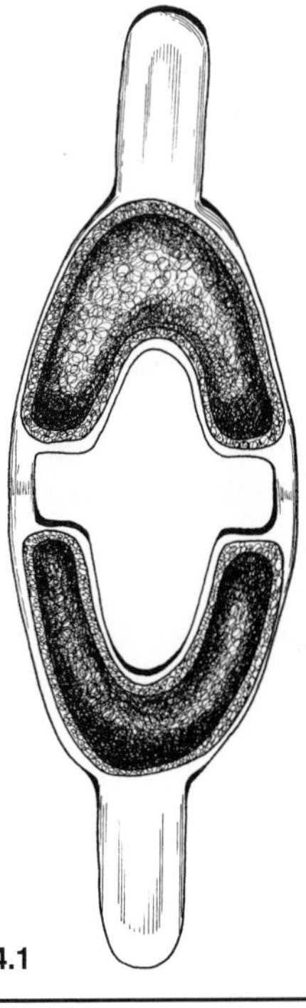

Fig. 4.1

At the end of treatment, advise the patient not to eat or drink for 1/2 hour, to prolong exposure of the teeth to fluoride; this results in greater fluoride uptake into enamel (Stookey et al 1986).

Various types of tray are available. Disposable trays with absorbent sponge linings are recommended because a small volume of gel suffices to saturate the sponge, which, when pressed against the teeth by finger pressure, coats the teeth with gel while preventing it from being squeezed out of the tray.

It should be remembered that APF contains a high concentration of fluoride (12.3 mg/ml); even a small bottle (200 ml) contains a potentially lethal dose (Table 4.1). The required quantity of gel should be dispensed directly into the tray and this should be kept out of the child's reach, because ingestion of small quantities (e.g. 1.6 ml by a 5-year-old child) may cause gastrointestinal symptoms. Care should be taken to avoid using unnecessarily large amounts of gel (not more than 5 ml), suction apparatus should be used during the 4-minute application period, and excess gel should be wiped from accessible tooth surfaces before asking the child to expectorate thoroughly. If these precautions are taken (as described in the technique section above), it is difficult to envisage how patients can possibly ingest the large amounts of gel ingested by some of the subjects in the study of Ekstrand et al (1981). This conclusion is supported by the results of studies which investigated the retention of fluoride following topical fluoride treatment (McCall et al 1983, LeCompte & Doyle 1985, Tyler & Andlaw 1987).

The effectiveness of topical fluoride treatment is well documented (Brudevold & Naujoks 1978, Ripa 1981, Ripa 1991). APF solution and gel appear to be equally effective. Of eight clinical trials in which APF solution was applied once or twice a year by the direct method to permanent teeth of children, two children showed no effect but the others showed 28–55% fewer carious surfaces after periods of 2 or 3 years. Similarly, studies with APF gel applied in trays showed reductions of 20–40%; no studies have been done of the direct application of gel. These percentage reductions reflected average differences of about one tooth surface per child per year; in no study was the difference as great as two surfaces per child.

Relatively few studies have tested the effectiveness of applying fluorides to the primary dentition. Neutral 2% sodium fluoride and 4% stannous fluoride solutions have been used, but not APF. In general, the results indicated modest reductions in caries incidence (McDonald & Muhler 1957).

Most topical fluoride studies have been conducted in areas served by water supplies containing low concentrations of fluoride. The few studies conducted in fluoridated areas have given conflicting results, and it may be concluded that topical fluoride treatment is not justified for lifelong residents of fluoridated areas, unless they show signs of caries activity and can be classified as 'high-risk' patients for this or other reasons (p. 50). When fluoride is introduced into a public water supply, topical fluoride treatment may be continued for 'high-risk' children whose teeth were erupted when fluoridation began.

Almost all toothpastes that are currently available contain fluoride, and it is uncertain whether topical fluoride treatment confers a significant additional benefit to children who use fluoride toothpaste. A 3-year study showed that twice-yearly applications of APF gel were of little benefit to 11–12-year-old children who used fluoride toothpaste (Mainwaring & Naylor 1978) but another study showed a significant benefit (Hagan et al 1985). Children with high caries incidence are most likely to benefit from topical fluoride application.

Newly erupted teeth derive more benefit from topical fluoride than more mature teeth; this indicates the importance of treating teeth soon after their eruption. Thus, topical fluoride treatment could be started at the age of about 3 years, soon after the primary molars erupt. However, because of the practical difficulties of performing the technique efficiently for such young children, and because systemic fluoride is of more value at this age (p. 48), topical fluoride treatment, if indicated, is often delayed until permanent teeth erupt at the age of 6 or 7 years. Thereafter, twice-yearly application may be continued up to late adolescence. Continuation into adult life generally is not justified; the few studies of fluoride application to adults' teeth give no clear evidence of its value. However, it can be justified for adults who show evidence of continued high caries activity.

Fluoride varnishes

Fluoride varnish remains in contact with enamel for longer periods of time than do solution or gel. Varnishes contain 5% sodium fluoride (Duraphat) or 0.7% fluorsilane (Fluor Protector).

Duraphat varnish is most frequently used in the

Table 4.1 Volumes of APF solution or gel (12.3 mg F/ml) required to cause gastrointestinal symptoms or lethal fluoride poisoning (based on data given in Table 4.6).

Age (years)	Gastint. Symptoms volume (ml)	Lethal poisoning volume (ml)
5	1.6	52
10	2.4	78
15	3.7	117

UK. Since it sets in contact with saliva, it is particularly useful when treating young children. It is also convenient to use when treating specific sites of caries activity, for example early enamel demineralization at the cervical margins of teeth in older children and adults.

The amount of varnish used when treating children has been estimated to range from 30 to 640 mg, containing 0.7 to 14.5 mg fluoride (Roberts & Longhurst 1987). Since the dose that might cause gastrointestinal symptoms is 1 mg F/kg body weight (Table 4.6), this amount is well within the acceptable limit.

Clinical trials of fluoride varnishes have indicated that they are effective in preventing dental caries (Clark 1982, Modeer et al 1984). Although the results have been variable and varnish has not been directly compared with solution or gel, the evidence suggests that varnish is at least as effective.

Prophylaxis paste

Various fluorides have been incorporated into prophylaxis pastes: sodium fluoride, stannous fluoride, APF, sodium monofluorophosphate, and stannous hexafluorozirconate. Clinical trials to test the efficacy of these pastes in preventing dental caries have given variable results (Horowitz 1970, Murray et al 1991) and therefore it is concluded that prophylaxis with such pastes should not be considered as an alternative treatment to the application of solution, gel or varnish. However, there are no contraindications to using a fluoride-containing paste to clean teeth before the application of solution, gel or varnish.

4.1.2 Methods administered by the patient (or parent)

Fluoride toothpaste

Since almost all toothpastes currently marketed in the UK contain fluoride, most people who use toothpaste give themselves a topical fluoride treatment when they brush their teeth.

Many clinical trials have been conducted to investigate the effects on children of toothpastes containing either sodium fluoride, stannous fluoride, amine fluoride, APF or sodium monofluorophosphate. The results are fairly consistent in showing reductions of about 15–30% in the number of tooth surfaces becoming carious over periods of 2–3 years; in most studies these reductions reflected the prevention of caries in about one surface per child per year (Fehr & Moller 1978). There is no firm evidence that any one type of fluoride toothpaste is more effective than others.

Most toothpastes contain 0.1% fluoride; therefore 1 g of toothpaste contains 1 mg fluoride. The average amount of toothpaste used by children below 7 years of age ranges from about 0.4 to 1.4 g, and the average proportion ingested ranges from 14 to 35% (Barnhart et al 1974). Thus, fluoride ingestion can be estimated to range from 0.06 to 0.5 mg at each brushing session. Low-fluoride toothpastes are now also available, one containing as little as 0.04 mg F/g.

Concern has been expressed about toothpaste ingestion by young children who do not rinse or expectorate efficiently after brushing. The great majority of children ingest less than 0.25 g of toothpaste (Barnhart et al 1974, Baxter 1980), but the occasional child ingests as much as 1 g of paste, containing 1 mg of fluoride (Hargreaves et al 1972). The concern centres on the possibility of causing mottling of developing enamel, because it has been estimated that daily ingestion by a small child of 0.04 mg fluoride per kg body weight can cause fluorosis of permanent teeth (Fejerskof et al 1988). Therefore, enamel fluorosis might result if a 2-year-old child weighing 12.5 kg ingests 0.5 mg fluoride daily, and this amount could possibly be ingested by a child brushing twice a day and swallowing 50% of the paste. Therefore, parents should be advised to supervise toothbrushing by young children and, especially if the child is already receiving systemic fluoride from tablets or from a public water supply, to use a low-fluoride paste and to limit the amount placed on the brush to the size of a small pea or to a light smear (Rock 1994).

However, there is no evidence that ingestion of fluoride toothpaste per se causes mottling; indeed, in a study investigating this possibility, fewer developmental defects of enamel were found in children who used a toothpaste containing more than twice the normal concentration of fluoride (0.24%) than in children who used a fluoride-free toothpaste (Houwink & Wagg 1979).

Fluoride tablets and drops

In areas served by low-fluoride water supplies, tablets and drops provide a method for systemic administration of fluoride. In theory, this form of administration has the advantage over water fluoridation that it allows specific doses of fluoride to be given. In practice, it is difficult to sustain the interest of even the most highly motivated families for the long-term consumption that is necessary.

Fluoride drops contain sodium fluoride, but the amount delivered in each drop varies; for example, one preparation delivers 0.125 mg fluoride per drop, and another 0.033 mg per drop.

Fluoride tablets contain either 0.5 mg fluoride (1.1 mg sodium fluoride) or 1 mg fluoride (2.2 mg sodium fluoride). Tablets are prepared with various flavours.

For delivering doses of 0.25 mg the drops are most convenient; the appropriate number of drops may be added each day to a baby's drink. When doses of 0.5 mg are required, drops may be continued, but when children are old enough to suck or chew tablets they should be encouraged to do so because there is strong evidence that fluoride in tablets can exert a topical as well as a systemic effect.

The dosage recommended for use in the UK is shown in Table 4.2. However, because there is evidence from several countries of an increased prevalence of mild fluorosis in permanent teeth, which is attributed at least in part to fluoride supplements taken during the first 4 years of life when the crowns of permanent anterior teeth are forming, it has been suggested that the lowest dose (0.25 mg) should be continued up to the age of 3 or 4 years (Riordan 1993, Ismail 1994).

In the past there was some controversy about the desirability of starting fluoride supplementation during pregnancy. Although fluoride passes through the placenta, the concentration that reaches the fetus is much lower than that in the maternal blood, and it is now generally agreed that there is no indication for starting fluoride administration before birth and that is should be delayed until the baby is at least 6 months old.

An important period for fluoride supplementation is the first 5 or 6 years of life, during which time the enamel of all primary and permanent teeth (other than third molars) is formed. Another important period is from the age of 5–6 years to the age of 12–14 years; this is the pre-eruptive maturation phase of premolars and second molars, during which time fluoride is taken up by the developing enamel of these teeth from the tissue fluids. However, some parents are reluctant to

Table 4.3 Volume of fluoride drops (3.8 mg F/ml) and number of tablets (1 mg F/tab) required to cause gastrointestinal symptoms or lethal fluoride poisoning (based on data given in Table 4.6).

Age (yrs)	Gastrointestinal symptoms		Lethal poisoning	
	Drops (ml)	Tablets	Drops (ml)	Tablets
2	3	10	84	320
5	5	20	168	640
10	8	30	252	960

continue giving tablets for so many years because they do not want their child to develop a habit of self-medication that might persist into adolescence and even into adult life. If the patient is classified as 'high risk' (p. 49), and if they live in a low water-fluoride area, encouragement to continue taking tablets is justified but, if not, it is reasonable to discontinue tablet administration and possibly to transfer to a mouthrinsing regimen when permanent teeth start to erupt (see below).

A serious drawback limiting the use of fluoride tablets and drops in dental practice is the need to have the intelligent cooperation of the child's parents. They must be highly motivated to administer fluoride daily for several years, and they must be careful and responsible in storing the tablets in a safe place, out of children's reach.

Fluoride drops are dispensed in bottles containing 30 ml of 0.38% fluoride, or 60 ml of 0.17% fluoride. Reference to Table 4.3 shows that gastrointestinal symptoms might be caused if a 5-year-old child consumes about one-sixth of the contents of a 30 ml bottle, or if a 10-year-old child consumes about a quarter; but there is a considerable safety margin before reaching the lethal dose.

Fluoride tablets are usually dispensed in quantities of 120 tablets, in bottles with child-proof lids. Again, reference to Table 4.3 shows that unpleasant symptoms could occur if an overdose were taken, but that it would be necessary to consume the contents of several bottles to reach a lethal dose.

Fluoride mouthrinses

Mouthrinsing with a fluoride solution is a simple and convenient method of topical fluoride application. Several proprietary anti-plaque mouthrinses also contain fluoride.

The solutions most commonly available are flavoured neutral sodium fluoride solutions; a 0.05%

Table 4.2 Recommended dosage of fluoride tablets and drops (mg F/day), related to the concentration of fluoride in the drinking water (British National Formulary 1995).

Age	Water F (ppm)		
	<0.3	0.3–0.7	>0.7
<6 months	0	0	0
6 months–2 years	0.25	0	0
2–4 years	0.5	0.25	0
>4 years	1.0	0.5	0

solution (0.023% fluoride) is recommended for daily use, and a 0.2% solution (0.09% fluoride) for weekly or fortnightly use.

Method. The child and parent should be given the following instructions:

1. Clean teeth thoroughly in the usual way.
2. Take about 10 ml of solution into the mouth and gently 'swish' the solution between the teeth for at least 1 minute.
3. Spit out the solution after the 1-minute period, do not swallow it.
4. Do not eat or drink for at least half an hour.

Whether the 0.05% sodium fluoride solution is used daily or the 0.2% weekly is for the child and parent to decide; there is no evidence that one or the other regimen is more effective. The parent should be advised to select a specific time every day or week, so that it is not forgotten.

Clinical trials of mouthrinsing have been conducted in schools, where it could be supervised. Various solutions have been tested, including neutral sodium fluoride, APF, stannous fluoride and amine fluoride solutions. Studies in several countries have shown that daily or weekly mouthrinsing reduces the incidence of dental caries by about 40% over periods of 2–3 years in non-fluoridated areas; these reductions reflect the prevention of caries in about one tooth surface per child per year (Birkeland & Torell 1978). It has also been shown that fluoride rinsing can benefit children living in a fluoridated area (Driscoll et al 1982).

Many of the early trials of fluoride mouthrinsing were conducted before fluoride toothpastes were widely available, but later studies have shown that rinsing with a fluoride solution reduced caries incidence in children who, it can be assumed, used fluoride toothpaste at home (Ripa 1983). However, in studies involving brushing with a fluoride toothpaste and mouthrinsing with a fluoride solution, little additional benefit was gained by children who rinsed after brushing compared to those who only either brushed or rinsed (Ashley et al 1977, Blinkhorn et al 1983); but it should be noted that children in the latter study rinsed for only 30 seconds. It is possible that only children with a high caries rate benefit significantly from using a fluoride mouthrinse in addition to brushing their teeth with a fluoride toothpaste.

Mouthrinsing may be introduced when a child is 6–7 years of age and able to rinse correctly; primary molars and, especially, newly-erupting permanent incisors and first molars, may benefit from this topical fluoride. However, the incidence of caries in children between the ages of 6 and 12 years is almost exclu-sively in the occlusal surfaces of permanent first molar teeth, and topical fluoride is less effective in preventing caries in these surfaces than in smooth surfaces. Therefore mouthrinsing is more useful during, and for a few years after, the eruption of premolars and permanent second molars, because their approximal surfaces are about as susceptible to caries as their occlusal surfaces. Mouthrinsing may then be continued until late adolescence, or into adulthood if caries activity remains high.

In common with fluoride tablet administration, a drawback to the use of the mouthrinsing method is that the child's and parent's interest must be maintained and the parent must be motivated enough to ensure that the child rinses conscientiously. The parent must also ensure that the stock bottle of solution is kept out of the child's reach. The 0.05% solution is supplied in 300 ml or 500 ml bottles, and the 0.2% solution in 150 ml bottles. Table 4.4 shows that gastrointestinal symptoms may occur if, for example, a 5-year-old ingests about 30 ml of 0.2% solution, or 130 ml of 0.05% solution. However, lethal doses can only be reached by ingesting the contents of many bottles.

4.1.3 Selection of methods for the child patient

The methods of using fluoride most commonly recommended in dental practice are topical applications (solution, gel or varnish), and home use of toothpaste, tablets or mouthrinses. The use of fluoride toothpaste should be recommended to all patients, but it must be decided which of the other methods to select for each patient. Obvious factors that affect this choice are the child's age and the fluoride concentration in the local water supply; but another important factor that should be considered is the degree of risk that caries presents to the child.

Patients may be classified either as 'high risk' or as

Table 4.4 Volumes of mouthrinse solutions required to cause gastrointestinal symptoms or lethal fluoride poisoning: 0.05% NaF solution (0.23 mg F/ml) and 0.2% NaF solution (0.9 mg F/ml). Based on data given in Table 4.6.

Age (yrs)	Gastint. symptoms		Lethal poisoning	
	0.05% soln (ml)	0.2% soln (ml)	0.05% soln (ml)	0.2% soln (ml)
5	86	22	2783	711
10	130	33	4174	1067
15	196	50	6261	1660

Table 4.5 An outline for selecting methods of using fluoride for a child patient (assuming use of fluoride toothpaste, and a low water-fluoride level).*

	6 months–6 years	6–12 years	12–18 years
Low-risk child favourable parental attitudes	Drops/tablets	Tablets (or mouth-rinse)	Mouthrinse or topical
unfavourable parental attitudes	—	Mouthrinse? or topical?	Mouthrinse? or topical?
High-risk child	Drops/tablets + topical	Tablets + topical + mouthrinse	Topical + mouthrinse

* Refer to text

'low risk'. The 'high risk' patient may be described as having one or more of the following characteristics:

1. A high caries susceptibility, as assessed by previous caries experience and present caries activity.
2. A medical condition (for example, congenital heart disease) that may be complicated by bacteraemia resulting from infection or from some forms of dental treatment.
3. A medical condition (for example, a bleeding disorder) that makes certain forms of dental treatment hazardous.
4. Mental handicap, which sometimes makes any treatment more than usually difficult.

The 'low risk' patient is one with low caries experience and no complicating medical condition.

An outline for selecting appropriate methods of using fluoride is presented in Table 4.5. The age ranges presented in the table simply represent convenient 6-year periods, to be used as a rough guide; there will, no doubt, be some overlap of method of fluoride usage from one age range to another.

Age 6 months–6 years

For preschool children systemic administration is the most effective and often the only practicable method. However, before recommending the use of tablets or drops it is important to assess whether the parents are interested enough to administer the daily dose for several years. A good indicator of parental attitudes is their response to oral hygiene instruction and diet counselling, which should be carried out before considering the use of fluoride. Drops or tablets may be recommended for a 'low-risk' child whose parents are keen to use all available preventive methods, but they should not be recommended if parental attitudes are unfavourable. For a 'high-risk' child, every effort should be made to gain the parents' interest and co-operation in administering drops or tablets, and topical fluoride (usually in the form of varnish) should also be applied if possible.

Age 6–12 years

From the age of 5 or 6 years to the eruption of pre-molars and second molars (age 12–14 years), tablet administration again is the most beneficial method.

For the 'low-risk' child taking fluoride tablets during this period (and, it may be assumed, using a fluoride toothpaste) the use of other methods cannot be justified. It could be argued that every available method that might help to prevent caries should be used, but this must be considered with reference to the time needed to apply topical fluoride and the expense incurred by the parents. However, proprietary mouth-rinses are not expensive, and a keen parent may be encouraged to buy them for home use. This would be inappropriate and impracticable if parental attitudes remained unfavourable, but some parents who are uninterested or who object to administering fluoride systemically may be agreeable to supervising their child using a mouthrinse. If it is assessed that mouthrinsing is done conscientiously, there is no justification for topical applications, and even if mouthrinsing is not done, topical application is not strongly justified for the 'low risk' child using fluoride toothpaste at home.

For the 'high-risk' child, full use of all available methods is strongly advocated.

Age 12–18 years

After the age of 12–14 years, tablet administration should be stopped but topical methods may be continued, especially for the 'high-risk' child.

4.2 TOXICITY

Fluoride is a potentially toxic substance. Since it is utilized in various forms for caries prevention, it is important to know the amount of fluoride used and the safety margins involved with each form of treatment (Heifetz & Horowitz 1984).

The information on toxic doses given in this chapter is based on the data presented in Table 4.6. The 'certainly lethal dose' of fluoride is generally accepted to be 32–64 mg fluoride per kg body weight

Table 4.6 The amount of fluoride required to cause gastrointestinal symptoms or lethal poisoning.

Age (years)	Weight (kg)	mg F to cause gastint. symptoms*	mg F to cause lethal poisoning†
2	10	10	320
3	14	14	448
4	18	18	576
5	20	20	640
8	25	25	800
10	30	30	960
15	45	45	1440

* Dose: 1 mg F/kg (Spoerke et al 1980)
† Dose: 32 mg F/kg (Hodge & Smith 1965)

(Hodge & Smith 1965); the calculations in Table 4.6 are based on the lower limit of 32 mg/kg.

The dose that might cause gastrointestinal symptoms (nausea, hypersalivation, abdominal pains, vomiting, diarrhoea) appears to be about 1 mg fluoride per kg body weight, although only very minor symptoms occur with doses below 5 mg/kg (Spoerke et al 1980).

The risk of overdosage is extremely small, but it is important to take appropriate action if it is suspected. If the amount of fluoride product that has been ingested can be estimated (e.g. number of tablets, or volume of mouthrinse), the amount of fluoride ingested can be calculated from the information given in Table 4.7.

Table 4.7 The amount of fluoride contained in various fluoride products (products available in February 1996).

Product	Amount of fluoride
Tablets	0.5 or 1.0 mg per tablet
Drops	
Fluorigard (Colgate Palmolive)	3.8 mg/ml
Fluordrops (Stafford Miller)	1.7 mg/ml
Rinses	
Fluorigard Daily (Colgate Palmolive)	0.23 mg/ml
Fluorigard Weekly	0.9 mg/ml
Fluorinse (Stafford Miller)*	9.0 mg/ml
Reach (Johnson & Johnson)	0.23 mg/ml
Mouthguard (Maclean)	0.23 mg/ml
Gel (APF)	12.3 mg/ml

* This product is diluted before use

When overdosage is suspected the following action is recommended (Bayless & Tinanoff 1985):

If less than 5 mg F/kg has been ingested: give the child milk to drink and keep the child under observation.

If more than 5 mg F/kg has been ingested: induce vomiting if possible, give milk and refer to hospital.

4.3 METHODS OF USING FLUORIDE IN THE COMMUNITY

It is clear that child patients may receive the benefits of fluoride in various ways. However, some children do not visit a dentist regularly and therefore cannot benefit (except by using a fluoride-containing toothpaste); a national survey in the UK (O'Brien 1994) showed that 10% of 5-year-old children had never attended a dentist. To reach these children, methods are required that can be applied to the community as a whole.

4.3.1 Systemic

Fluoridation of public water supplies

The adjustment of the fluoride concentration of public water supplies to 1 part per million (ppm) is the most effective method now available of preventing dental caries. Over 200 million people in about 40 countries live in areas where water supplies are fluoridated, and a further 40 million live in areas naturally rich in fluoride. About 135 million people in the USA drink fluoridated water (about 60% of the population), but only about 5.5 million (10% of the population) in the UK drink water that contains either added fluoride or natural fluoride at a level of more than 0.7 ppm (PHA/BFS 1994).

Most commonly, fluoride is added in the form of hexafluorosilicic acid or sodium hexafluorosilicate, but sodium silicofluoride and sodium fluoride have also been used. Fluoridation equipment delivers and maintains the level of fluoride between 0.9 and 1.1 ppm. The equipment has automatic devices which constantly monitor the concentration of fluoride in the water as it leaves the treatment plant, and a 'fail-safe' mechanism which would shut down the plant should the fluoride level exceed 1 ppm (Dept. of Environment 1987). At a concentration of 1 ppm, the added fluoride compounds dissociate into their constituent ions, which have identical properties to those of fluoride, silicon and other ions naturally present in water. Regular checks are made of the fluoride levels in local water supplies.

The relationship between the concentration of

fluoride in water supplies and the prevalence of dental caries was demonstrated in the USA by Dean et al (1942); their survey of over 7000 12–14-year-old children showed that children living in areas served by water supplies containing at least 1 ppm fluoride had about 50% fewer carious teeth than children living in low-fluoride areas. This relationship has since been confirmed in a large number of studies throughout the world; moreover, the benefits of fluoride are life-long (Murray 1971).

The safety of fluoridation has been extensively studied, and is beyond doubt (World Health Organization 1967, Royal College of Physicians 1976). Water fluoridation is an ideal public health measure because its benefits are not dependent on the interest and cooperation of the recipients, and because it is cheap.

Fluoride tablets

Fluoride tablet schemes have been administered in many countries, including several European countries, the USA and Australia. Some schemes have involved preschool children but the majority have been school-based. Fluoride tablets (1 mg fluoride) are administered daily, usually by the schoolteachers. In some schemes, efforts are made also to involve the parents, so that tablets may be administered at home during school holidays. Since safe storage of tablets at school cannot be guaranteed, they are supplied in limited quantities, for example 120 tablets, which is 1 week's supply for a class of 24 children. It is, of course, necessary to check that children are not already receiving systemic fluoride at home.

Studies of the effectiveness of fluoride tablet schemes have reported reductions in caries incidence in primary and permanent teeth (Binder et al 1978). The success of these schemes depends on long-term cooperation of the teachers; although little of their time is demanded it has not always been easy to maintain their interest.

A disadvantage of school-based schemes is that, by the time children start school, the crowns of all permanent teeth (except third molars) are already well developed; for maximum effect administration of systemic fluoride should begin much earlier.

Fluoridation of school water supplies

The fluoridation of school water supplies has been found to be feasible and effective. It has been tested in certain isolated rural schools in the USA that have independent water supplies. Since children at these schools drink fluoridated water only for a part of each day and not at weekends or during holidays, the amount of fluoride added was several times higher than the level that would be indicated for community water fluoridation in that area; thus, in Elk Lake Pennsylvania, the school water was fluoridated to 5 ppm, and in Seagrove, North Carolina, to 6.3 ppm. Results after 12 years in Elk Lake (Horowitz et al 1972) and in Seagrove (Heifetz et al 1983) indicate that the method is effective in reducing the prevalence of dental caries in children. It has the advantage over tablet administration that daily involvement of teachers is not necessary. However, the initial cost of the fluoridation equipment is a disadvantage.

It should be noted that the studies of school-based tablet and water-fluoridation schemes were conducted at a time when dental caries prevalence was higher than it is now. The cost-effectiveness of such schemes at the present time is therefore questionable, except in areas where caries prevalence remains high. Horowitz (1989) concluded that existing schemes should be continued.

Fluoridated salt

Fluoridated table salt was introduced in Switzerland in 1955. Much of the salt available in Switzerland today contains 90 ppm fluoride; in two cantons, salt containing 250 ppm fluoride is available. Studies conducted in Switzerland, Colombia, Spain and Hungary indicate that fluoridated salt is effective in preventing caries in children (Marthaler et al 1978). In recent years, fluoridated salt has been introduced in France, Jamaica, Colombia, Costa Rica and Mexico (Horowitz 1990).

Fluoridated milk

Milk has been proposed as a suitable vehicle for fluoride, and equipment to fluoridate milk has been designed (Davis 1972). Studies in Scotland (Stephen et al 1984) and in Hungary (Banoczy et al 1983) have demonstrated the effectiveness of milk fluoridation. In the former study, involving 5-year-old children, the fluoride concentration was 1.5 mg per 200 ml container (7.5 ppm); in the latter, 0.75 mg/200 ml for 6–9-year-olds and 0.4 mg/200 ml for 3-5-year-olds.

Although the idea of fluoridating milk is attractive because milk is a natural food for children, the method is less precise than tablet administration because milk consumption by children varies greatly (even more so than water consumption). This disadvantage could be overcome if the milk was given to children at school under supervision. However, the practical difficulties of obtaining the cooperation of dairies and of school authorities appear formidable.

4.3.2 Topical

Mouthrinse

Mouthrinsing by children with a fluoride solution, weekly or fortnightly at school, has been introduced in some countries, especially in Sweden. Usually, a 0.2% neutral sodium fluoride solution is used. The procedure is very simple to administer. Each child is given a disposable cup containing 5–10 ml of solution and is instructed to retain and rinse the solution gently in the mouth for at least 1 minute, after which the solution is expectorated into the cup. Although in fluoride tablet schemes the teachers dispense the tablets, supervising the mouthrinsing procedure must be the responsibility of the administering authority.

The disruption of normal school activities can be minimal if the procedure is carried out efficiently. However, it is essential for the dental team to establish and maintain good rapport with the school authorities.

Solution, gel or prophylaxis paste

Supervised 'brush-ins' at school, during which children brush their teeth with fluoride solution, gel or prophylaxis paste, is another method that has been investigated. This method has the advantage over mouthrinsing that it involves the children in toothbrushing, during which time oral hygiene instruction may be given. However, the procedure is more difficult and time-consuming to administer and requires staff trained to a higher standard.

Solutions containing 1% sodium fluoride (0.4% fluoride) have been tested in Sweden, APF solutions and gels (0.6% fluoride and 1.23% fluoride, respectively) in the USA, Canada and Brazil, and amine fluoride (1.25% fluoride) in Switzerland. Caries reductions obtained with as few as four or five 'brush-ins' a year have been comparable with those obtained with weekly or fortnightly mouthrinsing (Horowitz et al 1974). 'Brush-ins' with prophylaxis pastes have mostly employed a 9% stannous fluoride paste (2.18% fluoride), but an APF paste (1.23% fluoride) has also been tested. The results of either annual or semi-annual 'brush-ins' with these pastes have been inconclusive (Horowitz & Bixler 1976).

The effectiveness of frequent self-application of fluoride gel was shown by Englander et al (1967). Children aged 11–14 years living in a non-fluoridated area applied gel to their teeth in individually constructed trays under supervision at school for 6 minutes every school day for nearly 2 years. Children who used a sodium fluoride gel (0.5% fluoride) developed, on average, 3.50 fewer carious surfaces than children in a control group, and children using an APF gel (0.5% fluoride) developed 3.29 fewer carious surfaces; percentage reductions were 80% and 75% respectively, the highest reported for any topical fluoride method. However, less frequent applications (three times weekly) by children in a fluoridated area reduced caries by only 29% after 30 months (Englander et al 1971).

4.3.3 Selection of methods for community use

Water fluoridation is not only the most effective method known at present for preventing dental caries but it is also the most cost-effective (Horowitz & Heifetz 1979). It is widely believed that fluoridation should be the corner-stone for any local or national caries-preventive programme (Backer-Dirks et al 1978).

If water fluoridation is not feasible and a choice is to be made between other methods, the decision must be based, at least in part, on the relative cost-effectiveness of alternative methods. Calculating cost-effectiveness is complicated by a number of factors: for example, most of the information available about the effectiveness of different methods is based on clinical trials in which a method is tested on selected subjects for a limited number of years, under ideal conditions that do not necessarily exist in the community at large.

However, Horowitz & Heifetz (1979) estimated the cost-effectiveness of various methods and concluded that fluoride tablet administration is more cost-effective than school water fluoridation and that weekly mouthrinsing with 0.2% fluoride solution is the most cost-effective of topical methods.

REFERENCES

Ashley F P, Mainwaring P J, Emslie R D, Naylor M N 1977 Clinical testing of a mouthrinse and a dentifrice containing fluoride: a 2-year supervised study in schools. British Dental Journal 143: 333–338

Backer-Dirks O, Kunzel W, Carlos J P 1978 Caries-preventive water fluoridation. Caries Research 12 (suppl 1): 7–14

Banoczy J, Zimmerman P, Printer A, Hadas E, Bruszt V 1983 Effect of fluoridated milk on caries: 3-year results. Community Dentistry and Oral Epidemiology 11: 81–85

Barnhart W E, Hiller L K, Giles J L, Michaels S F 1974 Dentifrice usage and ingestion among four age groups. Journal of Dental Research 53: 1317–1322

Baxter P M 1980 Toothpaste ingestion during tooth-brushing by school children. British Dental Journal 148: 125–128

Bayless J M, Tinanoff N 1985 Diagnosis and treatment of acute fluoride toxicity. Journal of the American Dental Association 110: 209–211

Binder K, Driscoll W S, Schutzmannsky G 1978 Caries-preventive fluoride tablet programmes. Caries Research 12 (suppl 1): 22–30

Birkeland J M, Torell P 1978 Caries-preventive fluoride mouthrinses. Caries Research 12 (suppl 1): 38–51

Blinkhorn A S, Holloway P J, Davies T G H 1983 Combined effects of a fluoride dentifrice and mouthrinse on the incidence of dental caries. Community Dentistry and Oral Epidemiology 11: 7–11

Brudevold F, DePaola P F 1966 Studies on topically applied acidulated phosphate fluoride at Forsyth Dental Center. Dental Clinics of North America (July) 299–308

Brudevold F, Naujoks R 1978 Caries-preventive treatment of the individual. Caries Research 12 (suppl 1): 52–64

Clark D C 1982 A review on fluoride varnishes: an alternative topical fluoride treatment. Community Dentistry and Oral Epidemiology 10: 117–123

Davis J G 1972 Milk as a vehicle for fluoridation of the diet for children. In: The fluoridation of children's milk: Proceedings of a Scientific Symposium. Kimpton, London, pp 34–40

Dean H T, Arnold F A, Elvove E 1942 Domestic water and dental caries: V. Additional studies of the relation of fluoride domestic water to dental caries experience in 4425 white children aged 12–14 years of 13 cities in 4 states. Public Health Reports 57: 1155–1179

Department of Environment 1987 Code of practice – technical aspects of fluoridation of water supplies. Her Majesty's Stationery Office, London

Driscoll W S, Swango P A, Horowitz A M, Kingman A 1982 Caries-preventive effects of daily and weekly fluoride mouthrinsing in a fluoridated community: final results after 30 months. Journal of the American Dental Association 105: 1010–1013

Ekstrand J, Koch G, Lindgren L E, Petersson L G 1981 Pharmacokinetics of fluoride gels in children and adults. Caries Research 15: 213–220

Englander H R, Keyes P H, Gestwicki M, Sultz H A 1967 Clinical anticaries effect of repeated topical sodium fluoride applications by mouthpieces. Journal of the American Dental Association 75: 638–645

Englander H R, Sherrill L T, Miller B G, Carlos T P, Mellberg J R, Senning R S 1971 Incremental rates of dental caries after repeated topical sodium fluoride applications in children with lifelong consumption of fluoridated water. Journal of the American Dental Association 82: 354–358

Fehr F von der, Moller I 1978 Caries-preventive fluoride dentifrices. Caries Research 12 (suppl 1): 31–37

Fejerskov O, Manji F, Baelum V, Moller I J 1988 Dental fluorosis: a handbook for health workers. Munksgaard, Copenhagen

Gish C W, Muhler J C, Howell C L 1962 A new approach to the topical application of fluorides for the reduction of dental caries in children: results at the end of 5 years. Journal of Dentistry for Children 29: 65–71

Hagan P P, Rozier R G, Bawden J W 1985 The caries-preventive effects of full- and half-strength topical acidulated phosphate fluoride. Pediatric Dentistry 7: 185–191

Hargreaves J A, Ingram G S, Wagg B J 1972 A gravimetric study of the ingestion of toothpaste by children. Caries Research 6: 237–243

Heifetz S B, Horowitz H S 1984 The amounts of fluoride in current fluoride therapies: safety considerations for children. Journal of Dentistry for Children 51: 257–269

Heifetz S B, Horowitz H S, Brunelle J A 1983 Effects of school water fluoridation on dental caries: results in Seagrove, NC, after 12 years. Journal of the American Dental Association 106: 333–337

Hodge C, Smith F A 1965 Biological properties of inorganic fluorides. In: Simons J H (ed) Fluorine chemistry, vol 4. Academic Press, New York

Horowitz H S 1970 The current status of topical fluorides in preventive dentistry. Journal of the American Dental Association 81: 166–177

Horowitz H S 1989 Effectiveness of school water fluoridation and dietary fluoride supplements in school-aged children. Journal of Public Health Dentistry 49 (special issue): 290–296

Horowitz H S 1990 The future of water fluoridation and other systemic fluorides. Journal of Dental Research 69 (special issue): 760–764

Horowitz H S, Bixler D 1976 The effect of self-applied stannous fluoride-zirconium silicate prophylactic paste on dental caries in Santa Clara County, California. Journal of the American Dental Association 92: 369–373

Horowitz H S, Heifetz S B 1979 Methods for assessing the cost-effectiveness of caries-preventive agents and procedures. International Dental Journal 29: 106–117

Horowitz H S, Heifetz S B, Law F E 1972 Effect of school water fluoridation on dental caries: final results in Elk Lake, Pennsylvania, after 12 years. Journal of the American Dental Association 84: 832–838

Horowitz H S, Heifetz S B, McClendon B J, Viegas A R, Guimaraes L O C, Lopes E S 1974 Evaluation of self-administered prophylaxis and supervised toothbrushing with acidulated phosphate fluoride. Caries Research 8: 39–51

Houwink B, Wagg B J 1979 Effect of fluoride dentifrice usage during infancy upon mottling of the permanent teeth. Caries Research 13: 231–237

Ismail A I 1994 Fluoride supplements: current effectiveness, side-effects and recommendations. Community Dentistry and Oral Epidemiology 22: 164–172

Knutson J W 1948 Sodium fluoride solutions: technique for application to the teeth. Journal of the American Dental Association 36: 37–39

LeCompte E J, Doyle T E 1985 Effects of suctioning devices on oral fluoride retention. Journal of the American Dental Association 110: 357–369

McCall D R, Watkins T R, Stephen K W, Collins W J H, Smalls M J 1983 Fluoride ingestion following APF gel application. British Dental Journal 155: 333–336

McDonald R E, Muhler J C 1957 The superiority of topical application of stannous fluoride on primary teeth. Journal of Dentistry for Children 24: 84–86

Mainwaring P J, Naylor M N 1978 A 3-year clinical study to determine the separate and combined caries-inhibiting effects of sodium mono-fluorophosphate toothpaste and an acidulated phosphate fluoride gel. Caries Research 12: 202–212

Marthaler T M, Mejia R, Toth K, Vines J L 1978 Caries-preventive salt fluoridation. Caries Research 12 (suppl 1): 15–21

Mellberg J R, Ripa L W 1983 Fluoride in preventive dentistry. Quintessence, Chicago, ch 6

Modeer T, Twetman S, Bergstrand F 1984 Three-year study of the effect of fluoride varnish (Duraphat) on proximal caries progression in teenagers. Scandinavian Journal of Dental Research 92: 400–407

Murray J J 1971 Adult dental health in fluoride and non-fluoride areas. British Dental Journal 131: 391–395

Murray J J, Rugg-Gunn A J, Jenkins G N 1991 Fluorides in caries prevention, 3rd edn. Butterworth-Heinemann, Oxford, ch 11

O'Brien M 1994 Children's dental health in the United Kingdom 1993 Office of Population Censuses and Surveys. Her Majesty's Stationery Office, London, p 46

Public Health Alliance & British Fluoridation Society 1994 One in a million: water fluoridation and dental public health

Riordan P J 1993 Fluoride supplements in caries prevention: a literature review and proposal for a new dosage schedule. Journal of Public Health Dentistry 53: 174–189

Ripa L W 1981 Professionally (operator) applied topical fluoride therapy: a critique. International Dental Journal 31: 105–120

Ripa L W 1983 Supervised weekly rinsing with a 0.2% neutral sodium fluoride solution: final results of a demonstration program after six school years. Journal of Public Health Dentistry 43: 53–62

Ripa L W 1984 Need for prior toothcleaning when performing a professional topical fluoride application: review and recommendations for change. Journal of the American Dental Association 109: 281–285

Ripa L W 1991 A critique of topical fluoride methods (dentifrices, mouthrinses, operator- and self-applied gels) in an era of decreased caries and increased fluorosis prevalence. Journal of Public Health Dentistry 51: 23–41

Roberts J F, Longhurst P 1987 A clinical estimation of the fluoride used during application of a fluoride varnish. British Dental Journal 162: 463–466

Rock W P 1994 Young children and fluoride toothpaste. British Dental Journal 177: 17–20

Royal College of Physicians 1976 Fluoride, teeth and health. Pitman Medical, Tunbridge Wells

Spoerke D G, Bennett D L, Gullekson D J K 1980 Toxicity related to acute low dose sodium fluoride ingestions. Journal of Family Practice 10: 139–140

Stephen K W, Boyle I T, Campbell D, McNee S, Boyle P 1984 Five-year double-blind fluoridated milk study in Scotland. Community Dentistry Oral Epidemiology 12: 223–229

Stookey G K, Schemehorn B R, Drook C A, Cheetham B L 1986 The effect of rinsing with water immediately after a professional fluoride gel application on fluoride uptake in demineralised enamel: an in vivo study. Pediatric Dentistry 8: 153–157

Tyler J G, Andlaw R J 1987 Oral retention of fluoride after application of acidulated phosphate fluoride gel in air-cushion trays. British Dental Journal 162: 422–425

World Health Organization 1967 Fluorides and human health. World Health Organization, Geneva, ch 8, p 273–322

RECOMMENDED READING

Mellberg J R, Ripa L W 1983 Fluoride in preventive dentistry: theory and clinical applications. Quintessence, Chicago

Murray J J, Rugg-Gunn A J, Jenkins G N 1991 Fluorides in caries prevention, 3rd edn. Butterworth-Heinemann, Oxford, ch 11

Nikiforuk G 1985 Understanding dental caries: 2. Prevention: basic and clinical aspects. Karger, Basel, chs 2–6

Thylstrup A, Fejerskov O 1994 Textbook of cariology, 2nd edn. Munksgaard, Copenhagen

5 Pit and fissure sealants

5.1 BACKGROUND

The effect of systemic or topical fluorides in preventing dental caries is noted principally on the smooth surfaces of teeth; the effect on pit and fissure caries is relatively small. It is probable that the protected stagnation sites provided by pits and fissures offer such favourable conditions for the initiation of caries that fluoride is inadequate to combat it. Therefore there is a place in preventive dentistry for a method aimed specifically at preventing caries in these caries-prone sites.

The idea of sealing pits and fissures before they become carious is not new, but early attempts met with only limited success because the adhesion of tested materials to enamel was inadequate. The success of the current sealing technique is based on the discovery that adhesion of acrylic and composite resins to enamel is greatly increased if the enamel is first etched with acid (Buonocore 1955).

Phosphoric acid, in the concentration range of 30–50%, is normally used to etch enamel. A 1-minute application removes about 10 μm of surface enamel and etches the underlying surface to a depth of about 20 μm (Silverstone 1974). Etching produces a porous layer of enamel into which resin can flow; the porosity provides a large surface area for adhesion of resin and also excellent mechanical retention.

5.2 TYPES OF SEALANT

The resins currently used as sealants are based on the 'bis GMA' resin developed by Bowen (1963); 'bis GMA' is the reaction product of bis (4-hydroxyphenyl) dimethylmethane and glycidyl methacrylate. Two types are available: those that polymerize after mixing catalyst and 'universal' components (autopolymerizing types), and those that polymerize only after exposure to a suitable light source. Initially ultraviolet light (wavelength 365 nm) was used, but this has been superseded by visible (blue) light (wavelength 430–490 nm).

Most of the resins that have been used as fissure sealants are 'unfilled', that is, they do not contain filler particles. However, filled resins are also available; these are more resistant to abrasion in vitro but not in vivo (Jensen et al 1985), and their retention in fissures is comparable to that of unfilled resins (Stephen & Strang 1985). Most sealants now contain a colouring agent to aid detection of the sealant (Rock et al 1989).

Reviews of clinical trials of pit and fissure sealants have shown that the results have been consistent (with few exceptions) in demonstrating that sealants are well retained if applied correctly, and that they are highly effective in preventing dental caries (Ripa 1980, Mertz-Fairhurst 1984, Rock 1984, Stephen & Strang 1985, Weintraub 1989, Gordon & Nunn 1996). Fissure sealing should always be done as part of comprehensive preventive treatment, which includes diet counselling, oral hygiene instruction and use of fluorides.

5.3 SELECTION OF PATIENTS AND TEETH

Sealing of pits and fissures in all patients may be considered to be ideal treatment and is, indeed, justified for all patients classified as 'high risk' (page 50). However, financial and other constraints demand that guidelines for patient and tooth selection should be established. The following guidelines reflect the recommendations of the British Society of Paediatric Dentistry (1993):

1. The highest priority should be given to sealing permanent first molars soon after they erupt. However, if the occlusal fissures appear smooth and shallow, and if caries activity is low (indicated, for example, by a caries-free primary dentition), they may be kept under regular review. If one first molar becomes carious there would be strong justification for sealing the other three.

2. Premolars and, especially, permanent second molars, should be sealed if the patient's past caries experience (for example in first molars) suggests that these teeth will also be at risk.

3. Primary molars are generally given relatively low priority, but sealing can be justified, especially for 'high risk' patients.

4. Teeth should be sealed as soon as possible after they erupt.

5. Sealants should be kept under review, and repaired or replaced if they become defective.

Ideally, sealant is placed over pits and fissures that are diagnosed as caries-free. If there is doubt about the integrity of the occlusal surface a bite-wing radiograph should be taken. However, if sealant is inadvertently placed over an early carious lesion, it is reassuring to know that the lesion will probably not progress (Going 1984), presumably because it is sealed off from bacteria and further sources of carbohydrate. If a small lesion is diagnosed, a preventive resin restoration (sealant restoration) may be placed (p. 119).

Technique: pit and fissure sealing

Procedure	Method	Rationale	Notes
1. Clean the tooth surface	Dislodge debris from the pit or fissure with a sharp probe. Use a pumice-water slurry on a prophylaxis brush to clean the pit or fissure and surrounding tooth surface. Wash the surface with an air/water spray.	It has generally been considered that it is necessary to remove plaque and pellicle that might interfere with subsequent acid etching. Pumice is used instead of prophylaxis pastes because the latter contain fluoride and/ or oily constituents that may reduce the effectiveness of acid etching. Particles of pumice must be removed because they might prevent sealant flowing into the fissure.	There is evidence to suggest that this cleaning procedure is unnecessary (Donnan & Ball 1988). A reasonable compromise would be to use a brush but no pumice. Cleaning with an air-polishing unit is most efficient (Brocklehurst et al 1992). **Fig. 5.1a**
2. Isolate and dry the tooth	Isolate the tooth with cotton wool rolls and/or absorbent pads. Use a saliva ejector. When treating a mandibular tooth, use a flanged saliva ejector (Figs. 5.1a and 7.1). Dry the tooth surface with compressed air. With one hand, carefully maintain the position of saliva ejector, cotton wool rolls and/or absorbent pads until the treatment is completed. Do not attempt to isolate teeth in more than one quadrant at a time.	For successful bonding of resin to enamel to occur, it is essential that the tooth is kept isolated from saliva. Water or saliva on the tooth surface would dilute the acid etchant. Close control is necessary because any movement of the tongue or cheeks may displace the saliva ejector, cotton rolls or absorbent pads.	It is essential to have an oil-free air line. Since this task immobilizes one hand, it is essential to have assistance with the procedures that follow.

Technique: pit and fissure sealing *(contd)*

Procedure	Method	Rationale	Notes
3. Etch the enamel	Apply 30–50% phosphoric acid with a small cotton wool pledget or sponge pad, or with a small brush.	30–50% phosphoric acid produces the optimum degree of etching to ensure good bonding of resin.	The etchant or 'conditioner' supplied with commercial products is phosphoric acid in the concentration range of 30–50% either as solution or gel. Care must be taken to avoid dripping on to the patient—the eyes are particularly at risk, and protective spectacles should be worn.
	Extend the area of etching beyond the fissures up to the tips of the cusps (Fig. 5.1b) or to a radius of 3–4 mm around a pit.	Adequate extension of the etched area is essential to ensure that the margin of the sealant is placed on etched enamel.	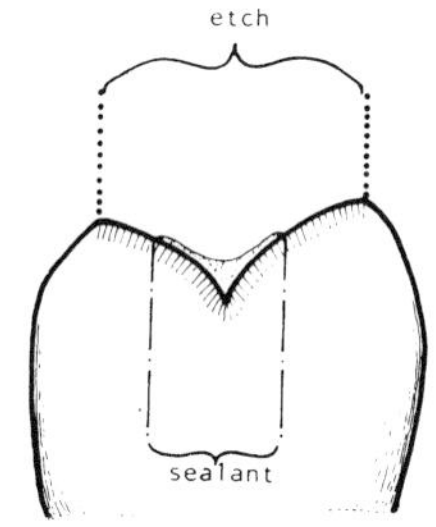 **Fig. 5.1b**
	Keep the enamel wet with acid for 1 minute.	A 1-minute application produces an etching pattern that ensures a strong bond with resin.	The need for a 1-minute application has been questioned, and there is evidence that a 20-second etching period is sufficient for permanent teeth (Stephen et al 1982, Eidelman et al 1988).
4. Wash and dry the enamel surface	With an assistant holding the tip of a high-volume aspirator tube close to the tooth, wash the acid off with a stream of water directed at the etched surface for 15 seconds (Fig. 5.1c). Do not allow the patient to rinse.	Efficient aspiration is important; if the considerable volume of water that is used is not removed, the patient may be forced to swallow and, in so doing, may displace saliva on to the etched surfaces. Inadequate washing, or contamination of the etched surface by saliva, inhibits resin bonding to enamel.	Aspiration also spares the patient the unpleasant taste of acid washed from the tooth. 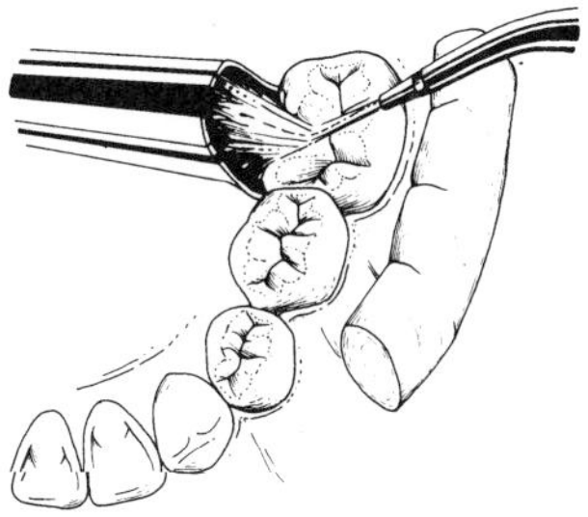 **Fig. 5.1c**
	Holding the cheek away from the tooth, remove wet cotton rolls and replace with dry ones.		Essential requirements for strong bonding of resin to enamel are: a. to etch enamel adequately b. to wash and dry the etched surface thoroughly c. to keep the etched surface absolutely free of any contaminants. If the etched surface does become contaminated, a further 1-minute etch is recommended.
	Dry the etched surface thoroughly with oil-free compressed air for 30 seconds.	Inadequate drying, or contamination by oil, also reduces the resin–enamel bond strength.	When the etched surface is dried it should appear 'chalky'. If it does not it should be re-etched.

Technique: pit and fissure sealing (*contd*)

Procedure	Method	Rationale	Notes
5. Apply the resin	Apply the resin (mixed according to the manufacturer's instructions) with any convenient dental instrument (e.g. a small excavator), or with the applicator provided with the commercial product. Place the resin at one end of the fissure (or pit) and encourage it to flow into and over the entire length of the fissure. Add further increments if required until the fissure is covered and the margin of the resin is about 2 mm up the cuspal inclines (Fig. 5.1b); the margin must be within the periphery of the etched area.	The manufacturer's instructions must be followed precisely to ensure a predictable setting time. Resin is retained principally on etched enamel of the cuspal inclines. The margin must be firmly based on etched enamel to prevent marginal leakage.	The type of applicator used is not important provided that the resin can be placed with precision. The outline of the sealant is dictated by the morphology of the fissure (Fig. 5.1d for mandibular molar, Fig. 5.1e for maxillary molar). Etched enamel remaining uncovered by resin soon remineralizes because saliva is supersaturated with calcium salts.
6. Allow the resin to polymerize	Maintain careful isolation for the polymerization time recommended by the manufacturer or, if using a light-cured resin, apply the polymerization light for the recommended time period.		The time required to polymerize a light-sensitive resin varies according to the light source used, but any of the currently available visible light sources will polymerize any of the resins within 60 seconds (Stephen & Strang 1985).
7. Check the sealant	Pass a blunt probe gently over the surface of the resin to check that it covers the entire fissure. If any part of the fissure is not sealed, add further resin immediately and allow it to polymerize (this addition may only be made if isolation has been maintained and the surface is therefore uncontaminated). Wipe away the thin, sticky surface film of unpolymerized resin with a cotton wool pledget.	Removal of the surface film is optional, but spares the patient its unpleasant taste.	

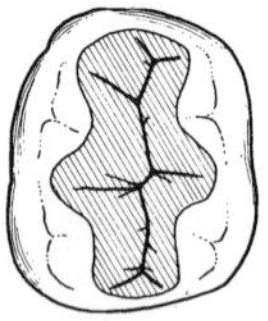

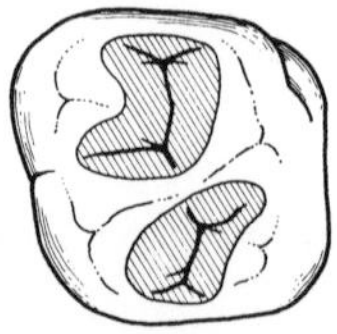

Fig. 5.1d   **Fig. 5.1e**

REFERENCES

Bowen R L 1963 Properties of a silica-reinforced polymer for dental restorations. Journal of the American Dental Association 66: 57–64

British Society of Paediatric Dentistry 1993. A policy document on fissure sealants. International Journal of Paediatric Dentistry 3: 99–100

Brocklehurst P R, Joshi R I, Northeast S E 1992 The effect of air-polishing occlusal surfaces on the penetration of fissures by a sealant. International Journal of Paediatric Dentistry 2: 157–162

Buonocore M G 1955 A simple method of increasing the adhesion of acrylic filling material to enamel. Journal of Dental Research 34: 849–853

Donnan M F, Ball I A 1988 A double-blind clinical trial to determine the importance of pumice prophylaxis on fissure sealant retention. British Dental Journal 165: 283–286

Eidelman E, Shapira J, Houpt M 1988 The retention of fissure sealants using twenty-second etching time: three-year follow-up. Journal of Dentistry for Children 55: 119–120

Going R E 1984 Sealant effect on incipient caries, enamel maturation, and future caries susceptibility. Journal of Dental Education 48: 35–41

Gordon P H, Nunn J H 1996 Fissure sealants. In: Murray J J (ed) The prevention of oral disease, 3rd edn. Oxford University Press, Oxford, ch 5

Jensen Ø E, Handelman S L, Perez Diez F 1985 Occlusal wear of four pit and fissure sealants over two years. Pediatric Dentistry 7: 23–29

Mertz-Fairhurst E J 1984 Current status of sealant retention and caries prevention. Journal of Dental Education 48: 18–26

Ripa L W 1980 Occlusal sealants: rationale and review of clinical trials. International Dental Journal 30: 127–139

Rock W P 1984 The effectiveness of fissure sealant resins. Journal of Dental Education 48: 27–31

Rock W P, Potts A J C, Marchment M D, Clayton-Smith A J, Galuszka M A 1989 The visibility of clear and opaque fissure sealants. British Dental Journal 167: 395–396

Silverstone L M 1974 Fissure sealants—laboratory studies. Caries Research 8: 2–26

Stephen K W, Kirkwood M, Main C 1982 Retention of a filled fissure sealant using reduced etch time. British Dental Journal 153: 232–233

Stephen K W, Strang R 1985 Fissure sealants: a review. Community Dental Health 2: 149–156

Weintraub J A 1989 The effectiveness of pit and fissure sealants. Journal of Public Health Dentistry 49 (special issue): 317–330

RECOMMENDED READING

Murray J J, Bennett T G 1984 A colour atlas of acid etch technique. Wolfe, London

Nikiforuk G 1985 Understanding dental caries: 2. Prevention: basic and clinical aspects. Karger, Basel, ch 7

Simonsen R J 1978 Clinical applications of the acid etch technique. Quintessence, Chicago, ch 2

Simonsen R J 1985 Pit and fissure sealant: theoretical and clinical considerations. In: Braham R L, Morris M E (eds) Textbook of pediatric dentistry, 2nd edn. Williams & Wilkins, Baltimore, ch 11

Treatment of dental caries—operative methods

Part 3

6 Local analgesia

It is the dentist's responsibility not only to provide treatment but also to ensure that the patient remains comfortable and relaxed. The elimination of pain is essential, particularly with children; whereas adults may tolerate discomfort and remain cooperative, many children become frightened if they are hurt and will not cooperate further. Not only is the elimination of pain important to the patient: it also allows the dentist to proceed with treatment relaxed in the knowledge that the patient will not be hurt. Only when the dentist and patient are relaxed can treatment proceed smoothly and be performed efficiently.

Although most people dislike injections of any kind, the great majority accept local analgesia for dental treatment if it is introduced properly. The technique of administration to a child patient is crucially important. If done carefully the procedure can be painless and therefore acceptable; if done carelessly it may be so unpleasant and frightening that the child may refuse to accept it again, with serious consequences for future dental treatment.

Before introducing local analgesia, it is essential to be aware of the child's attitudes towards it; gathering this information is an important part of history-taking (Ch. 1). The child who has had previous experience of injections and whose attitudes are favourable, or the child with no previous experience but whose behaviour is cooperative, may be introduced to local analgesia at any time (although it is always preferable, especially in the latter case, not to introduce local analgesia at the first visit). On the other hand, the frightened child must be approached in a different way: the first objective must be to allay the child's fears. A series of three or four short introductory appointments should be arranged (as outlined on p. 16), after which a decision is made either to proceed with the administration of local analgesia or, if the child remains apprehensive, to introduce some form of sedation or even general anaesthesia. If there is greater urgency to begin treatment, sedation or general anaesthesia may be introduced at an earlier stage. The important point is that the dentist must first know the child's attitudes towards local analgesia and then plan its introduction accordingly. An injection should be administered only to a cooperative child; to give it carelessly to a frightened child is bad practice, and to force it on a child can only be condemned as barbaric.

Local analgesia is not always essential for conservative dentistry. Although pain thresholds vary greatly, the general statement may be made that local analgesia is desirable if sound dentine needs to be cut in cavity preparation. However, it is a strong clinical impression, albeit unsupported by scientific evidence, that primary teeth are less sensitive to cavity preparation than permanent teeth. Certainly, small occlusal cavities in primary teeth can often be prepared without local analgesia, as can some large cavities that need little further extension; on the other hand, local analgesia is almost always essential if cavity preparation involves more than minimal cutting of sound dentine.

Local analgesia presents a special problem with preschool children because they are, in general, less tolerant of pain and discomfort than older children. With care and skill a painless injection can be given, but the strange sensations of local analgesia cannot be avoided and these cause some children considerable anxiety. Reassurances and explanations may not be understood or may be inadequate to allay this anxiety. Therefore, when introducing restorative treatment to a preschool child it is often preferable, and justifiable, to start without local analgesia (having selected a tooth requiring only minimal cavity preparation), proceeding very carefully and being prepared to stop at the first sign of the child experiencing any discomfort. Even if only a temporary restoration is placed, the child will be encouraged by the experience of having 'had a filling'. This simple operative procedure would therefore have served as a useful behaviour shaping exercise (p. 17), making local analgesia easier to administer at a future treatment session.

6.1 EQUIPMENT

An aspirating syringe should be used routinely. A possible hazard with any injection is the penetration of a blood vessel and intravascular injection of solution, which might have toxic effects; only by the use of an aspirating syringe can this hazard be eliminated. Although the risk of intravascular injection exists primarily when giving deep injections (e.g. inferior dental nerve block), and is minimal when giving infiltrations, the use of an aspirating syringe for all

injections is now routine practice. After the needle is inserted, slight retraction of the plunger aspirates a small volume of fluid into the cartridge; if this fluid is blood, the needle must be repositioned before injecting.

It is essential to use disposable needles to avoid any risk of conveying infection from one patient to another. 'Short' needles are used for most injections; these are 2 cm or 2.5 cm in length. 'Long' needles (3.0 cm) are used for inferior dental nerve blocks. Fine needles (gauge 30) are recommended for infiltrations, and thicker (gauge 27) needles for all other injections.

The solution most commonly used is 2% lignocaine with 1:80 000 adrenaline. Prilocaine (3%) with felypressin (0.31 i.u./ml) is also commonly used and is the solution of choice when there are reasons for avoiding the injection of adrenaline.

6.2 INFILTRATION

A solution deposited supraperiostally infiltrates through the alveolar bone to reach the root apex. Since alveolar bone in children is more permeable than it is in adults, less local analgesic solution suffices to produce analgesia of primary teeth, and analgesia of mandibular primary molars may usually be achieved by infiltration in children up to the age of about 5 years.

Technique: maxillary infiltration

Procedure	Method	Rationale	Notes
1. Organize equipment and materials	Have all the necessary equipment and materials ready for use before the patient enters the surgery.	For a successful technique it is important to be able to proceed smoothly from start to finish, without interruptions to prepare equipment.	
	Place equipment and materials on a clean surface behind the dental chair; it is especially important to keep the syringe out of sight.	The sight of a needle causes some anxiety to most patients (adults as well as children).	
2. Establish a good operating position	Adjust the chair and headrest position so that the child's line of vision is at least 45° from the horizontal.	Control of the child's field of vision is important so that the syringe will not be seen by the child.	
	Sit or stand in front of and facing the child ('8 o'clock' position for a right-handed dentist). Adjust the height of the chair to allow the injection site to be seen easily and comfortably.	Correct positioning of the dentist is important to provide optimal access and visibility.	Some dentists prefer to work from behind the patient ('11 o'clock' position for a right-handed dentist) when injecting on the left side.

Technique: maxillary infiltration *(contd)*

Procedure	Method	Rationale	Notes
3. Inform the child	Tell the child, clearly but casually, that to "clean decay" from the tooth it is best to "make the tooth go to sleep". Stress that only the tooth will go to sleep, and that it will "wake up" later.	Lengthy, detailed explanations are unnecessary and may arouse anxiety in the child. Proper selection of words is imperative. Avoid the use of "needle", "injection", "prick", "hurt", unless the child mentions them. "Make it go to sleep" is better than "put to sleep"—the latter may have unpleasant connotations in relation to pets or farm animals.	The precise method of informing the child will be influenced by the child's age and stage of psychological development, and also by attitudes to previous injections, evident from the dental history (p. 6).
4. Apply topical analgesic	Show the child a cotton roll on one end of which has been placed topical analgesic cream or solution, and let the child smell its "fruity" smell. Explain that this will start to make the tooth go to sleep.	The use of topical analgesics, while not essential, increases the chance of giving a completely painless injection, and is therefore strongly recommended. Suggestions of generally-acceptable fruity smells reduce the risk of objections to their taste.	If topical analgesic cream is used, care should be taken not to place too much on the end of the cotton roll, because it can be squeezed out when applied to the tissues, and run back into the throat. To minimize this problem, one end of the cotton roll may be pulled out, so forming a cup-shaped depression at the other end in which the cream is better localized when placed against the tissues.
	After checking that the child's seating and head positions are correct, retract the cheek with the left hand and dry the tissue at the muco-buccal fold above the tooth to be treated, using the dry end of the cotton roll. Then turn the roll around and hold the topical analgesic against the tissue for 2 minutes; distract the child during this period. Maintain the child's head position until the end of the injection procedure by continuing to hold the cheek with the left hand.	The surface analgesic will be most effective if applied to dry tissue, and allowed to act for at least 2 minutes.	Some dentists prefer to apply topical analgesic on a cotton pledget held in tweezers, especially for posterior teeth when access for cotton rolls is difficult. Jet injection also produces excellent topical analgesia (p. 75).
5. Prepare to give the injection	While still maintaining control of the child's head position with the left hand, remove the cotton roll after 2 minutes and receive the syringe from an assistant in the right hand. If the injection is to be given in the maxillary left quadrant, receive the syringe over the child's left shoulder. If the injection is for a maxillary right tooth, the assistant should pass the syringe from behind the patient, over the right shoulder The assistant should first carefully place the syringe in the dentist's hand so that it can be used immediately, and then remove the needle guard.	Maintenance of the child's head position, ensuring that the line of vision is towards the ceiling, is essential at this stage. It should not be necessary to hide the syringe — it can be handled comfortably below the child's line of vision. Receiving the syringe in this manner avoids passing it in front of the patient. Unnecessary movement and noise in transferring the syringe to the dentist might attract the child's attention. It should not be necessary to change the grip on the syringe before using it.	If the child becomes anxious at this stage and cannot be quickly reassured, it is usually better to return the syringe to the assistant, release control of the child's head and attempt, through further explanation, to obtain the child's consent to proceed. Forcing an injection on an unwilling child may succeed in obtaining analgesia but can only damage the good relationship on which further cooperation depends. If consent is not obtained quickly, it may be preferable to proceed without analgesia

Technique: maxillary infiltration (*contd*)

Procedure	Method	Rationale	Notes
			or to consider introducing some form of sedation; protracted discussion may only increase tension and anxiety.
6. Give the injection	With the left hand, pull the cheek outwards so that the mucous membrane is made taut (Fig. 6.1a). Position the tip of the needle at the muco-buccal fold just above the tooth to be treated, supporting the syringe against the left hand, which is stabilized by resting free fingers on the patient's face.	A needle penetrates taut tissue more easily. Supporting the syringe against a stable left hand gives better control in positioning and directing the needle.	When producing analgesia of permanent first molars, infiltrations are given mesial and distal to the tooth (i.e. over the 2nd molar and 2nd premolar), because the dense zygomatic arch lies over the 1st molar root apex. Alternatively, a modified posterior superior alveolar nerve block may be given (p. 70).
	Gently insert the tip of the needle into the tissue, or draw the taut tissue over the needle (Fig. 6.1b).		

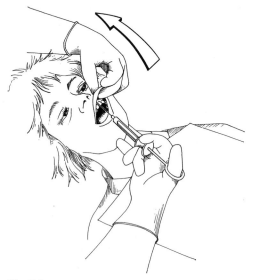

Fig. 6.1a

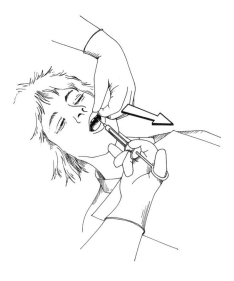

Fig. 6.1b

Immediately inject a few drops of solution, pause for a few seconds, then advance the needle carefully about 1 cm, 45° to the long axis of the tooth, to bring its tip close to the root apex.	A few drops of solution quickly produces analgesia of the soft tissue, thus reducing or eliminating pain during further penetration of the needle.
Inject slowly.	Fast injection invariably causes pain.
For primary teeth in children under about 6 years of age, about 1 ml of solution is sufficient. In older children, use a full cartridge.	The buccal plate of bone is more permeable in young children.

Technique: maxillary infiltration *(contd)*

Procedure	Method	Rationale	Notes
	Take about 30 seconds to give the injection. While injecting, casually inform the child that as the tooth "goes to sleep" it will "feel funny", and give reassurance that it will "wake up later".	The child's anxiety may be aroused by strange sensations that have not been explained.	
7. Withdraw the syringe and give post-operative instructions	When the solution has been injected, withdraw the needle but continue to maintain the child's head position with the left hand until the syringe has been passed to the assistant, *below* the child's field of vision, and the needle guard has been replaced on it.	A successful technique may be spoilt by careless manipulation of the syringe at this stage.	
	Ask the child to rinse.	Rinsing is not necessary, but by doing so the child's attention is distracted while the analgesic is taking effect, and the freedom of movement may be appreciated following the previous few minutes' restriction.	
	Warn the child and parent about the danger of cheek or lip biting. Reinforce the child's good behaviour.	A child may 'play' with an insensitive cheek or lip by biting it, sometimes causing severe injury.	It is important to emphasize this warning to the child and the parent before they leave the surgery.

Technique: mandibular infiltration (only suitable for primary molars in young children)

Procedure	Method	Rationale	Notes
1. Organize equipment and materials 2. Establish a good operating position 3. Inform the child 4. Apply topical analgesic	See 'maxillary infiltration'.		
5. Prepare to give the injection	For left or right mandibular infiltrations, receive the syringe from an assistant in the same way as for left or right maxillary infiltrations.		

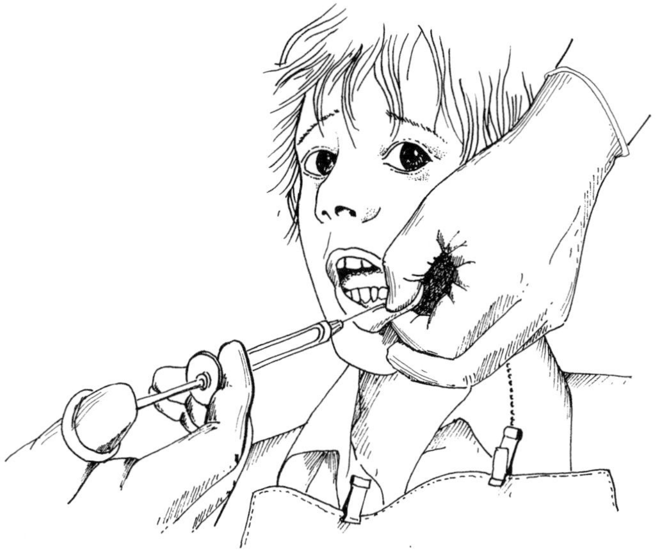

Fig. 6.2

Technique: mandibular infiltration (only suitable for primary molars in young children) **(contd)**

Procedure	Method	Rationale	Notes
6. Give the injection	With the left hand, pull the cheek outwards so that the mucous membrane is made taut. Holding the syringe in a horizontal position, take it carefully to the patient's mouth (Fig. 6.2). Position the tip of the needle at the muco-buccal fold just below the tooth to be treated. Proceed as outlined under 'maxillary infiltration' except that the syringe should be kept approximately parallel to the occlusal plane rather than being brought in line with the long axis of the tooth.	The child is least likely to see the syringe if it is kept horizontal. To give the injection in the same way as a maxillary infiltration, with the syringe 45° to the long axis of the tooth, would necessitate raising the syringe into the patient's line of vision; this is unnecessary.	
7. Withdraw the syringe and give postoperative instructions	See 'maxillary infiltration'.		

6.3 MODIFIED POSTERIOR SUPERIOR ALVEOLAR NERVE BLOCK (MAXILLARY MOLAR NERVE BLOCK)

It is sometimes difficult to achieve analgesia of maxillary permanent first molars by infiltration because solution does not easily penetrate the dense zygomatic bone over the first molar roots. Moreover, attempts to give a supraperiosteal injection in that region often cause pain because the needle contacts the prominent zygomatic process. These problems may be overcome by giving the infiltration distal to the zygomatic process, that is, over the permanent second molar; but an additional injection may be required over the second premolar (or second primary molar) because the mesio-buccal root of the maxillary first molar is sometimes innervated by the middle or anterior superior alveolar nerve.

An alternative approach is to block the main trunk of the posterior superior alveolar nerve. However, the conventional technique for the posterior superior alveolar nerve block requires a deep injection into a region containing a venous plexus, and therefore carries the danger of intravascular injection and of causing a haematoma; these dangers can be avoided by using the maxillary molar nerve block (Adatia 1976).

Technique: modified posterior superior alveolar nerve block (maxillary molar nerve block)

Procedure	Method	Rationale
1. Organize equipment and materials 2. Establish a good operating position 3. Inform the child 4. Locate anatomical landmarks	See 'maxillary infiltration'.	
	Palpate the zygomatic process and note its relationship to the teeth. Note the position of the distal root of the second molar (in a young child estimate this position). Pass the finger posteriorly along the muco-buccal fold and locate the maxillary tuberosity.	The injection will be given in line with the distal root of the second molar.

Technique: modified posterior superior alveolar nerve block (maxillary molar nerve block) *(contd)*

Procedure	Method	Rationale
5. Apply topical analgesic 6. Prepare to give the injection	See 'maxillary infiltration'.	
7. Give the injection	If injecting on the right side, retract the cheek with the left index or middle finger. If injecting on the left side, retract with the left thumb. Place the tip of the finger or thumb on the tuberosity. Insert the needle between the tip of the retracting finger and the distal surface of the zygomatic process, in line with the distal root of the second molar. Inject a few drops of solution. Advance the needle upwards and backwards about 1.5 cm, towards the alveolar bone. Aspirate and, if no blood is aspirated, slowly inject 1.5–2 ml of solution. While injecting, apply pressure to the alveolar mucosa with the finger or thumb; as solution accumulates it causes a bulge in the tissues anterior to the finger.	A few drops of solution produces analgesia of soft tissue, thus reducing or eliminating pain during further penetration of the needle. Penetrating about 1.5 cm takes the tip of the needle into the space above the attachment of the buccinator muscle. Injection of solution into a blood vessel may cause toxic reactions or may result in poor analgesia. Finger pressure localizes the solution, which facilitates the next step in the procedure.
8. Withdraw the syringe and massage the solution towards the posterior superior alveolar foramen	Withdraw the syringe as described previously (p. 69). Place a finger over the bulge at the injection site, ask the patient to close the mouth a little, and push the solution upwards, backwards and inwards towards the posterior superior alveolar foramen.	This method avoids the risk of causing a haematoma, which exists when a conventional posterior superior alveolar nerve block is given.

6.4 INFERIOR DENTAL NERVE BLOCK

The inferior dental nerve block is used to produce analgesia of mandibular teeth. However, for restorative dentistry, satisfactory analgesia of mandibular primary and permanent anterior teeth, and of mandibular primary molars in young children, can usually be produced by infiltration, thus avoiding the need for the potentially more unpleasant block injection.

Technique: inferior dental nerve block

Procedure	Method	Rationale	Notes
1. Organize equipment and materials 2. Inform the child	See 'maxillary infiltration'.		Ideally, an inferior dental block should be given to a child who has previously accepted a simple infiltration injection. Even with an excellent technique, a block injection may be painful. Together with the unpleasant numbness of face and tongue, this might cause a child to refuse any type of injection in the future, with far-reaching consequences for dental treatment.

Technique: inferior dental nerve block (*contd*)

Procedure	Method	Rationale	Notes
3. Establish a good operating position	Adjust the chair and headrest so that the child's line of vision is at least 45° to the horizontal.	Although when giving an inferior dental block it is more difficult to keep the syringe out of the patient's line of vision than when giving a maxillary infiltration, it is helpful to recline the patient.	
	If treating the mandibular left quadrant, sit or stand either behind the patient ('11 o'clock' position) or facing the patient ('8 o'clock' position). If treating the mandibular right quadrant, sit or stand facing the patient ('8 o'clock' position). Adjust the chair height to permit a comfortable view of the injection site.	Access to the injection site is obtained equally well from either position.	The positions described are for a right-handed dentist.
4. Locate the anatomical landmarks	Palpate the internal oblique ridge of the anterior border of the ramus, and note the pterygomandibular raphe and pterygomandibular triangle. The injection site is within the pterygomandibular triangle level with the occlusal surfaces of the molar teeth.		
5. Apply topical analgesic	Introduce the topical analgesic to the child as suggested under 'maxillary infiltration'. Ask the child to open the mouth wide, dry the injection site and apply the analgesic agent with a cotton roll or with a pledget held in tweezers. Attempt to keep the analgesic in place for 2 minutes without saliva contamination. If this is not practicable, prepare to give the injection sooner.	Effective surface analgesia is not usually produced in less than 2 minutes.	Some dentists do not use topical analgesic when giving an inferior dental nerve block because it often becomes quickly diluted and washed away by saliva, and patients may react to its unpleasant taste.
6. Prepare to give the injection	**Left quadrant** If positioned behind the patient, place the index or middle finger of the left hand on the internal oblique ridge at the level of the occlusal surfaces of the molar teeth, and support the mandible by placing the thumb on the posterior border of the ramus. If facing the patient, place the thumb on the internal oblique ridge and support the mandible posteriorly with the index finger. Receive the syringe from an assistant over the patient's left shoulder.	The position of the index finger or thumb is an important guide to the injection site (see below). Receiving the syringe as described avoids passing it within the patient's line of vision.	
	Right quadrant Place the thumb of the left hand on the internal oblique ridge and support the mandible posteriorly with the index finger. The assistant should pass the syringe behind the patient and hand it under the dentist's left arm, over the patient's right shoulder.		

Technique: inferior dental nerve block (*contd*)

Procedure	Method	Rationale	Notes
	As in the infiltration technique, the transfer of syringe should be done quietly and efficiently.		
7. Give the injection	**Indirect technique** Ask the patient to help by keeping the mouth open as wide as possible. Direct the needle towards the injection site, holding the syringe parallel to the occlusal plane and in line with the premolar and molar teeth. Insert the needle just medial to the thumb or index finger positioned on the internal oblique ridge, at the level of the occlusal surfaces of the molar teeth.	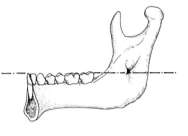	The use of the indirect or direct technique is dictated by the dentist's personal preference. In young children the position of the mandibular foramen is relatively low, in line with the cervical margins rather than the occlusal surfaces of the teeth (Fig. 6.3a). The direction of needle insertion should be modified accordingly.

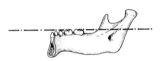

Fig. 6.3a

	Immediately on penetrating the tissue (a few millimetres only), inject a few drops of solution. Slowly advance the needle about 1.5 cm, then, keeping the tip of the needle in the same position, swing the syringe across the midline of the mouth, to lie over the opposite primary first molar (or first premolar) region (Fig. 6.3b).	A few drops of solution quickly produces analgesia of soft tissue, thus reducing pain during further penetration of the needle.	Small increments may be injected while advancing the needle gradually, thus moving the needle through anaesthetized tissue.

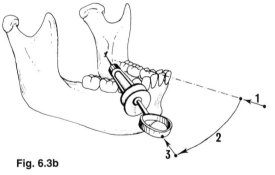

Fig. 6.3b

	Then advance the needle *gently* for about another 1 cm when it should contact bone. If bone is not contacted, do not insert the needle down to the hub of the syringe. Instead, withdraw it partly or completely, and reposition. When bone is contacted, aspirate; if blood is aspirated, withdraw the needle slightly and reposition.	Contacting bone with any force causes pain. Inserting the needle to the hub of the syringe is bad practice because should the needle break it would be difficult to recover. Aspiration of blood indicates that the needle has penetrated a blood vessel.	Breakage of a needle is, fortunately, a very rare occurrence.

Technique: inferior dental nerve block (*contd*)

Procedure	Method	Rationale	Notes
	If no blood is aspirated, inject about 3/4 of the cartridge *slowly*, over a period of about 30 seconds. Then withdraw the syringe slowly. If analgesia of lingual soft tissues is required, inject the remainder of the cartridge after withdrawing the syringe about half way. Inform and reassure the child about the "funny feeling".	Fast injection is painful.	
	Direct technique The technique is the same as the indirect technique except that the needle is directed towards the injection site while holding the syringe over the primary first molar (or first premolar) region of the opposite side of the mandible (Fig. 6.3c).		
8. Withdraw the syringe and give postoperative instructions	See 'maxillary infiltration'.		Fig. 6.3c

6.5 INTRAPAPILLARY INJECTION

The intrapapillary injection may be given to produce analgesia of palatal or lingual tissues, to avoid the need for the more painful injections directly into palatal or lingual tissues.

Technique: intrapapillary injection

1. Give a submucosal injection buccally using a short 30-gauge needle.
2. After about 1 minute, when soft tissue analgesia will have been obtained, inject into the interdental papilla mesial and distal to the tooth to be treated.
3. Pass the needle horizontally through the papilla from buccal to lingual (Fig. 6.4).

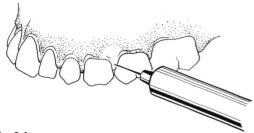

Fig. 6.4

4. Inject a small volume of solution.

6.6 INTRALIGAMENTARY INJECTION

The intraligamentary injection is given into the periodontal ligament using a syringe especially designed for the purpose. Several special syringes are available, one of which is illustrated in Fig. 6.5a. Intraligamentary injections can be given with a conventional needle and syringe, but the special syringes are preferred because they more easily produce the pressure that is required to inject into the periodontal ligament. As a safety feature, in case the pressure should break the glass cartridge containing the anaesthetic solution, the barrel of the special syringe completely encloses the cartridge.

A short or ultra-short (1 cm) 30-gauge needle is usually used, and the syringes accept standard 1.8 or 2.2 ml cartridges of anaesthetic solution. One complete pull of the trigger delivers 0.2 ml of solution. The pressure under which the solution is injected produces vasoconstriction in the periodontal ligament and, to minimize the risk of tissue damage due to vasoconstriction, it is recommended that solutions containing adrenaline are not used (Brännström et al 1982).

The intraligamentary injection has several advantages over conventional methods. It is usually considered to be less uncomfortable than either an inferior dental block injection, or a palatal injection, or a

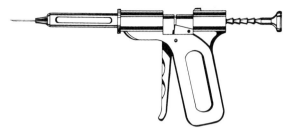

Fig. 6.5a An example of a special syringe for intraligamentary injection. A hard plastic cylinder within the metal barrel encloses the anaesthetic cartridge.

buccal infiltration in the premaxilla; analgesia is obtained very quickly and surrounding soft tissues are less affected. Since analgesia of mandibular teeth can be obtained, it is a useful injection when an inferior dental block injection must be avoided (e.g. for patients with bleeding disorders) or when a patient finds the block injection unacceptable.

The intraligamentary injection may be given to produce analgesia for restorative dentistry or for tooth extraction. However, after-pain has sometimes been reported following its use for restorative treatment. This pain is usually minor and subsides within a day or two, but can nevertheless be distressing to the patient.

Histological studies have, in the main, shown that tissue damage caused by intraligamentary injection is minor and resolves within a few weeks (Brännström et al 1982), but a more recent study reported considerable root resorption (Roahen & Marshall 1990). Concern has also been expressed about the possibility of forcing infected material from the gingival crevice into the periodontal tissues and (when the injection is given around a primary tooth) of the pressure damaging the developing permanent tooth, but there is no published evidence that these undesirable effects have actually occurred. However, because of these possible hazards and because of the lack of scientific knowledge concerning the mode of action of the injection, the American Dental Association (1983) recommended that the injection should be used only to supplement conventional methods when the latter fail, or in circumstances when an inferior dental block is impracticable or to be avoided.

6.7 JET INJECTION

It is possible to inject local analgesic solution into oral tissues without using a needle, by using an instrument that propels solution at high velocity through a fine orifice. Such instruments were first used to inject through skin, and later became available for oral use.

Early jet injection instruments were investigated by Stephens & Kramer (1964) and by Whitehead &

Technique: intraligamentary injection

1. Remove any calculus from the injection site, clean the gingival crevice with a rubber cup and apply hibitane or other disinfectant with a small cotton wool pledget. A surface anaesthetic paste or solution may be used instead of disinfectant solution, but the effectiveness of surface anaesthesia in this technique is uncertain.
2. Introduce the needle into the gingival crevice down the mesial or distal surface of the tooth, with the bevel of the needle facing away from the tooth (Fig. 6.5b).

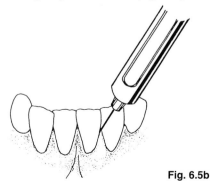

Fig. 6.5b

3. Squeeze a few drops of solution into the gingival crevice to anaesthetize tissues ahead of the needle.
4. Move the needle apically until it becomes wedged between the tooth and the alveolar crest—usually about 2 mm.
5. Squeeze the trigger slowly. If the needle is correctly placed there should be definite resistance to injection and the tissues around the needle should blanch. If resistance is not felt the needle is probably incorrectly placed, and injected solution will flow into the mouth.
   If a conventional syringe is being used, support the needle with fingers of the free hand before and during the injection.
6. Inject slowly. The injection of 0.2 ml should take at least 20 seconds.
7. For a posterior tooth, give an injection around each root.
8. Injections on the mesial and distal sides of a root may be given, but it is recommended that not more than 0.2 ml of solution is injected per root.
9. Despite the small volume of solution used, the cartridge must be discarded—it must not be used for another patient.

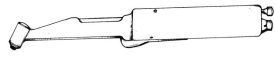

Fig. 6.6a   The Syrijet©

Young (1968). A more satisfactory instrument is the Syrijet© (Mizzy Inc., New York) (Fig. 6.6a). This incorporates a compressible spring which generates a pressure of 290 kPa (2000 pounds per square inch) when released, injecting solution through mucous membrane and into bone to a depth of about 1 cm. The instrument accepts standard 1.8 ml cartridges, and is calibrated to deliver volumes of between 0.05 and 0.2 ml.

Jet injection may be used not only to provide excellent soft tissue analgesia prior to needle injection but also to produce analgesia for dental procedures for which infiltrations are normally used. Blocks of the greater palatine, nasopalatine, long buccal and mental nerves also may be achieved, but not of the inferior dental, posterior superior alveolar or incisive nerves (Bennett & Monheim 1971).

Trauma to the mucosa is minimal when the injection is given into attached gingiva. The risk of causing slight injury is greater when injecting into loose tissue; if this is done at all not more than 0.5 ml should be injected.

Jet injection is particularly useful for producing soft tissue analgesia before those needle injections that normally tend to be painful even after application of topical analgesic; for example, infiltration in the maxillary incisor region, and palatal injections. It is also useful for producing analgesia for extraction of loose primary teeth, minor oral surgery, and the application of rubber dam clamps.

Unlike some previous jet injection instruments, the Syrijet©, when fired, is quiet and has little perceptible recoil. However, it is inevitable that patients should feel at least a sudden tap at the moment of injection, which may be considered slightly painful. Therefore, jet injection offers no advantage when a painless needle injection can be given (for example, to produce analgesia of maxillary premolars), except with a patient who has a phobia of needles. However, when using jet injection prior to potentially painful needle injection, it may be anticipated that the minor discomfort caused by the jet injection, followed by a painless needle injection, will be accepted better than a needle injection alone.

Despite its potentially useful applications in paediatric dentistry, the Syrijet© has not been widely used and is no longer available in the UK. No doubt its high cost has been a factor in limiting its use.

Technique: jet injection

1. Explain to the child that a "spray" is to be used "to make the gum (or tooth) go to sleep", and demonstrate by spraying a small volume into the air.
2. Clean the injection site with antiseptic solution and then dry with cotton wool or gauze.
3. Fit the detachable rubber sleeve, which is provided, over the nozzle of the instrument (except for palatal injections, when use of the rubber sleeve is not recommended).
4. Cock the spring mechanism.
5. Set the dosage.
   For analgesia of teeth: 0.1 ml for maxillary anterior teeth and premolars, 0.15 ml for mandibular incisors.
   For analgesia of soft tissues (prior to needle injection): 0.05 ml.
6. Grasp the instrument firmly, with the base of the index finger under the trigger.
7. Place the nozzle of the instrument at the injection site. Direct the long axis of the nozzle at right angles to the underlying bone, on attached gingiva near the root apex (Fig. 6.6b). Keep the tip of the nozzle in gentle contact with the tissue; do not exert pressure.
8. Warn the child that "the spray is coming".
9. Hold the instrument immobile while squeezing the trigger. If it is moved the jet may traumatize the mucosa; although this is slight and quickly resolves, it should be avoided if possible.

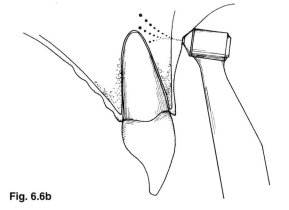

Fig. 6.6b

10. If analgesia of a tooth is found to be inadequate during cavity preparation, give a second jet injection or a needle injection. Soft tissue analgesia is always adequate to ensure a painless needle injection.

REFERENCES

Adatia A K 1976 Regional nerve block for maxillary permanent molars. British Dental Journal 140: 87–92

American Dental Association 1983 Status report: the periodontal ligament injection. Journal of American Dental Association 106: 224–242

Bennett C R, Monheim L M 1971 Production of local anaesthesia by jet injection. Oral Surgery, Oral Medicine, Oral Pathology 32: 526–530

Brännström M, Nordenvall K J, Hedström G 1982 Periodontal tissue changes after intraligamentary anaesthesia. Journal of Dentistry for Children 49: 417–423

Roahen J O, Marshall F J 1990 The effect of periodontal ligament injection on pulpal and periodontal tissue. Journal of Endodontics 16: 28–33

Stephens R R, Kramer I R H 1964 Intra-oral injections by high pressure jet. British Dental Journal 117: 465–481

Whitehead F I H, Young I 1968 An intra-oral jet injection instrument. British Dental Journal 125: 437–440

RECOMMENDED READING

Bennett C R 1984 Monheim's local anaesthesia and pain control in dental practice, 7th edn. Mosby, St Louis

Howe G L, Whitehead F I H 1990 Local anaesthesia in dentistry, 3rd edn. Butterworth Heinemann, Oxford

Mink J R, Spedding R H 1966 An injection procedure for the child dental patient. Dental Clinics of North America (July) 309–325

Roberts G J, Rosenbaum N L 1991 A colour atlas of dental analgesia and sedation. Wolfe, London, ch 3

Roberts D H, Sowray J H 1987 Local analgesia in dentistry, 3rd edn. Wright, Bristol

Wright G Z, Starkey P E, Gardner D E 1987 Child management in dentistry. IOP Publishing, Bristol, ch 11

7 Isolation of teeth

A prerequisite for successful restorative dentistry is that the teeth under treatment be adequately isolated from the cheeks, tongue and saliva. Isolation from cheeks and tongue is necessary to permit good access to, and a clear view of, the teeth; isolation from saliva is important because moisture affects the setting reactions and the physical properties of amalgam and other restorative materials, and reduces the adhesion of lining materials to dentine. In addition, contamination by salivary bacteria must be avoided when pulp treatment is being performed.

7.1 SALIVA EJECTORS

Common types of saliva ejector are illustrated in Figure 7.1. To ensure maximum patient comfort it is sensible to select the smallest saliva ejector that will suffice. For example, for treatment of a maxillary tooth, a flange-type ejector is not required and a simple tube ejector is preferable; for treatment of a mandibular tooth of a preschool child, the small rather than the large coil ejector should be selected.

7.2 COTTON WOOL ROLLS

Cotton wool rolls of various diameters are available, the smaller sizes being particularly useful for young children. Long cotton rolls are also available that can be bent so that they can be placed either buccal and lingual to mandibular teeth, or buccal to both maxillary and mandibular teeth; one type has a flexible central core that maintains the shape of the roll after it has been bent.

7.3 ABSORBENT PADS

Thin absorbent pads are available that may be used instead of, or in addition to, cotton wool rolls (Fig. 7.2). Usually they are used in the buccal sulcus, but they may also be placed lingually. They are particularly effective when treating maxillary molar teeth.

    The edges of the pads are sometimes rather rough;

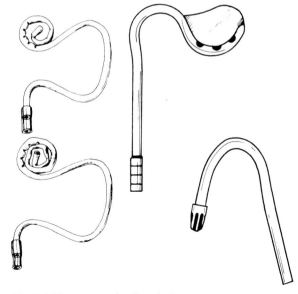

Fig. 7.1 Three types of saliva ejector.

79

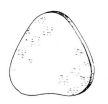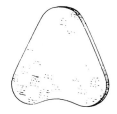

Fig. 7.2 Absorbent pads.

therefore they should be checked before use and trimmed with scissors if necessary. The pad must be placed properly, with its apex high in the sulcus posterior to the tooth to be treated. Since, when dry, it adheres to mucosa, it must be placed directly into the correct position; bending it slightly, so that it is convex on the cheek side, makes it easier to place. When treatment is complete the pad must be wetted thoroughly so that its removal does not damage the mucosa.

7.4 RUBBER DAM

The ideal method of isolating teeth is by the use of rubber dam. In the UK rubber dam is rarely used except to isolate teeth for endodontic treatment (Marshall & Page 1990); in some other countries (for example, the USA) it is more widely used.

Those who do not use rubber dam claim that it is awkward and time-consuming to place, that patients do not like it and that it is unnecessary. On the other hand, those who use it regularly claim that it is easy and quick to place, that patients accept it happily (assuming that they accept other dental procedures) and that, although not essential, its use is a great help in performing most restorative procedures (Elderton 1971, Curzon & Barenie 1973, Reuter 1983, Croll 1985, Reid et al 1991).

The principal advantages of using rubber dam are: 1. that it greatly improves visibility of posterior teeth by isolating them from the cheeks and tongue (this advantage is, of course, minimal at the front of the mouth where visibility is always good); 2. that it provides a dry operating field by isolating the teeth from saliva; 3. that it protects the patient from the risk of swallowing or inhaling instruments or materials that may inadvertently be dropped into the mouth; and 4. that it greatly reduces the microbial content of aerosols produced during operative dentistry. In addition, many patients appreciate the fact that tooth debris, water, dental materials and instruments are all excluded from their mouths. Rubber dam provides ideal working conditions which help the dentist to carry out treatment more efficiently and more safely.

7.4.1 Isolation of posterior teeth with rubber dam

The following materials and equipment are required:
Rubber dam material: Square 6 × 6 in or 5 × 5 in. 'Heavy' or 'extra heavy' thickness
Rubber dam frame: Young
Rubber dam punch: Ash or Ainsworth
Wedges and floss
Clamp forceps: Stokes
Clamps: The large variety of clamps available and the wide range of numbers by which they are identified often causes confusion. In an attempt to simplify the selection of clamps, a set has been introduced which is identified by letters ranging from A to K, with the addition of the letter 'W' to denote a wingless clamp (Ash Instruments, Dentsply). The recommended clamps are illustrated in Figure 7.3.

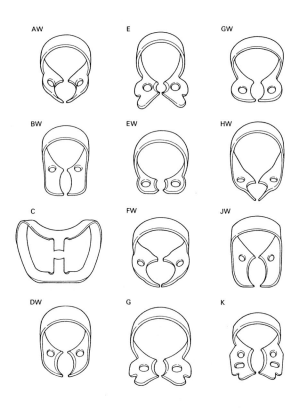

Fig. 7.3 The Ash Dentsply set of rubber dam clamps (reproduced by kind permission of Professor R. J. Elderton).

Technique: rubber dam application

Procedure	Method	Rationale	Notes
1. Prepare the dam	Mark a horizontal line across the middle of a square of rubber dam material and mark the line about 5 cm from the right border. Punch holes (the largest hole on the punch) about 5 mm apart (Fig. 7.4a). **Method 1**—Slit dam. With scissors, join holes 1, 2 and 3. The prepared dam now has a slit and a hole (Fig. 7.4b). **Method 2**—Separate holes. Punch a hole overlapping hole 1, to produce a larger hole. The prepared dam now has one large hole and three smaller ones (Fig. 7.4d).	Enlarging the hole makes it easier to pass the dam over the clamp at stage 8.	Methods 1 and 2 both provide excellent isolation of teeth from cheeks and tongue. Saliva control is less efficient with Method 1, but this is compensated by the easier application of the slit dam over the clamp (at stage 8), and by the absence of rubber interdentally when preparing deep Class II cavities. In addition, the slit technique is useful when preparing a tooth for a crown (Croll 1985). A rubber dam sheet prepared as shown in Fig. 7.4a or 7.4b can be used in any quadrant simply by turning it over from right to left, or from bottom to top (e.g. as in Fig. 7.4c for upper left quadrant). Chairside time can be saved if prepared sheets are always available. Use of a polythene or thin cardboard template ensures standard positioning of the holes.

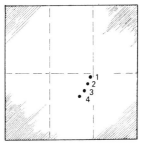

Fig. 7.4a

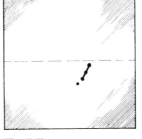

Fig. 7.4b

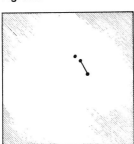

Fig. 7.4c

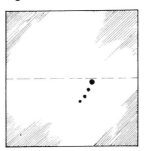

Fig. 7.4d

Procedure	Method	Rationale	Notes
	Method 3—One hole only. Punch one hole only and enlarge it by overlapping with a second hole.		Method 3 is sometimes suitable when only the clamped tooth is to be treated (see stage 3 below).
2. Attach the dam to the frame	Place the dam on a flat surface and position it according to the quadrant to be worked on (e.g. as in Fig. 7.4b or Fig. 7.4d for the lower left quadrant). Place the frame over the dam, with its transverse part towards the lower edge of the dam and with its convexity upwards (Fig. 7.4e).		

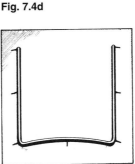

Fig. 7.4e

Procedure	Method	Rationale	Notes
	Attach the dam to the pegs at the corners of the frame (not to the other pegs). Do not stretch the dam tight between the pegs; keep it as loose as possible.	Attaching the dam loosely at this stage allows it to be stretched easily into the mouth when applying it at stage 8.	An alternative method is to attach the frame to the dam after the dam has been placed on the teeth.

Technique: rubber dam application (contd)

Procedure	Method	Rationale	Notes
3. Decide which tooth to clamp	Clamp primary second molars or permanent first molars only (premolars or second molars may be chosen in older patients). The decision on which tooth to clamp depends on the treatment to be done:	The morphology of primary second molars and permanent first molars enables clamps to be applied easily and securely.	

Restoration	Tooth to clamp
Occlusal primary first or second molar	primary second molar
Class II primary first molar	primary second molar
Class II primary second molar	permanent first molar
Occlusal permanent first molar	permanent first molar
Class II permanent first molar	permanent first molar

For Class II restorations it is preferable to clamp the tooth distal to the one being restored, as the clamp interferes with the placement of most types of matrix band.

It would be preferable to clamp a permanent second molar, but this is only present and erupted sufficiently in older children.

Procedure	Method	Rationale	Notes
4. Select a clamp	Recommended first choice clamps are as follows:		

	Ash* set	Other commonly-used clamps
Permanent molars		
partially erupted	AW†, FW, HW	Ivory 8A, 14A
fully erupted	BW, K	Ivory 3, 7, 14
Primary second molars	DW	Ivory 8A, 12A, 13A
Premolars	E/EW, G/GW	Ivory 2/2A
Permanent incisors & canines	C, E/EW	Ivory 6, 9

* Ash Dentsply
† W denotes a wingless clamp

Procedure	Method	Rationale	Notes
5. Introduce to the child	Explain that the dam is "a sort of raincoat". "It helps me to clean your teeth better and more quickly."	If good rapport exists between child and dentist, the child will want to help.	The form of introduction will, of course, depend on the age of the child.
6. Tie a length of floss to the clamp	Attach a length of floss (about 40 cm) to the arch of the clamp and slide it down the side that will be on the buccal of the tooth. The child's help may be enlisted in holding the clamp while the floss is is attached. The clamp may be described as the "clip" or "button" that will hold the "raincoat".	The floss will be held while placing the clamp on the tooth, as a precaution in case it should spring off the tooth. Attaching to the buccal side of the clamp ensures that it will not be in the way later on. It is desirable to allow the child to become familiar with an object that is to be placed in his/her mouth.	Although attachment of floss as shown in Fig. 7.4f is satisfactory to hold a clamp until it is firmly seated on the tooth, the method described by Reuter (1983), illustrated in Fig. 7.4g, can be recommended because it also secures the clamp should it fracture (though this is a very rare occurrence).
7. Place the clamp	Use clamp forceps to take the clamp to the tooth, holding the floss in your left hand (Fig. 7.4f). Place the clamp carefully just away from the gingival margin, releasing	With care, the clamp can be placed without causing discomfort to the child, even when a local analgesic has not been used. Ideally, local analgesia	In other methods of applying rubber dam, the dam is placed on the teeth first, or the dam is supported on a winged clamp which is then placed on the tooth.

Technique: rubber dam application *(contd)*

Procedure	Method	Rationale	Notes
	the forceps gradually. Still holding on to the floss with one hand, check the stability of the clamp with your fingers, making sure that it cannot be pulled off the tooth.	will have been administered for the planned restorative treatment, but pain could still be caused on the buccal gingival margin of a lower molar (innervated by the long buccal nerve), or on the palatal gingival margin of an upper tooth. Topical analgesia could be used but should not be necessary.	The advantage of placing the clamp first is that this can be done more easily, and therefore with less risk of causing discomfort, because there is a clear view of the tooth.

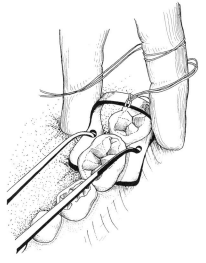

Fig. 7.4f

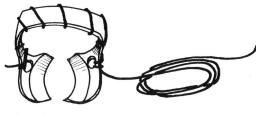

Fig. 7.4g

Procedure	Method	Rationale	Notes
	Ask the child to close slowly until the teeth gently touch the clamp.	It is important for the child to accept this limitation of mouth closure before proceeding to the next stage.	
8. Apply the dam	Sit (or stand) behind the patient's head and bring the dam, attached to the frame and in the correct position, to the mouth. Place the index fingers of both hands at the back of the slit, or of the most distal hole in the dam, and open it up widely. Holding the dam in this way, extend into the mouth with the index fingers, reaching for the clamp. When the arch of the clamp can be seen through the opening in the dam, carry the dam over and behind it (Fig. 7.4h). Then slide the dam under the wings of the clamp.		This procedure can be carried out while facing the patient, but it is more difficult, especially when applying dam to maxillary teeth.

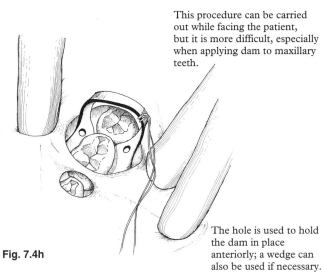

Fig. 7.4h

In *method 1*, slip the front end of the slit over one of the two teeth immediately mesial to the clamped tooth, and the hole over the next tooth (Figs 7.4i, j, k).

The hole is used to hold the dam in place anteriorly; a wedge can also be used if necessary.

In *method 2*, slide each hole in the dam over the appropriate tooth.

Technique: rubber dam application (*contd*)

Procedure	Method	Rationale	Notes
	Use a high-volume aspirator to remove water and debris during cavity preparation. Place a small saliva ejector under the dam if necessary, placing its tip in the lingual sulcus near the tooth to be treated. To remove the dam, remove the clamp first; the dam can then easily be lifted off.	The smallest possible saliva ejector should be used, to give the patient the greatest comfort and freedom of tongue movement. A flanged type is not required because the tongue is retracted by the dam.	A saliva ejector may not be required, especially when treating maxillary teeth; the patient can swallow when necessary with the dam in place.

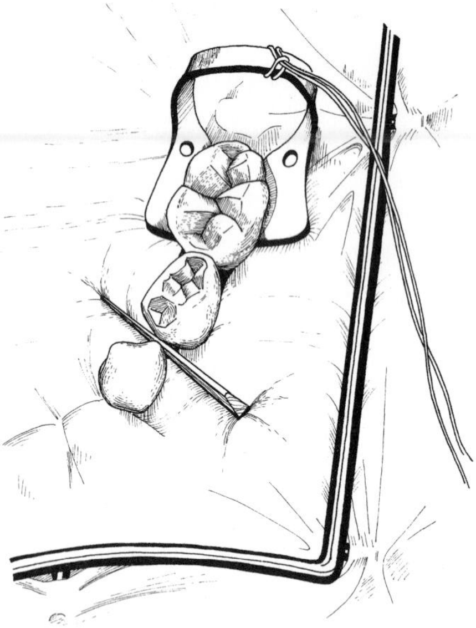

Fig. 7.4i 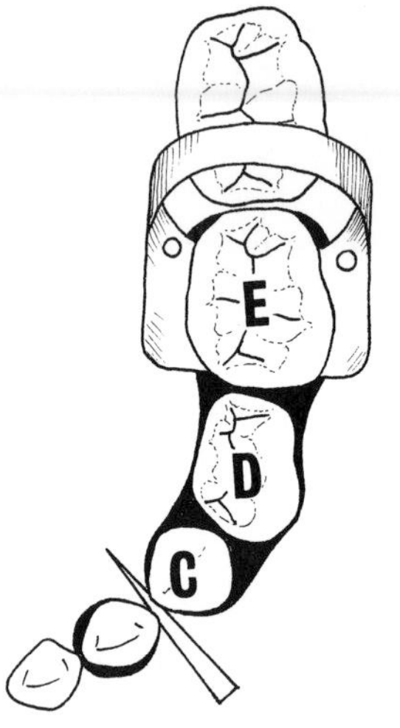   Fig. 7.4j 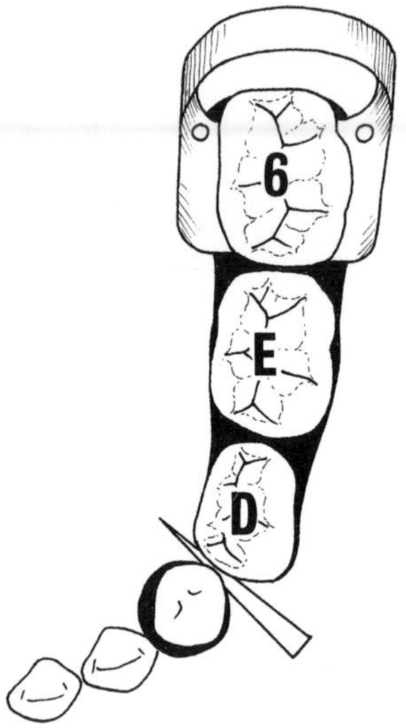   Fig. 7.4k

7.4.2 Isolation of the anterior teeth with rubber dam

Anterior teeth may be isolated with rubber dam to control saliva, which adversely affects the setting re-actions of restorative materials and which is a source of bacterial contamination during endodontic treatment, and to provide an effective barrier during endodontic treatment should a reamer or other small instrument be dropped accidentally into the mouth.

To isolate several anterior teeth, a premolar on one or both sides of the mouth may be clamped. However, if only one tooth is to be treated, it is often preferable to isolate that tooth only and secure the dam either with a floss ligature or with an incisor clamp. Some incisor clamps have large wings and it is therefore necessary either to place the dam on the tooth and then fit the clamp over it, or to support the dam on the wings of the clamp before placing it on the tooth.

REFERENCES

Croll T P 1985 Alternative methods for the use of the rubber dam. Quintessence International 16: 387–392

Curzon M E J, Barenie J T 1973 A simplified rubber dam technique for children's dentistry. British Dental Journal 135: 532–536

Elderton R J 1971 A modern approach to the use of rubber dam. Dental Practitioner 21: 187–193, 226–232, 267–273

Marshall K, Page J 1990 The use of rubber dam in the UK. A survey. British Dental Journal 169: 286–291

Reid J S, Callis P D, Patterson C J W 1991 Rubber dam in clinical practice. Quintessence, Chicago

Reuter J E 1983 The isolation of teeth and the protection of the patient during endodontic treatment. International Endodontic Journal 16: 173–181

RECOMMENDED READING

Duggal M S, Curzon M E J, Fayle S A, Pollard M A, Robertson A J 1995 Restorative techniques in paediatric dentistry. Martin Dunitz, London, ch 3

8 Treatment of carious primary teeth

During the last 20 years, a marked decrease in the prevalence of dental caries in children has been noted in the UK and many other countries. For example, surveys of child dental health in the UK in 1973, 1983 and 1993 have shown that the proportion of 5-year-old children in England and Wales with caries experience in primary teeth fell from 71% in 1973 to 48% in 1983 and to 43% in 1993 (O'Brien 1994a). Despite this reduction, the 1993 survey showed that, by the age of 9 years, 47% of children in England and 60% in Scotland, Wales and Northern Ireland had untreated caries in primary teeth (O'Brien 1994b). In addition to regional variations in caries experience there are considerable social class differences, children from lower social class families having higher caries experience (Bradnock et al 1984, O'Brien 1994c).

The principal reasons for restoring carious primary teeth are:

1. To eradicate disease and restore health. Disease of primary teeth should no more be ignored than disease of permanent teeth or, indeed, disease of any other part of the body.
2. To give the child the simplest form of treatment. When caries is treated early, a minimal restoration suffices; if, however, it is allowed to progress, treatment is likely to be more complex (e.g. pulpotomy) or more unpleasant (e.g. extraction).
3. To prevent the child suffering pain. Although untreated caries does not always cause pain, it is more likely to do so as it nears the pulp and, especially, if a pulpal or periradicular abscess is formed.
4. To avoid the infection that follows carious exposure of the pulp. Exposure of the pulp permits oral bacteria to gain access to the pulp chamber, root canals and periradicular tissues.
5. To preserve space that is required for the eruption of permanent teeth. However, retention of primary teeth until their normal exfoliation does not guarantee that the permanent teeth will erupt in good alignment.
6. To ensure comfortable and efficient mastication. Even the little mastication required by a soft diet can be painful and difficult if teeth are unhealthy.

During the primary dentition period, restoration of carious teeth is always desirable because the anterior teeth are important for aesthetic reasons and the posterior teeth are important for mastication and space maintenance. After the primary incisors are shed, space maintenance is the principal function of primary teeth; their function in mastication is diminished because permanent first molars are present. The benefit of restoring carious primary molars depends on the importance of maintaining space, and this varies greatly in different dentitions (Ch. 17).

8.1 PRINCIPLES OF CAVITY PREPARATION

The principles governing cavity preparation in primary teeth are similar to those that are applied in the treatment of permanent teeth. These may be summarized as follows:

1. The cavity outline should include the carious lesion and contiguous caries-susceptible pits and fissures. This principle should be followed with discretion; it is most important to avoid unnecessary destruction of sound tissue.
2. Whenever possible, but not when it necessitates excessive destruction of tooth substance, cavity margins should be placed where they are accessible to cleaning with a toothbrush and where they are least exposed to occlusal forces.
3. The cavity shape should be designed to provide the restoration with good resistance to masticatory forces and adequate retention against dislodgement.

Cavity preparations in primary teeth differ principally in their size and depth, because primary teeth have relatively thin enamel (about 1 mm thick) and relatively large pulps.

The techniques used throughout this century for cavity preparation in permanent and primary teeth have been based on principles laid down by Black in 1908, which involve preparing a cavity of standard shape for carious lesions on each tooth surface, the size and shape of a restoration thus being determined by the standard cavity design rather than by the extent of the carious lesion. During recent years, with the introduction of improved restorative materials and the adoption of a more preventive philosophy towards dental treatment, modifications in cavity preparation have been advocated. The emphasis now is first on removing the caries and then on designing a suitable cavity to retain the restoration (Elderton 1990, Kidd & Smith 1990).

The prime objective of this new approach is to conserve tooth structure, because studies have suggested that the survival time of amalgam restorations in permanent teeth is only 5–10 years (Elderton 1983), and each time a restoration is replaced more tooth substance is destroyed and the tooth becomes progressively weaker. However, the need for an ultra-conservative approach with primary teeth is less strong because the teeth exfoliate before multiple replacement of restorations is possible. Clearly it is undesirable to destroy more tooth substance than is necessary, but conservative versions of Black-type cavities, which might be considered unnecessarily destructive for permanent teeth, would be acceptable for primary teeth.

Elderton (1990) and Kidd & Smith (1990) did not consider primary teeth in their discussion of cavity preparation, but the general approach they present is adopted in the following description of cavity preparation in primary teeth. The procedures involved in 'modern' cavity preparation differ from those universally adopted in the past for preparation of Black-type cavities. The principal differences are as follows:

Black-type	'Modern'
1. Gain access (for cavity preparation, not necessarily to the caries).	1. Gain access to the caries.
2. Prepare the cavity—to the standard outline and shape.	2. Remove the caries.
	3. Plan the final cavity outline and shape.
3. Remove any remaining caries.	4. Complete the cavity preparation.

8.2 AMALGAM RESTORATIONS

Amalgam has long been the material of choice for restoring primary and permanent posterior teeth. Composite resin and glass-ionomer cement have been gaining popularity in recent years but amalgam is still the material most commonly used.

The toxicity of mercury has given rise to concern that amalgam restorations may present a health hazard to patients and that the use of amalgam contributes to environmental mercury pollution. However, the available evidence indicates that, although a very small minority of patients appears to suffer adverse reactions, amalgam cannot be considered a health hazard, and that modern methods of using and disposing of amalgam ensure adequate control of environmental pollution (Eley & Cox 1993).

The physical properties of modern dental amalgams are adequate for all but very large restorations, and the quality of the final restoration is less sensitive to minor deficiencies in clinical technique and less affected by moisture than are composite resin or glass-ionomer cement. The techniques involved in the use of amalgam are less demanding than with composite resin or glass-ionomer, and it is easier and quicker to condense firmly into prepared cavities. Therefore it is usually the restorative material of choice for posterior teeth, and is used for occlusal (Class I), approximal (Class II) and buccal or lingual (Class V) restorations.

Technique: occlusal (Class I) amalgam restoration

Procedure	Method	Rationale	Notes

1. Gain access to the caries	Recommended burs:
	for high-speed handpiece—
	    pear-shaped diamond 525
	    pear-shaped tungsten carbide 330
	for slow-speed handpiece—
	    round steel or tungsten carbide 1/2 or 1.
		A small bur conserves tooth substance.	Although a high-speed handpiece is generally preferred for restorative dentistry, young children may be alarmed by the noise and water spray; a slow-speed handpiece may therefore be used, at least initially. Miniature-head handpieces have obvious advantages in small mouths. The depth of penetration is most easily judged when using the pear-shaped diamond because its head is 1.5 mm long.

	Penetrate the occlusal surface within the carious area to a depth of about 1.5 mm (i.e. just into dentine) (Fig. 8.1a). The depth may be judged against the bur.	The enamel is penetrated most easily through the soft carious area.	
2. Remove the caries	Keeping the bur at the established depth, extend the cavity laterally from the centre of the lesion to remove caries from the enamel–dentine junction and walls of the cavity, until the periphery of the cavity is assessed by gentle probing to be caries-free.	Removing peripheral caries establishes the minimal lateral extension of the cavity.	

Fig. 8.1a

	Then, use a sharp excavator (Fig. 8.1b) or medium-sized round bur in a slow-speed handpiece (Fig. 8.1c) to remove caries from the floor of the cavity.	Excavators or burs are equally effective in removing caries.	After caries removal, the cavity floor may be irregular in depth, but a flat or slightly rounded floor will later be re-established by lining material.
	If a bur is chosen, use it at slow speed and with light pressure. If enamel at the cavity walls becomes undermined (Fig. 8.1d), it must be taken back to sound dentine with a fissure bur (Fig. 8.1e) or a chisel. If the cavity becomes very deep, proceed very gently with an excavator and assess the need for pulp capping or other pulp treatment (Ch. 9).	Excessive bur speed or pressure might endanger the pulp. Undermined enamel would probably fracture and create a defect at the margin of the restoration.	

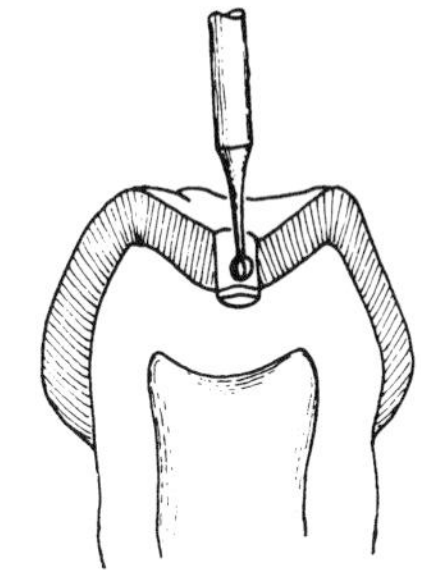

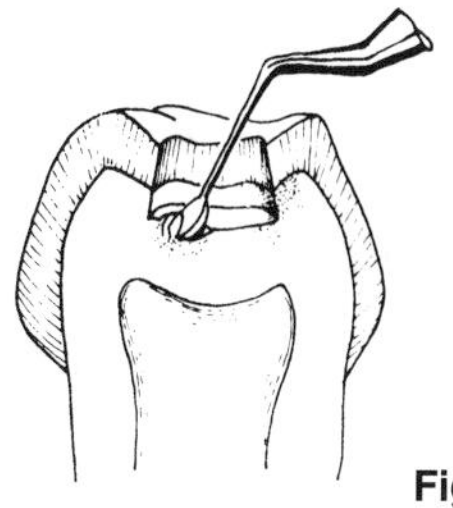

Fig. 8.1b

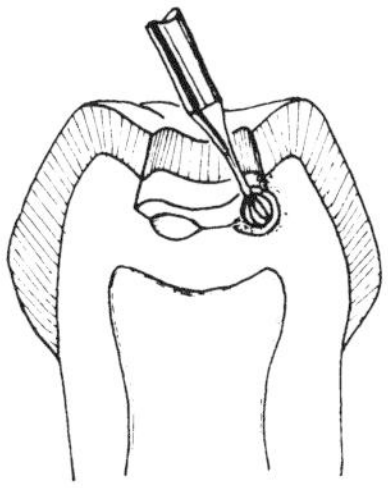

Fig. 8.1c

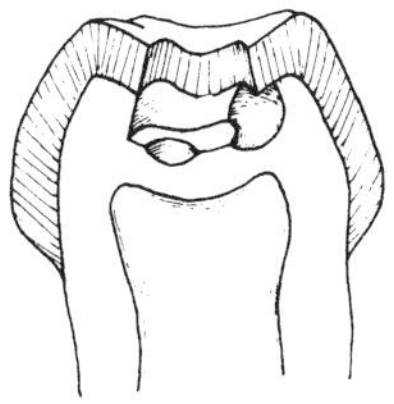

Fig. 8.1d

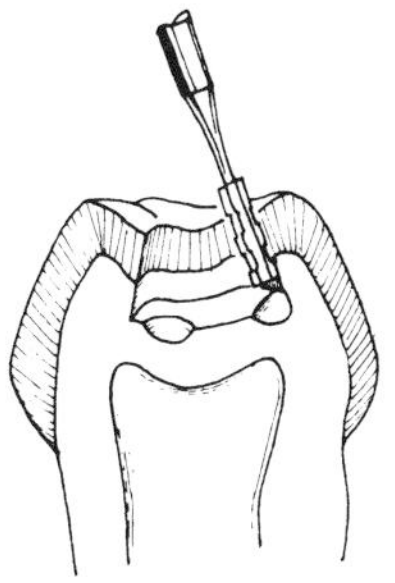

Fig. 8.1e

Technique: occlusal (Class I) amalgam restoration *(contd)*

Procedure	Method	Rationale	Notes
3. Plan the final cavity outline and shape	Consider the state of the remaining fissures and decide whether to extend the cavity into them. Make a final decision regarding the restorative material to be used. Consider whether the cavity needs further preparation to provide retention for the restoration.	The wish to eradicate fissures that appear deep and caries-susceptible must be balanced by the desire to preserve tooth substance. If the cavity is small and adjacent fissures sound, a sealant restoration (Ch. 10) may be preferred to amalgam. Retention of amalgam restorations is dependent entirely on the retentive features of the cavity. (Glass-ionomer adheres to enamel and dentine, and composite resin to acid-etched enamel.)	Black's principle of 'extension for prevention' is no longer strictly adhered to, but applied with discretion.

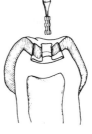

Fig. 8.1f

4. Complete the cavity preparation	(Assuming that it is decided to extend the cavity and that amalgam is the chosen restorative material.) If using a high-speed handpiece, continue with the same bur. If using slow-speed, change to a 1/2 or 1 flat fissure bur (Fig. 8.1f). Maintain the bur at the established cavity depth. Hold the pear-shaped bur parallel to the long axis of the tooth, or the straight bur at a slight angle.	The final cavity should have a flat or slightly concave floor, and walls diverging from the occlusal to provide retention for the restoration.	Pear-shaped burs produce a slightly concave floor and rounded cavity wall angles, which help to ensure that no voids remain when condensing the amalgam.
	In maxillary second molars and mandibular first molars, do not extend across the occlusal oblique ridges unless they are undermined by caries (Fig. 8.1g). If a fissure extends near to the mesial or distal marginal ridge, do not undercut the mesial or distal wall.	The oblique ridges are not caries-susceptible areas and should therefore be conserved if possible. Undercutting a wall near a marginal ridge would weaken the ridge and risk subsequent fracture.	
5. Wash, dry and assess the cavity preparation	Wash the cavity with water (Fig. 8.1h) and dry with compressed air. Using a probe, confirm that caries has been removed and that the cavity shape is satisfactory (Fig. 8.1i).		

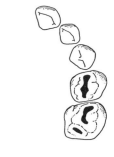

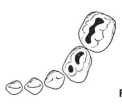

Fig. 8.1g

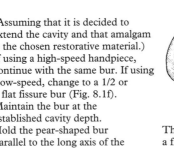

Fig. 8.1 h

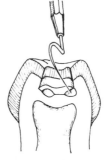

Fig. 8.1i

Technique: occlusal (Class I) amalgam restoration *(contd)*

Procedure	Method	Rationale	Notes
6. Line the cavity (if necessary)	No lining is required in minimal depth cavities (i.e. just into dentine).	Clinical experience has shown no undesirable after-effects when shallow cavities in primary teeth are not lined.	

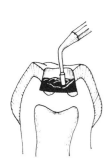

Fig. 8.1j

Procedure	Method	Rationale	Notes
	In deeper cavities apply a quick-setting calcium hydroxide lining to the dried dentine on the floor of the cavity (Fig. 8.1j). After the material has set, remove any excess from the enamel walls of the cavity with an excavator.	Calcium hydroxide is a thermal insulator protecting the pulp. Adjacent to pulp, it stimulates the formation of secondary dentine.	Various calcium hydroxide preparations are available. After lining, copal resin varnish may be applied to the walls, and cavo-surface margin, to reduce marginal leakage (Silva et al 1985). Two layers of varnish are recommended, each blown dry.
7. Condense amalgam into the cavity	Mix amalgam according to the manufacturer's instructions and carry it to the cavity in an amalgam carrier. Eject no more than about one-third of the amount required to fill the cavity, and condense it firmly with an amalgam plugger into the deepest parts of the cavity (Fig. 8.1k). Add further similar-sized increments and condense each with overlapping strokes covering the entire surface, until the cavity is overfilled by about 1 mm (Fig. 8.1m). Condense the overfilled amalgam over the margin of the cavity.	Adding amalgam in small increments ensures efficient condensation. Overlapping strokes help to ensure good condensation. Overfilling allows carving to the original tooth contour and permits removal of the mercury-rich surface layer of amalgam. Strong amalgam at the cavity margins is essential to prevent breakdown and leakage.	A small plugger should be used; pluggers suitable for permanent teeth are often too large. Mechanical condensers are available that ensure consistently efficient condensation, but many children find the vibration unpleasant. The strength of amalgam is markedly reduced when its mercury content exceeds 55% (Nadal et al 1961).

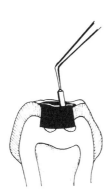

Fig. 8.1k   Fig. 8.1m

Technique: occlusal (Class I) amalgam restoration *(contd)*

Procedure	Method	Rationale	Notes
8. Carve the amalgam	With a carver (e.g. Ward's or Hollenbach), remove excess amalgam from the margin of the restoration by sweeping the instrument along the margin, supporting it on the adjacent enamel (Fig. 8.1n). Produce a contour similar to that of the original tooth surface, but do not attempt to reproduce deep fissures.	Supporting the carver on enamel prevents over-carving, which would leave a thin, weak edge of amalgam at the margin.	 **Fig. 8.1n**
9. Lightly burnish the amalgam margin	Run a burnisher lightly over the margin of the amalgam, again supporting the instrument on the adjacent enamel (Fig. 8.1p).	Light burnishing of the margin is beneficial but heavy burnishing would tend to bring mercury into the surface amalgam, thus weakening it.	Light burnishing improves the marginal adaptation and reduces corrosion of amalgam restorations (Kato & Fusayama 1968, Svare & Chan 1972, Lavadino et al 1987).
10. Smooth the restoration	Remove any loose particles with a cotton wool pledget (Fig. 8.1q) and lightly burnish the surface of the restoration.	 **Fig. 8.1p**	 **Fig. 8.1q**
11. Check the occlusion	Remove the rubber dam (if used) and ask the patient to "tap the teeth together gently on the back teeth". Check the surface for any shiny 'high' spots; if present, remove them with the carver and re-check the occlusion.		Premature contacts could cause fracture of the restoration.
12. Finish the restoration	Delay finishing for at least 24 hours. Pass a probe carefully around the entire margin of the restoration to detect any edges that may exist. Pass the probe alternately from amalgam to enamel and from enamel to amalgam, to detect either amalgam or enamel edges. Check also for marginal voids, when both enamel and amalgam edges would be detected. Use a pear-shaped finishing bur to remove amalgam or small enamel edges (Fig. 8.1r). Move the bur along the margin, resting on adjacent enamel. Use the same bur, or a stone, to make minor modifications to the surface contour of the restoration, if necessary.	Amalgam does not attain its final hardness until about 24 hours after mixing. The detection and removal of edges is important because they encourage the accumulation of plaque and recurrence of caries at the margin.	An amalgam edge indicates that carving was inadequate. An enamel edge indicates that the cavity was under-filled or that carving was excessive. A marginal void suggests that the amalgam was underpacked or poorly condensed. Gross enamel edges or marginal voids cannot be corrected, except by replacement of the restoration. If carving and burnishing were carried out efficiently at the previous visit, little additional finishing will be required. Various types of abrasive stone are available that may be used for trimming and polishing amalgam.

Technique: occlusal (Class I) amalgam restoration *(contd)*

Procedure	Method	Rationale	Notes

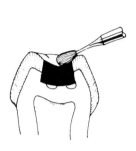

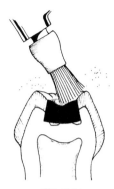

Fig. 8.1r   **Fig. 8.1s**

	Finally, polish the restoration using a rubber cup or bristle brush mounted in a slow-speed handpiece (Fig. 8.1s). Use a slurry of pumice and water or a proprietary prophylaxis paste. For a final polish a slurry of zinc oxide powder in water or alcohol may be used.	Polishing reduces surface corrosion and tarnish, and produces a smooth surface that discourages the retention of food debris and is easy to clean.	A well-finished and burnished amalgam restoration should need hardly any polishing.

Technique: approximal surface (Class II) amalgam restoration

Procedure	Method	Rationale	Notes
1. Gain access to the caries	Use a small round or pear-shaped bur (see p. 89) to penetrate the occlusal surface just inside the marginal ridge (Fig. 8.2a), to reach the caries.		If the adjacent tooth is not present direct access can be made through the approximal surface.
2. Remove the caries	With the same bur, or with a small fissure bur, gradually widen the cavity bucco-lingually and extend it gingivally until firm dentine is reached. On the buccal and lingual walls, slant the bur to make the walls converge slightly towards the occlusal surface (Fig. 8.2b). With a sharp excavator or medium-sized round bur in a slow-speed handpiece remove caries first from the walls and gingival floor of the cavity; then, very carefully with an excavator, remove deeper caries on the axial wall. If the cavity becomes very deep, assess whether pulp capping or other pulp treatment will be required (Ch. 9).	Convergent walls will provide resistance against vertical displacement of the restoration.	Ideally the approximal enamel wall remains intact at this stage, and protects the adjacent tooth from damage by burs. However, this sliver of enamel often breaks down and special care must then be taken not to damage the adjacent tooth.

Fig. 8.2a   **Fig. 8.2b**

Technique: approximal surface (Class II) amalgam restoration *(contd)*

Procedure	Method	Rationale	Notes
3. Plan the final cavity outline and shape	Make a final decision regarding the restorative material to be used.	If the cavity is small, glass-ionomer cement may be preferred to amalgam. If the cavity is large bucco-lingually, a stainless steel crown would be the restoration of choice.	The final cavity outline and shape will be influenced by the type of restorative material chosen.
	Consider the cavity design necessary to retain the restoration. For an amalgam restoration prepare an occlusal cavity to link up with the approximal part.	Resistance against horizontal displacement of approximal surface amalgam restorations in primary teeth must be provided by an occlusal 'lock'. In permanent teeth an occlusal 'lock' may not be required because retention grooves may be placed at the junctions of the axial-lingual and axial-buccal walls, but similar grooves placed in primary teeth would endanger the pulp.	An occlusal extension may not be necessary for a glass-ionomer restoration because of the adhesive properties of the material.
	Decide on the optimal final position of the gingival floor and of the buccal and lingual walls of the cavity.	In the past it was considered that the gingival floor should be placed just subgingivally and the margins of the buccal and lingual walls just into the embrasures (so that these margins of the restoration should be accessible to toothbrush bristles). It is now considered that there is no benefit in placing the gingival margin subgingivally and that more than minimal widening of the cavity buccally or lingually is not justified.	The position of the cavity margin is primarily dictated by the extent of the carious lesion. When the gingival floor must be extended subgingivally problems arise because the cervical constriction characteristic of primary molars results in a gingival floor that is very narrow mesio-distally (Fig. 8.2c). If the width is increased the pulp becomes endangered, especially at the buccal and lingual aspects of the axial wall.

Fig. 8.2c

| 4. Complete the cavity | Prepare the occlusal cavity as described on page 90. If the occlusal fissure is sound, extend the cavity only a few millimetres from the approximal cavity and widen it slightly at its furthest point (Fig. 8.2d). If the fissure is carious extend the cavity into it (Fig. 8.2e). | | |

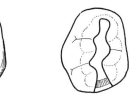

Fig. 8.2d   **Fig. 8.2e**   **Fig 8.2f**

| | Bevel the central part of the junction of occlusal floor and axial wall, removing about 1 mm of dentine (Fig. 8.2f). | Deepening the cavity increases the strength of the restoration at a point of potential weakness. The deepening must be restricted to the central part because extending laterally might endanger pulp horns. | A common cause of failure of Class II amalgam restorations in primary molars is fracture at the junction of the occlusal and approximal parts. |

Technique: approximal surface (Class II) amalgam restoration *(contd)*

Procedure	Method	Rationale	Notes
	If it has been decided to widen the approximal part of the cavity slightly so that the buccal and lingual margins of the restoration will be accessible to toothbrushing, this should be done with a fissure or pear-shaped bur, keeping the walls slightly convergent towards the occlusal surface. If the approximal enamel wall is still intact, break it away now by gently twisting or levering against the wall with an excavator or chisel (Fig. 8.2g). Plane the margin of the cavity with a chisel or gingival margin trimmer to remove any unsupported enamel. Ensure that the buccal and lingual walls of the approximal part of the cavity form angles of about 90° with the enamel surface (Fig. 8.2h).	A cavo–surface angle of 90° ensures that there are no unsupported enamel prisms at the margin and that the amalgam margin will be strong. The cavo–surface angle must not exceed 110° because this would leave a weak amalgam margin (Fig. 8.2i).	
	The gingival floor should be flat, but the margin need not be bevelled.	Enamel prisms in the cervical region of primary molars slope occlusally from the enamel–dentine junction; therefore none are left unsupported at the gingival margin of an approximal cavity (Fig. 8.2j).	In permanent teeth, enamel prisms slope cervically from the enamel–dentine junction; therefore it is normal practice to bevel the gingival margin (Fig. 8.2k).
	Ensure that the junctions of the gingival floor with the buccal and lingual walls are rounded (this will have been achieved if a pear-shaped bur was used for preparing the cavity—Fig. 8.2m).	Avoidance of sharp corners in the cavity helps to ensure that no voids remain when condensing amalgam into the cavity.	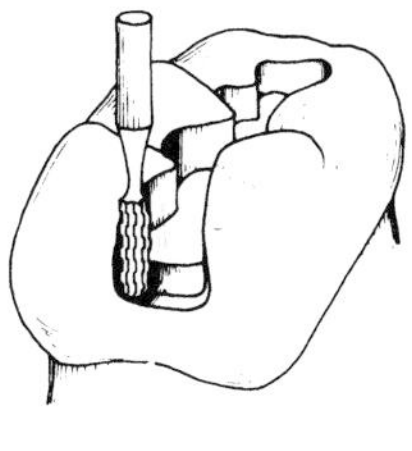

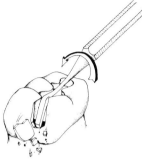

Fig. 8.2g

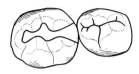

Fig. 8.2h

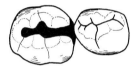

Fig. 8.2i

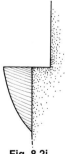

Fig. 8.2j

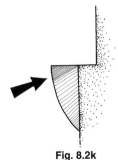

Fig. 8.2k

Fig. 8.2m

Technique: approximal surface (Class II) amalgam restoration *(contd)*

Procedure	Method	Rationale	Notes
5. Wash, dry and assess the cavity preparation 6. Line the cavity	See 'occlusal (Class I) amalgam restoration', pages 90–91.		
7. Fit a matrix	Adjust the diameter of the matrix band to approximately the size of the tooth crown. Slide the band down the crown until it passes the gingival margin of the cavity, then tighten the band firmly. Place a wedge either from the buccal or lingual side to press against the band at the gingival margin of the cavity, ensuring that the wedge does not push the band into the cavity.	If the band is too large, gingiva may be trapped between it and the tooth when the band is tightened; this might prevent close adaptation of the band and cause gingival bleeding, and may also be painful if the gingiva is not anaesthetized. Since primary molars have marked constrictions at their cervical margins, wedging is desirable to prevent amalgam from being pushed past the gingival floor of the cavity.	Several types of matrix band holder are available.
8. Condense amalgam into the cavity	See 'occlusal Class I amalgam restoration', page 91. Place the first small increment into the floor of the approximal part of the cavity and condense it firmly into the corners (Fig. 8.2n). Build up with several additional increments and overfill by about 1 mm. Pay particular attention to condensing the area next to the matrix band that will form the marginal ridge of the restoration (Fig. 8.2p).	It is important to obtain close adaptation of amalgam to the cervical margin of the cavity. Inadequate condensation of the amalgam close to the matrix band may result in its fracture when the band is removed.	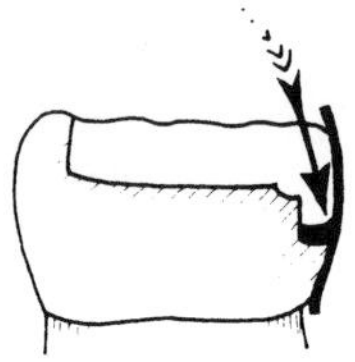 **Fig. 8.2n** 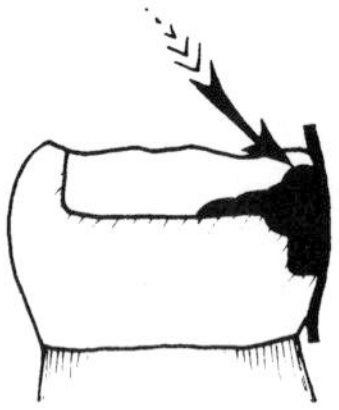 **Fig. 8.2p**
9. Carve the amalgam	Establish the level of the marginal ridge by directing the tip of a probe against the matrix band at the desired level, and moving the probe buccally and lingually to remove excess amalgam. Start carving with the matrix band in place. Remove the wedge, loosen the matrix band and carefully remove it. Trim excess amalgam from the buccal and lingual margins of the approximal part with a sharp carver, supporting the instrument on the adjacent enamel. Complete carving as described on page 92.	Delaying the removal of the matrix band allows the amalgam to harden; this reduces the risk of fracture when the band is removed.	
10. Lightly burnish the amalgam margin 11. Smooth the restoration 12. Check the occlusion 13. Finish the restoration	See 'occlusal (Class I) amalgam restoration', pages 92–93.		

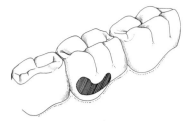

Fig. 8.3 Buccal cervical amalgam restoration.

Cavity preparation for a buccal or lingual (Class V) amalgam restoration is similar to that described for an occlusal (Class I) restoration. Having gained access to the carious lesion, the cavity is enlarged only as far as necessary to remove caries (Fig. 8.3), and the enamel margin is planed with a chisel or gingival margin trimmer. Because a buccal or lingual restoration is not subject to occlusal forces, composite resin or glass-ionomer are often preferred to amalgam.

8.3 COMPOSITE RESIN RESTORATIONS

Composite resins have been developed specifically for restoring posterior teeth, and satisfactory results have been obtained with occlusal and approximal surface restorations in primary molars (Oldenburg et al 1987). Occlusal wear is greater in composite than in amalgam restorations, but this only becomes significant after several years.

However, a disadvantage of using composite resin for posterior teeth is that the techniques involved are more demanding than with amalgam. Composite resin is more sensitive to moisture and the use of rubber dam is therefore mandatory. The marginal seal of the restoration is dependent on good adhesion of the resin to acid-etched enamel at the margin of the cavity, and effective etching is difficult to achieve at the gingival margin of a Class II cavity. Defects at the gingival margin are common (Eidelman et al 1989, Fuks et al 1990).

The only clear advantage that composite resin has over amalgam as a restorative material for posterior teeth is its appearance, and this is not usually an important consideration for primary molars.

Modifications of conventional cavity preparations have been tested. One simple modification was to bevel the enamel margin of the conventional amalgam cavity. Another, more radical, modification was to remove only enough enamel and dentine to eliminate caries, and to bevel the enamel margin: no attempt was made to provide retention. Composite restorations placed in the latter type of cavity were less successful that those placed in conventional or enamel-bevel cavities (Oldenburg et al 1987).

Technique: approximal surface (Class II) composite resin restoration

Procedure	Method	Rationale	Notes
1. Prepare cavity as for amalgam	See pages 93–96.	Modified cavity preparations that have been tested have not proved successful.	The enamel margin of the cavity may be bevelled.
2. Line the cavity	Use a quick-setting calcium hydroxide material to line the floor of the cavity.		Alternatively, glass-ionomer cement may be used as a base, using calcium hydroxide only to line very deep parts of the cavity.
3. Place a matrix	Use a thin metal matrix material, contour it with a burnisher so that it contacts the adjacent tooth, and place a wedge at the cervical margin (Fig. 8.4a). Alternatively, use a polyester matrix.	The pressure exerted on the matrix when condensing resin is not sufficient to shape the matrix, as it is when condensing amalgam.	The difficulty of obtaining a satisfactory approximal surface contour and a good contact with the adjacent tooth is one of the disadvantages of using composite resin rather than amalgam.

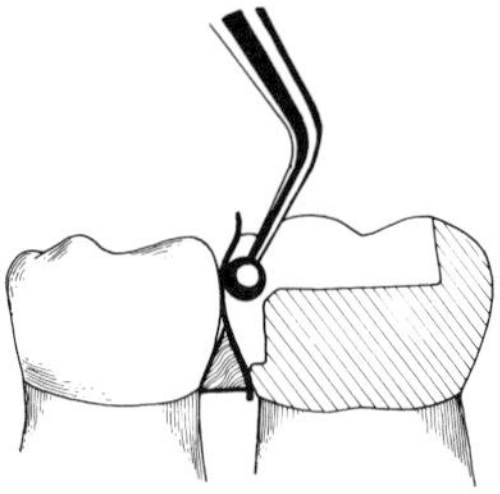

Fig. 8.4a

Technique: approximal surface (Class II) composite resin restoration *(contd)*

Procedure	Method	Rationale	Notes
4. Etch the enamel at the margin of the cavity	With a cotton wool pledget, sponge pad or small brush, apply 30–50% phosphoric acid to the enamel of the cavity walls and margin. After 1–$1\frac{1}{2}$ minutes, wash for 15 seconds and dry for 30 seconds.	Etching is required to ensure bonding of the composite resin to enamel. Enamel of primary teeth requires a longer etching period than enamel of permanent teeth.	It is preferable to use etchant in gel form to avoid the risk of acid flowing into the cavity and possibly irritating the pulp. A coloured gel is available which aids precise placement.
5. Apply unfilled resin to the etched enamel	Use a small brush to apply unfilled resin (bonding agent) to the etched enamel. Alternatively, use a dentine adhesive, and apply it in the same manner to the dentine wall of the cavity and to the enamel margin. Allow the resin to polymerize, or polymerize with a light source, depending on the type of resin used.	The low-viscosity unfilled resin penetrates into the etched enamel. Dentine adhesive is especially useful to provide additional retention in a large cavity.	Although use of unfilled resin has not been shown to be essential, it is generally used.
6. Insert composite resin restorative material	Mix the material according to the manufacturer's instructions (if using an autopolymerizing material). Carry the first increment into the deepest part of the cavity on the tip of a small hand instrument, or by using a special syringe (Fig. 8.4b). Condense with an amalgam plugger (Fig. 8.4c). Add further increments and condense. If using a light-sensitive material polymerize each increment before adding further material.	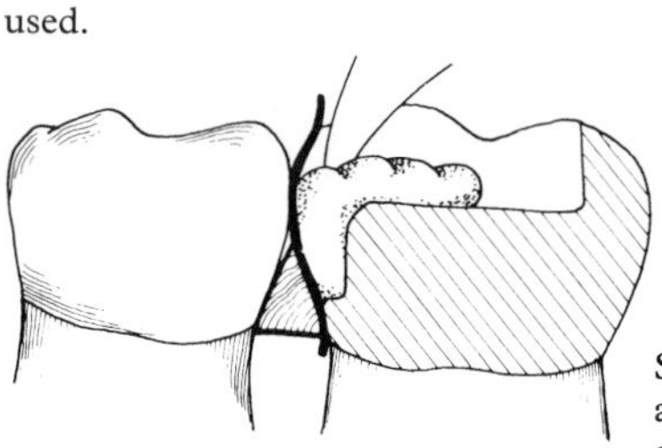	Several types of syringe are available for delivering composite or other material.
7. Remove the matrix, trim excess and polish	After the material has polymerized, remove the matrix, trim excess and polish the restoration with fine diamond and tungsten carbide burs, and abrasive discs.	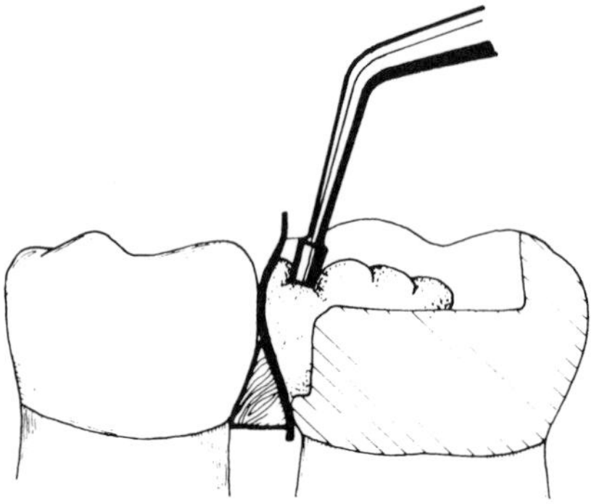	

Fig. 8.4b

Fig. 8.4c

8.4 GLASS-IONOMER RESTORATIONS

The most important property of glass-ionomer cements is adhesion to enamel and dentine. For this reason it has been suggested, ever since these cements were introduced, that they would be useful materials for restoring primary teeth, especially when it is difficult to prepare a retentive cavity. They have been used for Class II restorations in primary molars (but not for similar restorations in permanent teeth) despite lacking the strength desirable for such restorations, and clinical trials have confirmed that they are not as durable as amalgam restorations (Fuks 1984, Welbury et al 1991, Papathanasiou et al 1994).

To improve the physical properties of glass-ionomer cement, silver powder has been incorporated; the silver is sintered at high temperature to form a silver-cermet cement (McLean & Gasser 1985). Results of clinical studies of silver-cermet restorations in primary molars have been equivocal: for example, Croll & Phillips (1986) reported encouraging results, but Hung & Richardson (1990) reported that 40% of their restorations had fractured within one year. Kilpatrick et al (1995) found a silver-cermet less satisfactory than a glass-ionomer cement.

Glass-ionomer and silver-cermet cements leach fluoride, which can have a useful effect not only in preventing recurrence of caries at the margin of a restoration but also in preventing caries, or promoting remineralization of early caries, in the approximal surface of the adjacent tooth. Fluoride leached from Class II silver-cermet restorations has been shown to reduce *Streptococcus mutans* counts on adjacent enamel surfaces (Berg et al 1990).

Thus, although glass-ionomer cements are not as durable as amalgam, they have some useful applications; for example, when a patient's cooperation is limited and it is desirable to simplify operative procedures as much as possible, or when, in a child with previous high caries experience, the approximal surface adjacent to that to be restored is sound or shows signs of surface demineralization. However, they are not strong enough to be used for a large Class II restoration that presents a large surface area to masticatory forces.

Technique: approximal surface (Class II) glass-ionomer restoration

Procedure	Method	Rationale	Notes
1. Prepare a cavity as for amalgam	See pages 93–96.	Although glass-ionomer cement adheres to enamel and dentine, it is better, if possible, to provide mechanical retention within the cavity.	
2. Line the cavity only if it is deep	Place quick-setting calcium hydroxide over the deep part of the cavity only.	It is desirable to cover only the minimum area of dentine consistent with protecting the pulp, so as to leave the greatest possible dentine area for adhesion of cement.	
3. Place a matrix	See 'approximal surface (Class II) composite resin restoration', page 98.		
4. Clean the cavity walls	Use the conditioning solution supplied by the manufacturer, (usually 10% poly (acrylic acid), applying it with a cotton wool pledget to the cavity floor and walls for 10–15 seconds, followed by washing with water and light drying.	The surface of enamel and dentine cut during cavity preparation is covered by fine debris (the 'smear layer'), which is removed by the acid cleanser, enhancing adhesion.	It is not necessary to dry thoroughly; poly (acrylic acid) is a constituent of the cement and any residual acid left after washing will therefore not interfere with the setting reaction.
5. Insert the glass-ionomer cement	Mix the material according to the manufacturer's instructions (if using an 'auto-cure' material). Maintain excellent isolation to prevent moisture contamination while filling the cavity. Carry the first increment into the deepest part of the cavity on the tip of a small hand instrument, or by using a special syringe. Condense with an amalgam plugger.	Hydration during setting adversely affects the physical properties of the material.	'Light-cure' glass-ionomer cements may also be used. The technique is the same as for composite resin (pages 98–99).

Technique: approximal surface (Class II) glass-ionomer restoration *(contd)*

Procedure	Method	Rationale	Notes
	Add further increments quickly, and condense. When the cement has hardened apply a layer of special varnish or of light-curing unfilled composite resin over the surface of the restoration (do not polymerize the resin at this stage).	The working time of 'auto-cure' material is only $1\frac{1}{2}$ –2 minutes. Dehydration after the material has set adversely affects its physical properties.	Silver-cermets set more rapidly than glass-ionomer cement, and need to be protected with varnish or resin only if they would otherwise become subject to dehydration (e.g. if the mouth segment is isolated for further treatment).
6. Remove the matrix and trim excess	After the material has set, remove the matrix and trim excess with a sharp carver. Apply further varnish or unfilled resin over newly-exposed material.		
7. Polish the restoration	Delay polishing for several minutes, as recommended by the manufacturer. Polish with fine diamonds lubricated with unfilled resin or under air-water spray. Finally apply another thin layer of unfilled resin and polymerize it.	The final application of unfilled resin will fill any porosities in the surface.	Ideally, polishing of glass-ionomer restorations should be delayed until the patient's next visit, and the restoration protected until then with a layer of polymerized unfilled resin. Silver-cermet restorations can be polished immediately and do not need a protective seal.

8.4.1 Glass-ionomer tunnel restoration

A possible alternative to a conventional Class II cavity preparation is the 'tunnel' preparation, which leaves the marginal ridge of the tooth intact. It is only feasible for a small approximal surface lesion that has not severely undermined the marginal ridge. A radiopaque glass-ionomer cement, or a silver-cermet cement, is used to fill the cavity.

The advantage of this preparation is that it is very conservative, but disadvantages are that caries removal may be incomplete because access to the caries down a narrow tunnel is limited, and that the marginal ridge may be weakened and subsequently fracture. However, fluoride leach from the cement may inhibit the progress of residual caries, and, if a marginal ridge fractures, the cement can be left in place as a base (if it is satisfactory) and the tooth restored with composite resin without further cavity preparation.

No reports have yet been published of long-term clinical studies of tunnel restorations, but favourable results have been obtained in clinical practice (Croll 1988).

8.5 STAINLESS STEEL CROWNS FOR PRIMARY MOLARS

When caries in a primary molar is extensive, restoration with amalgam, composite resin or glass-ionomer cement is often impracticable. A preformed stainless steel crown is the ideal restoration in these cases (Full et al 1974, Croll 1986). Stainless steel crowns have been shown to be more durable than amalgam restorations (Roberts & Sherriff 1990) and are certainly more satisfactory than large Class II restorations.

Six sizes of crown (3M Nichrome®) are made for each primary molar. The crowns are shaped to conform with the gingival contour of the teeth and are contoured inwards at the gingival margin.

Technique: tunnel restoration

1. Administer local analgesic and, ideally, place rubber dam.
2. With a small round bur, make a small occlusal cavity just inside the marginal ridge, just into dentine. Widen the cavity bucco-lingually to allow reasonable access to the caries.
3. Place a segment of metal matrix strip between the carious surface and the adjacent tooth. Do not wedge it.
4. From the occlusal cavity, proceed with a round bur at slow speed, at an angle towards the caries (Fig. 8.5).

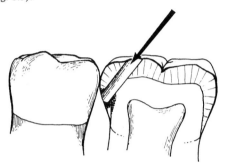

Fig. 8.5

5. After reaching the carious cavity, continue with the slowly rotating bur to remove caries and to break through the approximal surface; the breakthrough becomes apparent by a sudden movement of the metal strip and is confirmed by a bur mark on its surface.
6. Remove any further caries with a small excavator and check the walls of the cavity carefully with a probe. If in doubt, widen the tunnel slightly with a fissure bur. Wash the cavity thoroughly to remove debris.
7. Place a matrix band and wedge it in the usual manner.
8. 'Condition' the dentine surface (as recommended by the manufacturer of the restorative material being used).
9. Inject the glass-ionomer or silver-cermet into the cavity, using a syringe with a nozzle narrow enough to enter the 'tunnel'.
10. Condense the material and slightly overfill the cavity.
11. After the cement has hardened, brush on to the surface either special varnish or light-curing unfilled composite resin, to prevent dehydration of the cement while removing excess and smoothing the surface (do not polymerize the resin at this stage). Silver-cermet does not require protection with varnish or resin.
12. After trimming and smoothing the restoration under air-water spray, brush on another layer of either varnish or unfilled resin (this time polymerizing it); again, silver-cermet does not require this.

Technique: stainless steel crown

Procedure	Method	Rationale	Notes
1. Prepare equipment	Fine tapered diamond, e.g. 582 Straight diamond, 541 Pear-shaped diamond 525 or 526 Dividers Contouring plier, Johnson 114 or 3M Unitek 800–108 Curved crown scissors Fine abrasive stone ⎫ to use in slow- Rubber polishing wheel ⎬ speed handpiece Wooden tongue blade. ⎭		
2. Remove caries	Administer local analgesia and, ideally, place rubber dam.	Although the preparation of a tooth for a crown is fairly superficial, local analgesia is usually required for caries removal, and because gingival trauma may be caused during tooth preparation and when fitting the crown. Use of rubber dam is ideal, especially if caries is deep and pulp exposure possible.	Local analgesia may not be required if caries has previously been removed and the cavity has been filled with cement or amalgam; but application of topical analgesic may not be sufficient to avoid discomfort from gingival trauma.
	Remove caries using excavators or a large round bur at slow speed. If caries is superficial the shape of the resulting cavity is not important. If caries is deep and a pulp exposure possible, prepare a retentive cavity first before proceeding to remove deep caries. Fill the cavity with cement or, after lining, with amalgam.	The cavity left after excavating superficial caries is later filled with the material used to cement the crown. If pulpotomy is required, a retentive cavity is needed to seal medicaments in the pulp chamber.	If preferred, caries may be removed after rather than before crown preparation.

Technique: stainless steel crown *(contd)*

Procedure	Method	Rationale	Notes
3. Prepare the tooth	Use a high-speed handpiece with water coolant.		

Occlusal surface: Penetrate the occlusal fissure with the straight or pear-shaped diamond to a depth of 1.0–1.5 mm. Extend through the pits and fissures at this depth, passing through any oblique ridges and extending to the buccal, lingual and approximal surfaces (Fig. 8.6a). Grooves may also be made to the same depth running from the fissures up the cuspal inclines (Fig. 8.6b). Then reduce the whole surface to the depth of the grooves.

A reduction of 1.0–1.5 mm is required to allow placement of the crown without opening the bite.

The order in which the tooth surfaces are prepared is not important but reduction of the occlusal surface first is generally preferred.
The cutting head of the pear-shaped bur acts as a depth gauge.

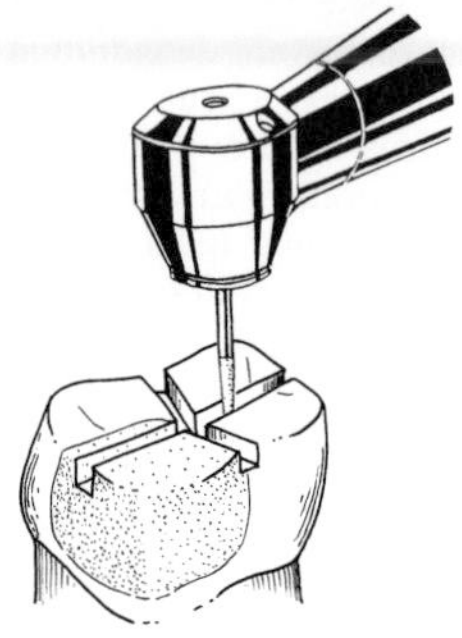

Fig. 8.6a

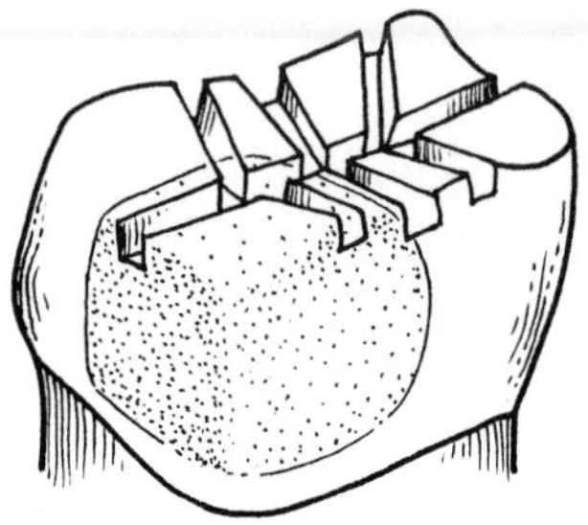

Fig. 8.6b

Approximal surfaces: Place the tapered diamond in contact with the tooth at the buccal or lingual embrasure, angled about 20° from vertical and with its tip at the gingival margin (Fig. 8.6c). Keep the instrument in this position while slicing across the tooth. After progressing about 2 mm, check that the cut is satisfactory and that a shoulder is not being produced.

Angling the diamond reduces the risk of damaging the adjacent tooth. It is better to slice from lingual to buccal (or vice versa) than from occlusal to gingival; the latter is more likely to produce a shoulder which might prevent the proper seating of the crown.

The retention of a stainless steel crown depends primarily on a tight fit at the gingival margin. Since, unlike a cast gold crown, it need not fit the tooth closely elsewhere, the shape of the preparation is relatively unimportant.

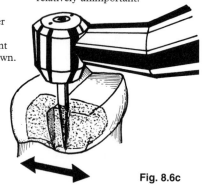

Fig. 8.6c

Buccal and lingual surfaces: With the tapered diamond, reduce first the buccal and then the lingual surface, to the level of the gingival margin, by not more than 1 mm, and round off the edges between these surfaces and the occlusal and approximal surfaces. It is not essential to eradicate all undercut at the gingival margin.

Some undercut may be useful in retaining the crown, e.g. mesiobuccally in a mandibular primary first molar.

Reduction of buccal and lingual surfaces may be minimal —sufficient only to allow the crown to be fitted. Sometimes reduction of only the buccal surface suffices.

Do not smooth the preparation as is recommended in finishing a preparation for a cast gold crown.

Smoothing is not necessary because the technique does not involve taking an impression of the preparation.

Technique: stainless steel crown *(contd)*

Procedure	Method	Rationale	Notes
4. Select the crown	Place the points of the dividers on the mesial and distal surfaces of the tooth at the level of the gingival margin. From the six sizes available, select a crown with the same mesio-distal dimension as that indicated by the dividers. Try the crown on the tooth to confirm that it is a close fit. If no crown fits exactly, choose one that is slightly large.	Use of dividers helps in the selection of the correct size of crown. A slightly large crown can be made to fit well by crimping its edge (see below).	
5. Fit the crown	Try the selected crown on the tooth. With a probe, check that the edge of the crown is within the gingival crevice; if it is resting on the gingival margin, turn in the edge of the crown with a contouring plier. Gently press the crown into place. If the crown is over-extended the gingiva will blanch; if so, cut the crown in that area with crown scissors or reduce it with a stone, and try it again. (If the crown is cut with scissors, smooth with the stone before replacing it on the tooth.) When the crown appears to be seated satisfactorily, check the occlusion (rubber dam, if used, must be removed at this stage). If the crown is still high, remove it and re-check that there is sufficient clearance when the teeth are in occlusion. Further reduce either the occlusal surface of the tooth or the periphery of the crown to permit the crown to be seated properly.		When trying on the crown, care should be taken to avoid the possibility of it being swallowed or inhaled should it slip from the fingers. A piece of gauze may be held behind the tooth. (These precautions are unnecessary if rubber dam has been placed.) Since crowns are manufactured with occluso-gingival dimensions equal to average clinical tooth crown heights, reduction of the crown may not be required. Many crowns are incorrectly fitted with margins that are over-extended sub-gingivally (Spedding 1984).
6. Contour the crown	Check the gingival margin of the crown with a probe and use a contouring plier where necessary to achieve a close fit. Place the crown on the tooth again, check the margin and eliminate any edges by further contouring. Use an excavator or scaler to remove the well-fitting crown. Check the contacts of the crown with adjacent teeth. If necessary, use an Abel 112 plier to expand the crown and produce better contacts.	The margin of the crown must be shaped to produce a tight fit on the tooth. Ideally the crown should snap into place and not be very easy to remove.	Sometimes it is difficult to place a well-fitting crown directly from the occlusal; it may be easier to place the lingual margin first and then rotate the crown buccally until it is fully seated.
7. Polish the margin of crown	Polish the margin of the crown with a fine stone followed by a rubber wheel.	A rough surface will irritate the gingiva and favour the accumulation of plaque.	
8. Cement the crown	Wash and dry the tooth and the crown, and isolate the tooth with saliva ejector and cotton rolls.	The tooth and crown must be clean and dry for good adhesion of cement.	

Technique: stainless steel crown *(contd)*

Procedure	Method	Rationale	Notes
	Use an adhesive cement (e.g. polycarboxylate), mixing to a creamy consistency and flowing it down the inside walls of the crown until the crown is almost full. Seat the crown on the tooth from lingual to buccal (Fig. 8.6d) and press it firmly into place first with finger pressure and then by inserting a wooden tongue blade and asking the patient to bite firmly on it. When the cement is set, remove all excess, particularly from the gingival crevice and from interdental areas, using a probe and dental floss respectively.	Flowing cement down the walls of the crown reduces the risk of trapping air in it. Seating the crown from lingual to buccal allows excess cement to flow out buccally.	 **Fig. 8.6d**

8.6 RESTORATION OF PRIMARY ANTERIOR TEETH

Caries of primary anterior teeth is less common than caries of posterior teeth. When it occurs, it is often associated with rampant caries in the dentition as a whole. In young infants this is usually related to the frequent and prolonged consumption of sweet drinks from a feeding bottle or reservoir-type pacifier (Winter 1980). In such cases, caries progresses very rapidly, starting on the labial surfaces of maxillary anterior teeth and quickly involving all surfaces; often it is impossible to prepare satisfactory cavities to retain restorations, and crowning is required if the teeth are to be conserved.

In children over 3 or 4 years of age, new lesions of primary incisors are not usually associated with the use of pacifiers and do not progress so rapidly, although they are, nevertheless, indicative of high caries activity. These lesions appear first in mesial and distal surfaces of the teeth rather than in labial surfaces, and it is feasible to prepare satisfactory cavities to restore them. Because these lesions are less common in primary teeth than in permanent teeth, techniques for cavity preparation and tooth restoration are described in Chapter 10.

Either glass-ionomer cement or composite resin may be used to restore primary anterior teeth. Glass-ionomer lacks the translucency of composite resin, but has the useful advantages of being adhesive and of not requiring a lining unless the cavity is very deep.

Several types of crown may be considered for the restoration of grossly carious primary anterior teeth: stainless steel, composite resin, and polycarbonate crowns.

8.6.1 Stainless steel crown

Stainless steel crowns provide strong, durable restorations for primary incisors. Minimal or no tooth preparation is required other than for the removal of caries. Although their appearance can be improved by cutting out the labial surface and replacing with acrylic or composite resin (Hartmann 1983, Helpin 1983), this type of restoration is rarely used.

8.6.2 Composite resin crown ('strip crown')

Aesthetic restorations may be made with composite resin, using cellulose acetate crown forms (3M Strip Crowns). This method has the disadvantage that some tooth reduction is required to provide space for the restorative material, but the reduction is minimal in a tooth with gross caries.

8.6.3 Polycarbonate crown

Polycarbonate crowns (3M) are made in a range of sizes and make aesthetic restorations for primary incisors (Mink & Hill 1973, Stewart et al 1974).

The tooth is prepared and the enamel etched as described above, and the crown is cemented with acrylic resin. The inside surface of the selected crown should be roughened with a bur to increase adhesion of the resin, and a small hole should be drilled in its palatal surface to allow excess resin to escape.

Technique: composite resin 'strip' crown

1. Use a fine tapered diamond in a high-speed handpiece to reduce the incisal edge and all tooth surfaces, finishing the preparation in a chamfer below the gingival margin (Fig. 8.7a). Only minimal reduction is required.

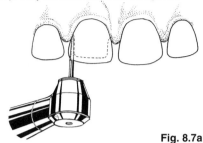

Fig. 8.7a

2. Make a groove with a small round or inverted cone bur on the labial surface, near the gingival margin (Fig. 8.7b); this provides additional retention.

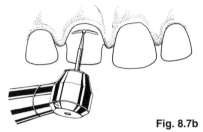

Fig. 8.7b

3. Remove any remaining caries.
4. Line dentine with quick-setting calcium hydroxide or with glass-ionomer cement.
5. Select and trim a crown form with fine scissors so that it fits accurately around the gingival margin. Punch two small holes in the incisal edge with a probe; these will allow air and composite resin to escape when placing the crown.
6. Isolate the tooth, etch enamel for $1-1\frac{1}{2}$ minutes, wash and dry. Apply bonding agent to the etched enamel.
7. Fill the crown form with an appropriate shade of composite resin, and place it carefully on the tooth.
8. Remove the excess resin that extrudes beyond the margin of the crown and through the holes in the incisal edge (Fig. 8.7c).

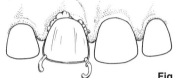

Fig. 8.7c

9. After the resin has set, remove the crown form after cutting it on the palatal side with an excavator or scaler, and smooth the margin of the restoration with a fine diamond.

If several teeth are to be crowned, chairside time may be reduced by preparing the crown forms beforehand on a plaster/stone cast of the child's dentition.

REFERENCES

Berg J H, Farrell J E, Brown L R 1990 Class II glass ionomer/silver cermet restorations and their effect on interproximal growth of mutans streptoccoci. Pediatric Dentistry 12: 20–23

Bradnock G, Marchment M D, Anderson R J 1984 Social background, fluoridation and caries experience in a 5-year-old population in the West Midlands. British Dental Journal 156: 127–131

Croll T P 1986 Primary molar stainless steel crown preparation. Quintessence International 17: 221–226

Croll T P 1988 Glass ionomer–silver cermet Class II tunnel-restorations for primary molars. Journal of Dentistry for Children 55: 177–182

Croll T P, Phillips R W 1986 Glass ionomer–silver cermet restorations for primary teeth. Quintessence International 17: 607–615

Eidelman E, Fuks A, Chosack A 1989 A clinical, radiographic and SEM evaluation of Class II composite restorations in primary teeth. Operative Dentistry 14: 58–63

Elderton R J 1983 Longitudinal study of dental treatment in the General Dental Service in Scotland. British Dental Journal 155: 91–96

Elderton R J 1990 The dentition and dental care. Heinemann, Oxford

Eley B M, Cox S W 1993 The release, absorption and possible health effects of mercury from dental amalgam: a review of recent findings. British Dental Journal 175: 355–362

Full C A, Walker J D, Pinkham J R 1974 Stainless steel crowns for deciduous molars. Journal of the American Dental Association 89: 360–364

Fuks A B 1984 Clinical evaluation of a glass ionomer cement used as Class II restorative material in primary molars. Journal of Pedodontics 8: 393–399

Fuks A B, Chosack A, Eidelman E 1990 Assessment of marginal leakage around Class II composite restorations in retrieved primary molars. Pediatric Dentistry 12: 24–27

Hartmann C R 1983 The open face stainless steel crown: an esthetic technique. Journal of Dentistry for Children 50: 31–33

Helpin M L 1983 The open face steel crown restoration in children. Journal of Dentistry for Children 50: 34–36

Hung T W, Richardson A S 1990 Clinical evaluation of glass ionomer–silver cermet restorations in primary molars: one-year results. Journal of the Canadian Dental Association 56: 239–240

Kato S, Fusayama T 1968 The effect of burnishing on the marginal seal of amalgam restorations. Journal of Prosthetic Dentistry 19: 393–398

Kidd E A M, Smith B G N 1990 Pickard's manual of operative dentistry, 6th edn. Oxford University Press, Oxford

Kilpatrick N M, Murray J J, McCabe J F 1995 The use of a reinforced glass-ionomer cermet for the restoration of primary molars: a clinical trial. British Dental Journal 179: 175–179

Lavadino J R, Ruhnke L A, Consani S 1987 Influence of burnishing on amalgam adaptation to cavity walls. Journal of Prosthetic Dentistry 58: 284–291

McLean J W, Gasser O 1985 Glass-cermet cements. Quintessence International 5: 333–343

Mink J R, Hill C J 1973 Crowns for anterior primary teeth. Dental Clinics of North America 17: 85–92

Nadal R, Phillips R W, Swartz M L 1961 Clinical investigation of the relation of mercury to the amalgam restoration. Journal of the American Dental Association 63: 488–496

Oldenburg T R, Vann W F, Dilley D C 1987 Composite restorations for primary molars: results after 4 years. Pediatric Dentistry 9: 136–143

O'Brien M 1994 Children's dental health in the United Kingdom 1993 Office of Population Censuses and Surveys. Her Majesty's Stationery Office, London, a) p 12; b) p 5; c) p 47–48

Papathanasiou A G, Curzon M E J, Fairpo C G 1994 The influence of restorative material on the survival rate of restorations in primary molars. Pediatric Dentistry 16: 282–288

Roberts J F, Sherriff M 1990 The fate and survival of amalgam and preformed crown molar restorations placed in a specialist paediatric dental practice. British Dental Journal 169: 237–244

Silva M, Messer L B, Douglas W, Weinberg R 1985 Base-varnish interactions around amalgam restorations: spectrophotometric and microscopic assessment of leakage. Australian Dental Journal 30: 89–95

Spedding R M 1984 Two principles for improving the adaptation of stainless steel crowns to primary molars. Dental Clinics of North America 28: 157–175

Stewart R E, Luke L S, Pike A R 1974 Preformed polycarbonate crowns for the restoration of anterior teeth. Journal of the American Dental Association 88: 103–107

Svare C W, Chan K L 1972 Effect of surface treatment on the corrodibility of dental amalgam. Journal of Dental Research 51: 44–47

Welbury R R, Walls A W G, Murray J J, McCabe J F 1991 The 5-year results of a clinical trial comparing a glass polyalkenoate (ionomer) cermet restoration with an amalgam restoration. British Dental Journal 170: 177–181

Winter G B 1980 Problems involved with the use of comforters. International Dental Journal 30: 28–38

RECOMMENDED READING

Duggal M S, Curzon M E J, Fayle S A, Pollard M A, Robertson A J 1995 Restorative techniques in paediatric dentistry. Martin Dunitz, London, chs 5, 6

Curzon M E J, Roberts J F, Kennedy D B 1996 Kennedy's Paediatric operative dentistry, 4th edn. Butterworth Heinemann, Oxford

Mount G J 1994 An atlas of glass-ionomer cements – a clinician's guide, 2nd edn. Martin Dunitz, London

Van Beek G C 1983 Dental morphology: an illustrated guide, 2nd edn. Wright, Bristol

9 Pulp treatment of primary teeth

Exposure of the pulp is caused most commonly by caries, but may also occur during cavity preparation or by fracture of the crown. Pulp exposures caused by caries occur more frequently in primary than in permanent teeth because the former have relatively large pulp chambers, more prominent pulp horns, and thinner enamel and dentine.

Exposure of the pulp by caries is invariably accompanied by infection of the pulp, and a traumatic exposure may quickly become infected by carious debris or saliva. The infected pulp becomes inflamed, and necrosis may result; if infection spreads to the alveolar bone the developing permanent tooth may be affected. Furthermore, although the inflammation may remain sub-acute or chronic and therefore give the patient little or no pain, the process may become acute at any time. For these reasons, a primary tooth with a pulp exposure should not be left untreated; a choice must be made between conservation by some form of pulp treatment, or extraction, perhaps accompanied either by a 'balancing' extraction or by space maintenance (Ch. 17).

Primary molars require pulp treatment much more commonly than do primary anterior teeth. The methods of treatment include pulp capping, pulpotomy and pulpectomy.

9.1 INDIRECT AND DIRECT PULP CAPPING

The aim of pulp capping is to maintain pulp vitality by placing a suitable dressing either directly on the exposed pulp or on a thin residual layer of slightly soft dentine; in the latter case the method is known as indirect pulp capping.

Calcium hydroxide is usually used for pulp capping because it stimulates the formation of secondary dentine more effectively than do other materials. Clinical studies have shown that the technique is successful when strict criteria are applied in selecting cases for treatment (Jeppeson 1971). Pulp capping is not recommended if the diameter of the exposure is greater than that of a pin-point, if there is more than gentle bleeding from the exposure site, or if there is a history of spontaneous pain.

Less commonly, preparations containing antibiotic and anti-inflammatory drugs are used instead of calcium hydroxide. The rationale of using these materials is that they suppress infection and inflammation. Clinical success has been reported in the treatment of small, symptomless pulp exposures in permanent teeth (Cowan 1966) and in primary teeth (Hansen et al 1971). However, slow pulp necrosis and abscess formation tend to occur in teeth treated with these materials, without causing symptoms. Because these changes develop slowly the use of these materials in primary teeth is not contraindicated, but in permanent teeth it is recommended that they are used only temporarily, to alleviate symptoms before treating by pulpectomy (Fédération Dentaire Internationale 1968, Watts & Paterson 1988).

Technique: pulp capping (indirect or direct)

Procedure	Method	Rationale	Notes
1. Prepare instruments and materials	Ideally, use a sterile, pre-packed tray containing cotton wool pledgets, burs and hand instruments required for pulpotomy.		Before starting to treat a tooth with a large carious lesion, it is important to prepare for pulp treatment so that it can be started without delay should the need arise.
2. Isolate the tooth	Apply rubber dam. If rubber dam cannot be used, isolate with cotton rolls and a saliva ejector, and maintain them in position throughout the treatment.	An essential condition for successful pulp treatment is that the pulp should not become contaminated by saliva.	Rubber dam also protects the patient should materials or instruments be inadvertently dropped into the mouth.
3. Prepare the cavity	Prepare a cavity in the normal way (Ch. 8).	It is important to complete the cavity preparation before removing deep caries so that the tooth can be quickly restored after pulp treatment, thus reducing the risk of contamination.	Before commencing treatment of a vital tooth suspected of having a pulp exposure, adequate local analgesia must be provided.
4. Excavate deep caries	Gently remove caries with an excavator, first removing peripheral caries, then proceeding towards the pulp. If, in a very deep cavity, it is assessed that the pulp is nearly exposed, and the overlying dentine is only very slightly soft, do not proceed to expose the pulp. Removal of caries may, however, expose the pulp. If the pulp is vital and the exposure is not more than a pin-point in diameter, direct pulp capping may be performed.	Indirect pulp capping is the treatment of choice in such cases. The prognosis after direct pulp capping is poor unless the exposure is very small.	Direct pulp capping should only be undertaken if strict criteria are satisfied. (p. 107).
5. Apply calcium hydroxide	Dry the cavity with a cotton wool pledget. Cover the deep parts of the cavity, including the pulp exposure (if present), with hard-setting calcium hydroxide paste.	The capping material will not adhere to a wet surface. Calcium hydroxide stimulates the formation of secondary dentine. A hard-setting material is more convenient to use than a non-setting type.	Compressed air should not be used to dry the cavity because this might irritate the pulp. Many calcium hydroxide preparations are available. If a non-setting paste is used it must be covered with a cement base before restoring the tooth with amalgam. A cement base should also be placed over hard-setting calcium hydroxide if the exposure is on the floor of the cavity, subject to direct pressure during condensation of amalgam.
6. Restore the tooth	See Chapter 8.		

Although direct pulp capping can be justified if the criteria outlined above are strictly applied, it is generally considered that pulpotomy is the treatment of choice for all categories of pulp exposure in primary teeth.

9.2 PULPOTOMY (PARTIAL PULPECTOMY)

Pulpotomy is a procedure in which the entire coronal pulp is removed, with the aim of removing all infected pulp tissue; the radicular pulp is then treated in different ways, according to the technique employed. Pulpotomy is performed mainly in vital teeth with pulp exposures larger than those considered suitable for pulp capping.

In permanent teeth, the classical pulpotomy technique involves placing calcium hydroxide in the base of the pulp chamber after having removed the coronal pulp. This technique has been used with success in the treatment of vital pulps in premolars and molars (Masterton 1966, Santini 1983). However, in primary teeth this method has been found to be relatively unsuccessful, often being accompanied by internal resorption of the roots (Magnusson 1970, Schroder 1978). Therefore, other pulpotomy methods have been developed for primary molars: *vital pulpotomy* using formocresol, and *devitalization pulpotomy*. These are alternative methods for teeth with vital pulps.

For non-vital pulps, pulpectomy and root canal therapy is the ideal treatment, but since this is often not practicable for primary molars, a non-vital pulpotomy method is also advocated.

9.2.1 Vital pulpotomy (formocresol pulpotomy)

After removal of coronal pulp, formocresol solution is applied to the radicular pulp for 4 or 5 minutes, after which an antiseptic dressing is placed over the radicular pulp stumps before restoring the tooth (Redig 1968). The use of this technique has been reviewed by Teplitsky & Grieman (1984). The formocresol solution that was used initially had the following composition:

Formalin (37%)	19 ml	Glycerin	25 ml
Cresol	35 ml	Water	21 ml

However, a 1 to 5 dilution of this solution has generally been used since Morawa et al (1975) showed it to be equally effective.

Formocresol solution releases formaldehyde, which diffuses through the pulp and, by combining with cellular protein, fixes the tissues. Histological and histochemical studies have shown that the pulp closest to the pulp chamber becomes well fixed; more apically, fixation may not be complete, and the most apical tissue may remain vital (Berger 1965, Mejare et al 1976, Rolling & Lambjerg-Hansen 1978). The fixed pulp tissue may later become replaced by vital granulation tissue. It is not known whether the strongly antiseptic properties of cresol play an essential part in the success of the method.

The effectiveness of the method, judged by clinical criteria, is high (Morawa et al 1975, Fuks & Bimstein 1981, Roberts 1996). Judged by histological criteria, however, the technique cannot be considered ideal because it does not promote pulp healing (Magnusson 1978).

Because formaldehyde is potentially mutagenic and carcinogenic, its use in dentistry has been questioned (Lewis & Chestner 1981), but a review of the evidence suggests that formocresol presents no health hazard in the quantities used in pulpotomy techniques (Ranly 1984). Glutaraldehyde has been considered a possible alternative to formocresol, but clinical trials have reported conflicting results (Garcia-Godoy 1986, Fuks et al 1990); further evidence is required before it can be recommended instead of formocresol (Feigal & Messer 1990, Ketley & Goodman 1991).

Technique: vital (formocresol) pulpotomy

Procedure	Method	Rationale	Notes
1. Prepare instruments and materials 2. Isolate the tooth 3. Prepare the cavity 4. Excavate deep caries	See 'pulp capping'. To provide easy access to the pulp chamber for pulpotomy, it is important to extend the occlusal part of the cavity across the whole of the occlusal surface, extending across the oblique ridges on the occlusal surfaces of maxillary second molars and mandibular first molars.		
5. Remove roof of pulp chamber	Use a sterile fissure bur (about No. 2) in a slow-speed handpiece. Insert it into the exposure and move it mesially and distally as required to remove the roof of the pulp chamber (Fig. 9.1a). Remove any overhanging ledges of dentine.	Pulp tissue under ledges may be not easy to remove.	Opening the pulp chamber with a bur at slow speed is simple since only a thin shelf of dentine needs to be removed (assuming a normal cavity has been prepared previously). A high-speed handpiece may be used, but care must be taken not to perforate the base of the pulp chamber.

Technique: vital (formocresol) pulpotomy *(contd)*

Procedure	Method	Rationale	Notes
6. Remove the coronal pulp	Remove the coronal pulp with a large excavator (Fig. 9.1b) or with a slowly rotating round bur.		

Fig. 9.1a   Fig. 9.1b

| 7. Wash and dry the pulp chamber | Syringe the pulp chamber with sterile water or saline; a disposable syringe with a sterile needle is ideal for this purpose (Fig. 9.1c). Dry and control bleeding with sterile cotton wool pledgets. | Syringing washes debris and pulp remnants from the pulp chamber. | |

| 8. Apply formocresol | Dip a cotton pledget in formocresol solution, remove excess by dabbing on a cotton roll, and place it in the pulp chamber, covering the radicular pulp stumps, for 4–5 minutes (Fig. 9.1d). Do not allow solution to leak on to the gingiva. | Formocresol solution must not be allowed to drip on to facial or oral soft tissues. | |

Fig. 9.1c

| 9. Apply antiseptic dressing | Prepare an antiseptic paste by mixing equal parts of eugenol and formocresol with zinc oxide. Remove the pledget containing formocresol and place just enough paste to cover the radicular pulp stumps (Fig. 9.1e). Dab the paste lightly into place with a moist cotton wool pledget. | The antiseptic dressing is used to combat any residual infection. Pressure on the vital radicular pulp should be avoided. | It has been suggested that, to reduce further the risk of a toxic effect, formocresol should not be included in the antiseptic dressing (Ketley & Goodman 1991). Other antiseptic pastes may be equally effective. |
| 10. Restore the tooth | Place quick-setting cement base before restoring with amalgam (Fig. 9.1f), or fill with cement before preparing the tooth for a stainless steel crown. Take a periapical radiograph to check whether the pulp chamber has been adequately filled. | Since the antiseptic paste sets slowly, a cement base is required before restoring the tooth. | A stainless steel crown is the ideal restoration because the crown of a tooth treated by pulpotomy is weak and may fracture. |

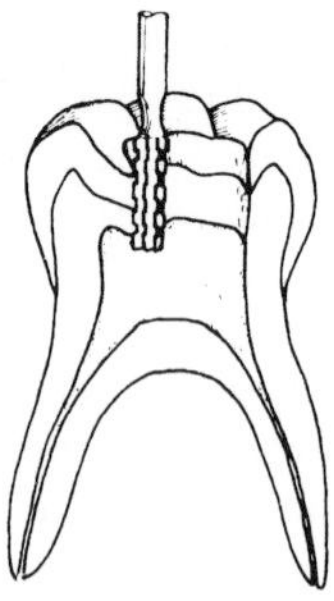

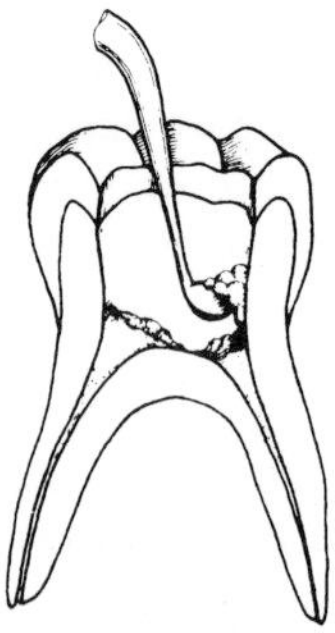

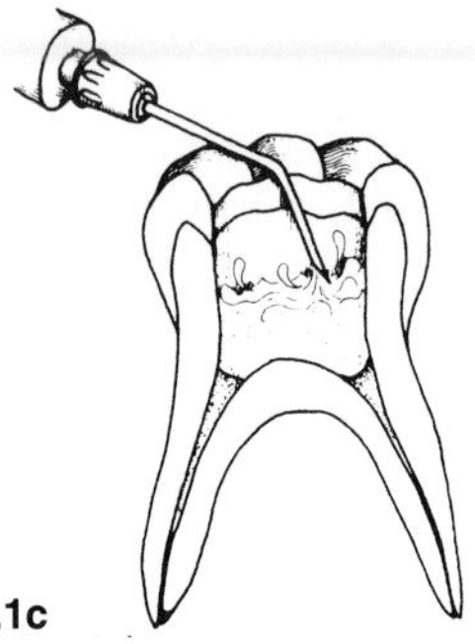

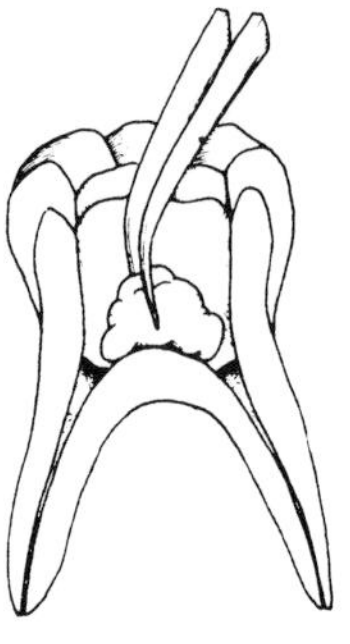

Fig. 9.1d 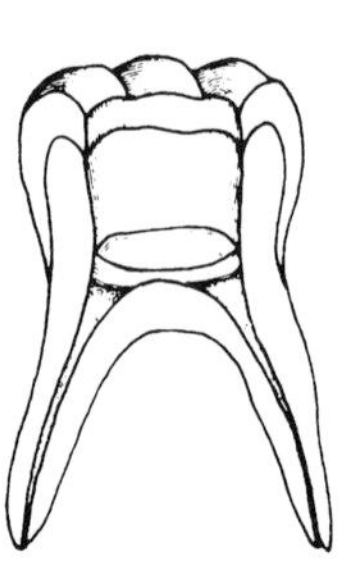   Fig. 9.1e 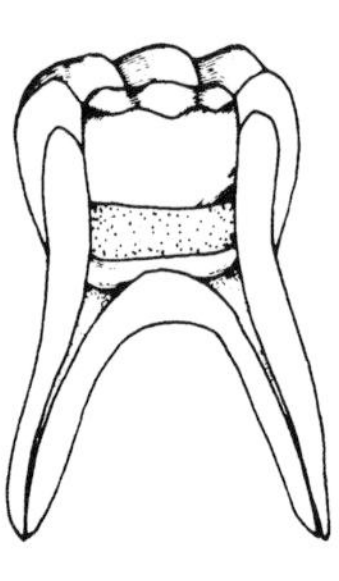   Fig. 9.1f

9.2.2 Devitalization pulpotomy

The generally-accepted pulpotomy treatment for vital primary molars is the 'formocresol pulpotomy' described above. However, there are occasions when it is not convenient or possible to proceed immediately with this treatment. For example, pulp involvement may not have been anticipated when treatment of the tooth started and sufficient time may not have been allocated for a pulpotomy procedure; or inflammation of the pulp may make it difficult to achieve adequate depth of analgesia for pulp amputation; or the patient's cooperation may be limited. In such circumstances the devitalization pulpotomy technique may be employed, which is convenient because the first stage involves only the placement of a devitalizing paste over the pulp exposure.

The devitalization paste (Boots, Specials Manufac-turing, number E 13498), has the following compo-sition:

Paraformaldehyde	1.0 g
Lignocaine	0.06 g
Carmine (colour)	0.01 g
Carbowax 1500	1.3 g
Propylene glycol	0.5 ml

The paste is placed over the pulp exposure and sealed in the tooth for 1–2 weeks. Formaldehyde gas liberated from the paraformaldehyde permeates through the coronal and radicular pulp, fixing the tissues. On the second visit, the pulpotomy is carried out (without the need for local analgesia) and an antiseptic paste is placed over the radicular pulp before restoring the tooth. Hobson (1970) reported a success rate of 77% after 3 years.

Technique: devitalization pulpotomy

Procedure	Method	Rationale	Notes

First visit:

Procedure	Method	Rationale	Notes
1. Prepare instruments and materials 2. Isolate the tooth 3. Prepare the cavity 4. Excavate deep caries	See 'pulp capping'. To provide easy access to the pulp chamber for pulpotomy, it is important to extend the occlusal part of the cavity across the whole of the occlusal surface, extending across the oblique ridges on the occlusal surfaces of maxillary second molars and mandibular first molars.		
5. Apply paraform-aldehyde paste	Ensure that the exposure site is free of debris. If the tooth is anaesthetized, enlarge the exposure with a round bur. Prepare a cotton pledget large enough to cover the exposure but small enough to be clear of cavity margins. Incorporate paraformaldehyde paste into the pledget, pick it up on the tip of a probe and place it gently over the exposure (Fig. 9.2a).	Adequate exposure of the pulp is essential for the devitalizing paste to be effective; formaldehyde gas liberated from paraformal-dehyde permeates the pulp tissue and fixes it. Leakage from the cavity would cause fixation of adjacent gingival tissues.	Paraformaldehyde paste may be applied to the exposure directly rather than on a cotton wool pledget. However, use of a pledget will minimize pressure on the pulp and reduce the risk of after-pain.

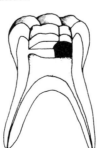

Fig. 9.2a

Technique: devitalization pulpotomy *(contd)*

Procedure	Method	Rationale	Notes
6. Seal the cavity with temporary dressing	Seal the paraformaldehyde paste into the cavity with a thin mix of quick-setting zinc oxide-eugenol (Fig. 9.2b).	A thin mix avoids causing pressure on the pulp.	The child and parent should be warned of the possibility of temporary discomfort, and advised to take an analgesic if necessary.

Second visit (1–2 weeks later)

7. Remove temporary dressing	Local analgesia should not be required. Isolate the tooth. Remove temporary dressing and paraformaldehyde paste. Probe the pulp at the exposure site—it should not bleed or be sensitive. If vital pulp is found, either re-dress with paraformaldehyde paste for a further 1–2 weeks, or perform a vital pulpotomy under local analgesia.	The pulp should be non-vital if the paste has been effective.	

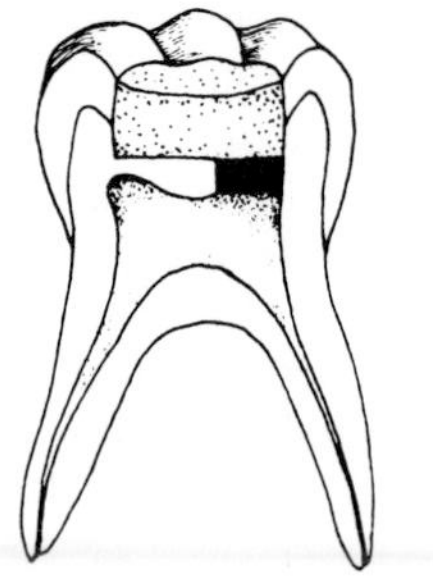

Fig. 9.2b

8. Remove roof of pulp chamber 9. Remove the coronal pulp 10. Wash and dry the pulp chamber 11. Apply antiseptic dressing 12. Restore the tooth	See 'vital (formocresol) pulpotomy'.		The pulpotomy procedure is relatively simple compared with vital pulpotomy because there is no bleeding.

9.2.3 Non-vital pulpotomy

Ideally, a non-vital tooth should be treated by pulpectomy and root canal filling (see below). However, pulpectomy of a primary molar is often impracticable and a two-stage pulpotomy technique is therefore more commonly used. Necrotic coronal pulp is first removed and the infected radicular pulp is treated with a disinfectant solution, which is applied on a cotton pledget and sealed in the pulp chamber for 1–2 weeks. Beechwood creosote (a mixture of cresol, guaicol and other phenols) has generally been used in the UK (Hobson 1970), but other medicaments may be equally effective; for example formocresol (Droter 1963, Roberts 1996) and camphorated monochlorophenol (Palmer 1971). At the second visit, the disinfectant solution is replaced by an antiseptic paste that is placed over the radicular pulp remnants before restoring the tooth. Hobson (1970) reported a success rate of 66% after 3 years, and Roberts (1996) 85% after nearly 2 years.

The presence of a sinus associated with a chronic abscess, or of some degree of tooth mobility, is not necessarily a contraindication for this method; a sinus is expected to disappear following control of the infection, and a mobile tooth becomes firm as periapical bone reforms. A tooth with an acute abscess may be treated by this method, after draining the pus and controlling the infection.

9.3 PULPECTOMY

Pulpectomy of primary molars is often considered impracticable because of the difficulty of obtaining adequate access to the root canals in the small mouths of children, and because of the complexity of root canals in primary molars. The canals are ribbon-shaped (narrow mesio-distally and wide bucco-lingually) and their complexity increases as physiological root resorption progresses; when root calcification ends at about the age of 3 years there is

Technique: non-vital pulpotomy

Procedure	Method	Rationale	Notes

First visit:

1. Prepare instruments and materials
2. Isolate the tooth
3. Prepare the cavity
4. Excavate deep caries

See 'pulp capping'.

Since the pulp is necrotic, local analgesia is not required.

5. Remove roof of pulp chamber
6. Remove the coronal pulp
7. Wash and dry the pulp

See 'vital (formocresol) pulpotomy'.

If access to the root canals is good, radicular pulp may be removed and the canals cleaned (see 'pulpectomy').

8. Apply disinfectant solution

Prepare a cotton wool pledget that will fit into the pulp chamber. Dip the pledget in disinfectant solution (e.g. formocresol, beechwood creosote or camphorated mono-chlorophenol), by dabbing on a sterile cotton wool roll and place it in the pulp chamber over the radicular pulp (Fig. 9.3a).

The strong disinfectant combats infection in the radicular pulp. The solution must not be allowed to drip on to the patient's face or oral soft tissues.

9. Seal the cavity with a temporary dressing

Seal the cotton wool pledget into the cavity with any temporary cement (Fig. 9.3b).

Since the radicular pulp is necrotic, no precautions need to be taken to avoid pressure.

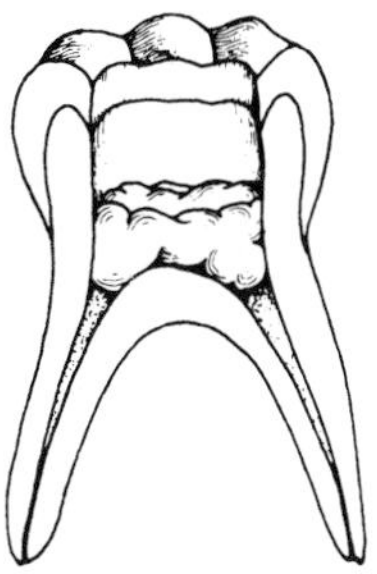

Fig. 9.3a 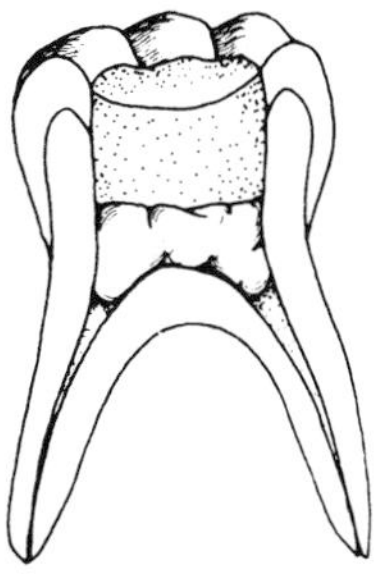   **Fig. 9.3b**

Second visit: 1–2 weeks later

10. Remove temporary dressing

Isolate the tooth. Remove the temporary dressing and the cotton wool pledget.

If symptoms persist, or if there are no signs of resolution of a sinus, a decision must be made either to repeat the treatment or to attempt pulpectomy or to extract the tooth.

Technique: non-vital pulpotomy *(contd)*

Procedure	Method	Rationale	Notes
11. Apply a resorbable antiseptic dressing	Use pure zinc oxide mixed with eugenol, or an iodoform paste. Press it firmly into the root canals with a cotton pledget or amalgam plugger (Fig. 9.3c).	Pressure forces the paste down the root canals, compressing the pulp tissue apically where residual infection is more accessible to the periapical blood supply.	Pure zinc oxide resorbs more readily than proprietary zinc oxide preparations. Formocresol has normally been incorporated into the zinc oxide paste but since the paste is forced towards and sometimes into the periapical tissues, this is now not recommended. Iodoform has been shown to be a satisfactory alternative (Ranly & Garcia-Godoy 1991).

Fig. 9.3c

12. Restore the tooth and take a radiograph	As in vital pulpotomy.		

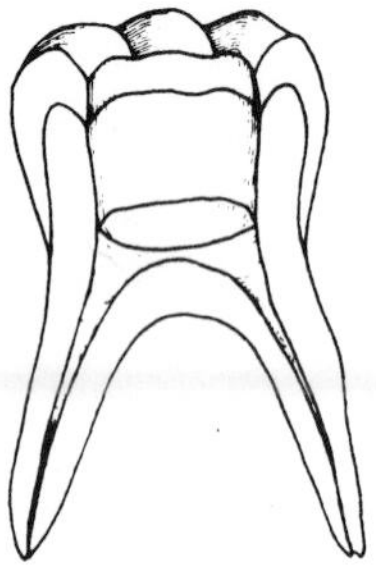

usually only one canal in each root, but later each root may have several intercommunicating canals (Hibbard & Ireland 1957). Thus, when the canals are least complex the patients are young and least likely to tolerate root canal treatment; in older patients the canals are too complex to be cleaned adequately. Because of these difficulties the non-vital pulpotomy technique is often used even for a tooth with a necrotic pulp, though pulpectomy may be attempted if conditions are favourable (Coll et al 1985, Duggal & Curzon 1989).

After opening the pulp chamber, removing coronal pulp and locating the root canals, the radicular pulp must be removed and the canals filed. If the apical radicular pulp shows signs of vitality, and if the tooth has been symptomless, treatment can be completed at the same visit. A radiograph to show the position of files in the root canals is desirable but not essential. Formocresol on a pledget of cotton wool may be left in the pulp chamber for 4–5 minutes before filling the canals with a zinc oxide or iodoform paste, using a spiral root canal filler.

If all the radicular pulp is necrotic, or if there is clinical or radiographic evidence of periradicular infection, a two-stage treatment is recommended, leaving formocresol in the pulp chamber for 1–2 weeks before filling the root canals.

9.4 SELECTION OF METHOD

The decision about which method to use is based mainly on the assessment of whether the pulp is vital or non-vital, and this is based on preoperative signs and symptoms and on the appearance of the pulp at the exposure site. Factors that should be considered, and their influence on the selection of treatment method, are outlined in Table 9.1.

Vital (formocresol) pulpotomy and devitalization pulpotomy are alternative methods of treatment. Normally, if local analgesia is adequate, the one-stage vital pulpotomy is preferred but, if analgesia is inadequate or if the necessary time is not available, the two-stage devitalization method may be chosen.

Table 9.1 Factors in the selection of treatment for a pulp-exposed primary molar

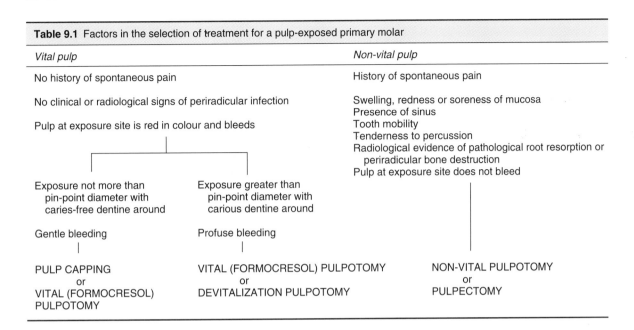

Vital pulp	Non-vital pulp
No history of spontaneous pain	History of spontaneous pain
No clinical or radiological signs of periradicular infection	Swelling, redness or soreness of mucosa Presence of sinus
Pulp at exposure site is red in colour and bleeds	Tooth mobility Tenderness to percussion Radiological evidence of pathological root resorption or periradicular bone destruction Pulp at exposure site does not bleed

Exposure not more than pin-point diameter with caries-free dentine around | Exposure greater than pin-point diameter with carious dentine around

Gentle bleeding | Profuse bleeding

PULP CAPPING
or
VITAL (FORMOCRESOL) PULPOTOMY
| VITAL (FORMOCRESOL) PULPOTOMY
or
DEVITALIZATION PULPOTOMY
| NON-VITAL PULPOTOMY
or
PULPECTOMY

9.5 INDICATIONS AND CONTRA-INDICATIONS FOR PULP TREATMENT OF PRIMARY MOLARS

The indications and contraindications for pulp treatment may be summarized as follows:

Indications

General

1. A cooperative patient.
2. A patient with a bleeding abnormality (e.g. haemophilia) for whom extraction would require hospitalization. Any bleeding accompanying the pulp treatment can easily be controlled.
3. A patient with an unhappy experience of tooth extraction; pulp treatment may be preferable to extraction for psychological reasons, and may be justified even if there is no dental indication for conserving the tooth.

Dental

1. A primary dentition in which all molars are present, or in which the effects of previous extractions have been controlled either by balancing extraction or by space maintenance (Ch. 17).
2. A mixed dentition in which it is assessed that there is just enough space for the eruption of permanent canines and premolars. Space maintenance is very important in this type of case, and the primary tooth is preferable to an artificial space maintainer.
3. A mixed dentition in which it is assessed that there is a gross shortage of space for the eruption of permanent canines and premolars. Again, space maintenance is very important in such a case.

Contraindications

General

1. A patient from a family having unfavourable attitudes towards dental health and the conservation of teeth (unless these attitudes can be changed).
2. A patient with inadequate cooperation for pulp treatment (unless this can be improved by successful behaviour management).
3. A patient with congenital heart disease or a history of rheumatic fever. Although pulp treatment could be performed under antibiotic cover, it is not certain that infection is eliminated during treatment; any residual infection would be a potential source of bacteraemia that might be a hazard to the patient in the future.
4. A patient in poor general health (e.g. diabetes, chronic kidney disease, leukaemia); these patients have poor resistance to infection and poor healing qualities.

Dental

1. A dentition in which the effects of previous extraction have not been controlled. Extraction is usually preferable to pulp treatment if the contralateral tooth is missing.
2. A mixed dentition in which it is assessed that there is mild shortage of space for the eruption of permanent canines and premolars. In such a case, extraction of primary first molars is not critical because space for the unerupted permanent teeth is usually provided later by extraction of a permanent tooth unit (commonly the first premolar), and this provides more space than is actually required. Extraction of primary first molars often allows crowded permanent incisors to align, and the small amount of mesial drift of posterior teeth that can be expected to occur is acceptable, and often advantageous. Primary second molars, however, should be conserved if possible, because of the greater amount of space loss that generally follows their extraction (p. 161).
3. A tooth with an acute abscess. However, in some cases it is possible to drain the pus and then treat as a chronic abscess. Drainage may be obtained by making as large an opening as possible into the pulp chamber and by passing a blunt probe down the gingival crevice to the root furcation where the abscess is usually located.
4. A dentition in which more than two or three teeth have pulp exposures. Such a dentition is probably neglected and does not justify pulp treatment unless the prognosis for improving home care is good.
5. A tooth with such gross coronal breakdown that restoration would be impossible following pulp treatment.
6. A tooth with caries penetrating the floor of the pulp chamber.
7. A tooth close to natural exfoliation.
8. A tooth with advanced pathological root resorption.

REFERENCES

Berger J E 1965 Pulp tissue reaction to formocresol and zinc oxide-eugenol. Journal of Dentistry for Children 32: 13–27

Coll J A, Josell S, Casper J S 1985 Evaluation of a one-appointment formocresol pulpectomy technique for primary molars. Pediatric Dentistry 7: 123–129

Cowan A 1966 Treatment of exposed vital pulps with a corticosteroid antibiotic agent. British Dental Journal 120: 521–523

Droter J A 1963 Formocresol in vital and non-vital teeth: a clinical study. Journal of Dentistry for Children 30: 239–242

Duggal M S, Curzon M E J 1989 Restoration of the broken-down primary molar: I Pulpectomy technique. Dental Update 16: 26–28

Fédération Dentaire Internationale 1968 The use of corticosteroids in endodontic therapy. International Dental Journal 18: 471–472

Feigal R J, Messer H H 1990 A critical look at glutaraldehyde. Pediatric Dentistry 12: 69–71

Fuks A B, Bimstein E 1981 Clinical evaluation of diluted formocresol pulpotomies in primary teeth of schoolchildren. Pediatric Dentistry 3: 321–324

Fuks A B, Bimstein E, Guelmann M, Klein H 1990 Assessment of a 20% buffered glutaraldehyde solution in pulpotomized primary teeth of schoolchildren. Journal of Dentistry for Children 57: 371–375

Garcia-Godoy F 1968 A 42-month clinical evaluation of glutaraldehyde pulpotomies in primary teeth. Journal of Pedodontics 10: 148–155

Hansen H P, Ravn J J, Ulrich D 1971 Vital pulpotomy in primary molars. A clinical and histologic investigation of the effect of zinc oxide-eugenol cement and Ledermix®. Scandinavian Journal of Dental Research 79: 13–23

Hibbard E D, Ireland R L 1957 Morphology of the root canals of the primary molar teeth. Journal of Dentistry for Children 24: 250–257

Hobson P 1970 Pulp treatment of deciduous teeth. Part 2: Clinical investigation. British Dental Journal 128: 275–283

Jeppesen K 1971 Direct pulp capping on primary teeth: a long term investigation. Journal of the International Association of Dentistry for Children 2: 10–19

Ketley C, Goodman J R 1991 Formocresol toxicity: is there a suitable alternative for primary molar pulpotomy? International Journal of Paediatric Dentistry 1: 67–72

Lewis B B, Chestner S B 1981 Formadelhyde in dentistry: a review of mutagenic and carcinogenic potential. Journal of the American Dental Association 103: 434–489

Magnusson B 1970 Therapeutic pulpotomy in primary molars: a clinical and histological follow-up. Odontologisk Revy 21: 415–431

Magnusson B O 1978 Therapeutic pulpotomies in primary molars with the formocresol technique. Acta Odontologica Scandinavica 36: 137–165

Masterton J B 1966 The healing of wounds of the dental pulp of Man: a clinical and histological study. British Dental Journal 120: 213–224

Mejare I, Hasselgren G, Hammarstrom L E 1976 Effect of formaldehyde-containing drugs on human dental pulp evaluated by enzyme histochemical technique. Scandinavian Journal of Dental Research 84: 29–36

Morawa A P, Straffon L H, Han S S, Corpron R E 1975 Clinical evaluation of pulpotomies using dilute formocresol. Journal of Dentistry for Children 42: 360–363

Palmer J 1971 Treatment of non-vital deciduous teeth in general practice. Dental Practitioner 21: 150–152

Ranly D M 1984 Formocresol toxicity: current knowledge. Acta Odontologica Pediatrica 5: 93–98

Ranly D M, Garcia-Godoy F 1991 Reviewing pulp treatment for primary teeth. Journal of the American Dental Association 122: 83–85

Redig D F 1968 A comparison and evaluation of two formocresol pulpotomy techniques using 'Buckley's' formocresol. Journal of Dentistry for Children 35: 22–32

Roberts J F 1996 Treatment of vital and non-vital primary molar teeth by one-stage formocresol pulpotomy: clinical success and effect upon age of exfoliation. International Journal of Paediatric Dentistry 6: 111–116

Rolling I, Lambjerg-Hansen H 1978 Pulp condition of successfully formocresol-treated primary molars. Scandinavian Journal of Dental Research 80: 267–272

Santini A 1983 Assessment of the pulpotomy technique in human first permanent mandibular molars. British Dental Journal 155: 151–154

Schroder 1978 A two-year follow-up of primary molars pulpotomized with a gentle technique and capped with calcium hydroxide. Scandinavian Journal of Dental Research 83: 273–278

Teplitsky P E, Grieman R 1984 History of formocresol pulpotomy. Journal of the Canadian Dental Association 50: 629–634

Watts A, Paterson R C 1988 The response of the mechanically-exposed pulp to prednisolone and triamcinolone acetonide. International Endodontic Journal 21: 9–16

RECOMMENDED READING

Duggal M S, Curzon M E J, Fayle S A, Pollard M A, Robertson A J 1995 Restorative techniques in paediatric dentistry. Martin Dunitz, London, ch 4

10 Treatment of carious permanent teeth

The prevalence of dental caries has decreased markedly during the last 20 years in many developed countries. Nevertheless, the most recent national survey in the UK showed that the proportion of children with experience of caries in permanent teeth was 28% of 9-year-olds, 52% of 12-year-olds and 63% of 15-year-olds (O'Brien 1994).

10.1 PREVENTIVE RESIN RESTORATION (SEALANT RESTORATION)

The ideal preventive treatment for a tooth that has a pit or fissure is to seal it before it becomes carious (Ch. 5). However, it is not uncommon when examining a pit or fissure to remain uncertain about whether it is caries-free, because it is difficult or impossible to explore its base. Also, it is not uncommon to detect a small, discrete carious lesion in an otherwise sound surface. Although sealing over an early lesion may be a justifiable form of treatment, because the lesion will probably become arrested under the sealant (Going 1984), the preferred treatment is to open up, very conservatively

Technique: preventive resin restoration (sealant restoration)

Procedure	Method	Rationale	Notes
1. Investigate the pit or the suspect part of the fissure, or the small carious lesion	With a small round bur (e.g. No. 2) in a slow-speed or high-speed handpiece, penetrate the pit or the suspect part of the fissure, or the carious lesion, to a depth of about 1 mm (Fig. 10.1a, b). Examine and gently probe the resulting cavity. If it is assessed as caries-free proceed to 2 below.	Removal of about 1 mm of enamel allows a better assessment to be made of whether the pit or fissure is carious.	Local analgesia is not required because only enamel is penetrated.

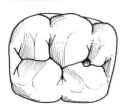

Fig. 10.1a

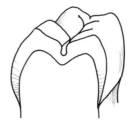

Fig. 10.1b

Technique: preventive resin restoration (sealant restoration) *(contd)*

Procedure	Method	Rationale	Notes
	If doubt persists, or if caries remains, proceed deeper with a slightly larger bur (Fig. 10.1c).	As the cavity becomes deeper it must be widened so that its base can be explored.	If caries is deeper than expected and involves dentine, it may be necessary to administer local analgesia and to extend the cavity further.

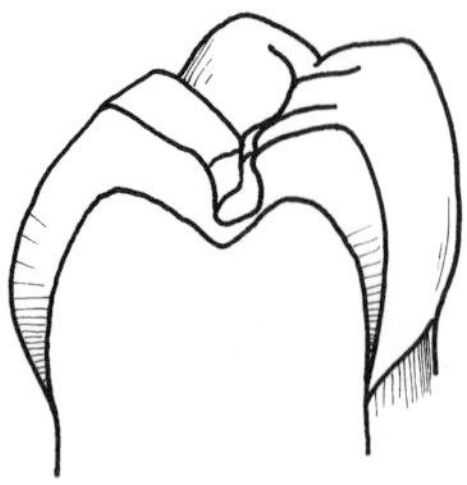

Fig. 10.1c

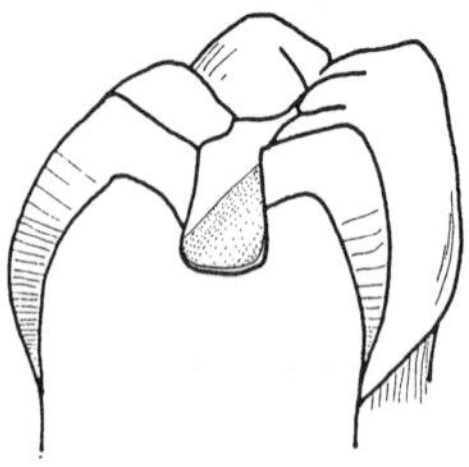

Fig. 10.1d

Procedure	Method	Rationale	Notes
	When the cavity is caries-free, undercut its walls slightly.

If dentine has been exposed, line with hard-setting calcium hydroxide (Fig. 10.1d). | It is not essential to produce a retentive cavity, but it is a simple procedure which increases the retention of the restoration. Since it is planned to use acid to etch the enamel, any exposed dentine should be lined. | The preventive resin restoration is retained primarily by the bonding of resin to acid-etched enamel. |
| 2. Isolate the tooth
3. Etch
4. Wash
5. Dry | See 'fissure sealing' (Ch. 5). | | |
| 6. Place the sealant restoration | If the cavity produced in enamel is minimal, apply resin as described for fissure sealing (Figs 10.1e, f). | | |

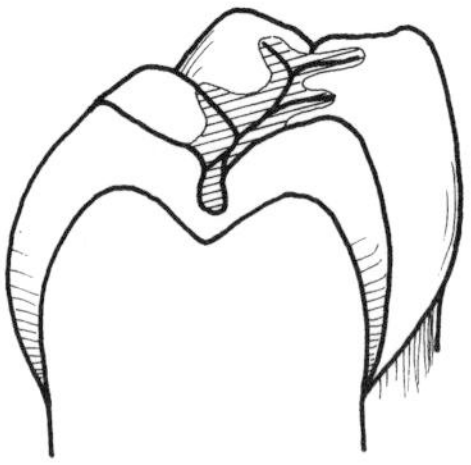

Fig. 10.1e

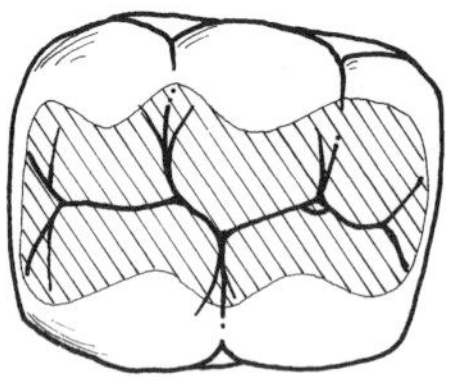

Fig. 10.1f

Procedure	Method	Rationale	Notes
	If a deeper cavity has been made, fill the cavity first with composite resin restorative material (i.e. filled resin); then cover it and the adjacent fissures with unfilled resin (Figs 10.1g, h, i, j).	Composite restorative material is stronger and more resistant to abrasion than unfilled resin and is therefore more appropriate to use in a large cavity.	Glass-ionomer cement may be used instead of composite resin restorative material to fill the cavity.

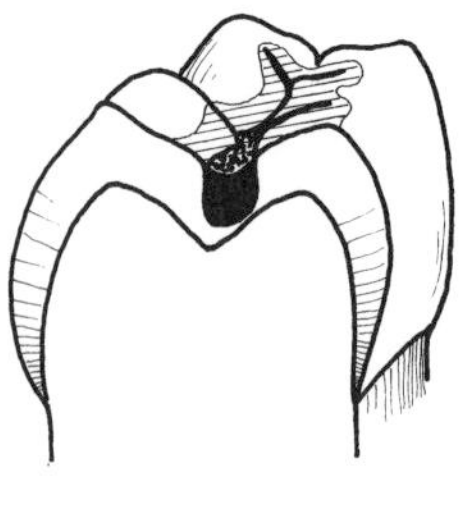

Fig. 10.1g

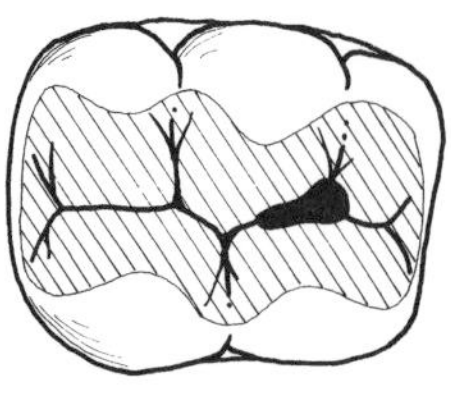

Fig. 10.1h

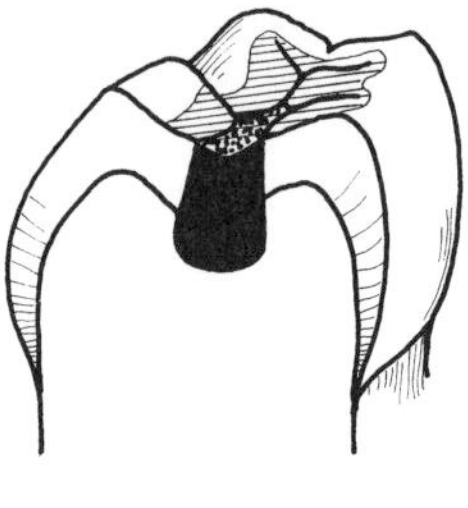

Fig. 10.1i

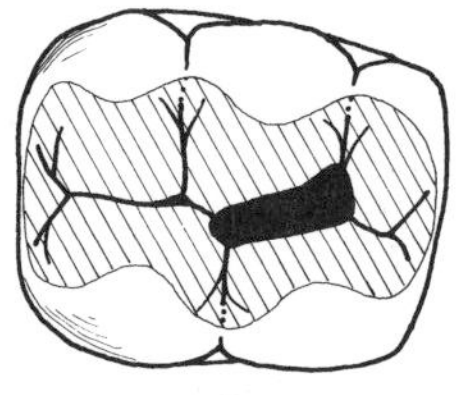

Fig. 10.1j

with a bur, the part of the fissure where diagnosis is uncertain or where early caries exists, to fill the resulting small cavity with composite resin and to seal the adjacent fissures. This type of restoration was originally called a sealant restoration (Simonsen & Stallard 1977) but is now also referred to as a preventive resin restoration (Simonsen 1985). It has been shown in clinical trials to be effective (Raadal 1978, Simonsen 1980, Houpt et al 1988, Welbury et al 1990).

10.2 RESTORATIONS FOR POSTERIOR TEETH

Amalgam is still the material most commonly used for the restoration of Class I and II cavities in permanent teeth, but the continued development of composite resins suggests that these materials may provide an acceptable alternative to amalgam. Composite resin or glass-ionomer cement is often preferred to amalgam for Class V cavities.

The techniques for cavity preparation and restoration of posterior teeth will not be described here; they are similar to those described for primary teeth in Chapter 8, and further details may be obtained from textbooks of operative dentistry.

The use of stainless steel crowns for primary molars has been described in Chapter 8. These crowns are also available in sizes suitable for permanent first molars and are particularly useful for restoring very carious or hypoplastic teeth in children aged 7–9 years. They may serve only as temporary restorations for a year or two before extracting the teeth at the most appropriate stage of dental development (Ch. 19), or

they may last satisfactorily until adolescence, when a permanent type of crown may be considered.

10.3 RESTORATIONS FOR ANTERIOR TEETH

The most common sites for carious attack in permanent anterior teeth are the approximal and labial surfaces (Class III and V lesions respectively). Approximal lesions may undermine and cause fracture of incisal corners (Class IV lesions).

Composite resin is normally used to restore these types of cavity in permanent anterior teeth. Glass-ionomer cement may be used for Class III and V cavities but the material is less translucent and therefore less aesthetic than composite resin (and it is not strong enough for incisal corner restorations).

Cavity preparation for a Class V lesion simply involves removing the caries, extending the cavity to sound dentine and enamel walls, and bevelling the enamel margin. It is not essential to make the cavity retentive. If composite resin is to be used, either a dentine-bonding agent is first painted on the cavity floor and walls, or glass-ionomer cement is used to line the dentine; the composite resin then adheres to the dentine-bonding agent or to the glass-ionomer and the acid-etched enamel walls of the cavity. Glass-ionomer restorations are retained by their adhesion to enamel and dentine.

A matrix is required when placing a Class V restoration. Several types are available, of which two are illustrated in Figure 10.2. A clear matrix must, of course, be chosen when using a light-curing material.

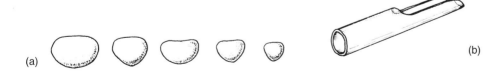

(a)   (b)

Fig. 10.2 Matrices for Class V restorations: (a) coated tin, (b) cellulose acetate.

Technique: Class III composite resin restoration

Procedure	Method	Rationale	Notes
1. Gain access to the caries	Recommended burs are: *for high-speed handpiece—* small round diamond 520 small round tungsten carbide 1 *for slow-speed handpiece—* round steel No. 1/2 or 1.		
	Whenever possible, gain access to the cavity from the palatal/lingual aspect (Fig. 10.3a). If the cavity is large, enter through the surface most destroyed by caries. Penetrate the enamel as close as possible to the interdental space without risking damage to the adjacent tooth.	Best appearance is achieved if the labial surface is preserved. In the mandible, however, access is usually made through the labial surface because this is much easier and because restorations in mandibular incisors are hidden behind the lower lip.	

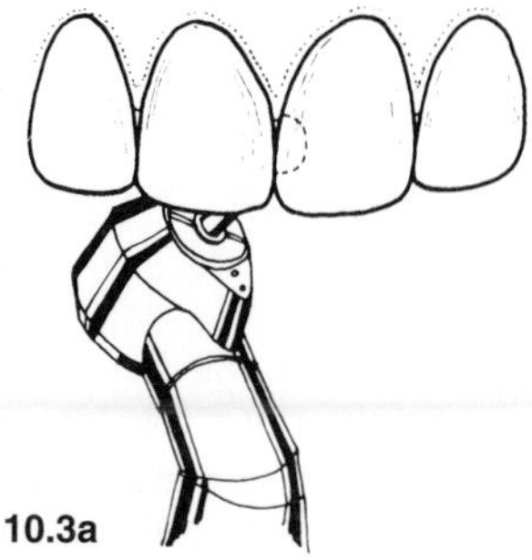

Fig. 10.3a

2. Remove the caries	(The method is described for a maxillary incisor, assuming that access is made through the palatal surface). As soon as the bur enters the cavity, change to a $\frac{1}{2}$ or 1 flat fissure bur in the slow-speed handpiece (Fig. 10.3b), enlarge the cavity from incisal to gingival, and shape the palatal wall so that it becomes almost semi-circular in outline.	Preparing the cavity outline with a slow-speed handpiece is recommended because the cavity is usually small and the pulp may easily be exposed by an inadvertent movement of a high-speed instrument. Creating a semi-circular outline permits adequate access for removal of caries and for subsequent insertion of restorative material.	
	Do not extend the cavity outline more than is necessary to remove caries and to provide access for lining and restorative materials. Use an excavator or a round bur in a slow-speed handpiece to remove caries from the floor and/or walls of the cavity (Fig. 10.3c). If a bur is chosen, run it at a slow speed and with light pressure.		

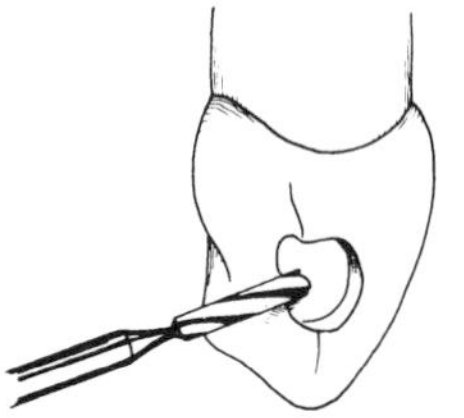

Fig. 10.3b   **Fig. 10.3c**

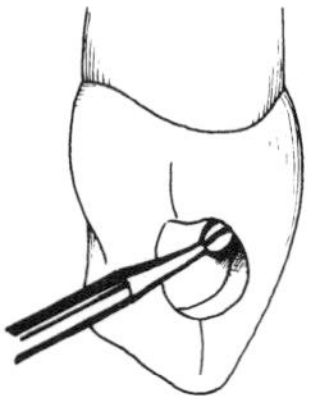

3. Plan the final cavity outline and shape	Consider whether the cavity outline, following caries removal, needs to be modified. Consider whether the cavity needs further preparation to provide retention for the restoration.	Labial or palatal margins may have to be taken back if the walls are very thin and weak. Although retention of the restoration will be aided by acid-etching the enamel margin and can be further enhanced by using a dentine-bonding agent, it is prudent to provide mechanical retention if possible.	In small cavities, a slight general undercut of the walls is sufficient; this may be more pronounced on the gingival and incisal aspects.

Technique: Class III composite resin restoration *(contd)*

Procedure	Method	Rationale	Notes
4. Complete the cavity preparation	Define the cavity margin using a small chisel or margin trimmer (Fig. 10.3d), gaining access through the cavity.	Hand instruments are preferred to burs for defining the margin of the cavity because access with appropriate burs may be difficult and the burs might damage the adjacent tooth.	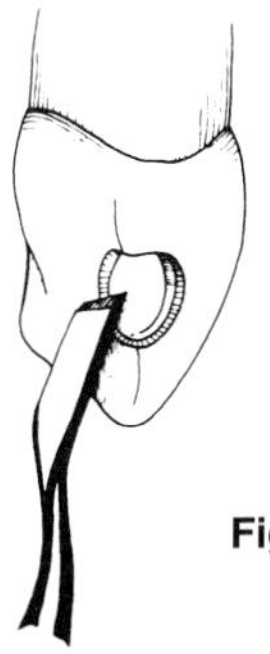 **Fig. 10.3d**
	If retention is considered inadequate (particularly in a large cavity), use a No. 1/2 or 1 round bur to produce a groove in the dentine of the gingival floor (Fig. 10.3e) and a pit in the incisal corner (Fig. 10.3f).	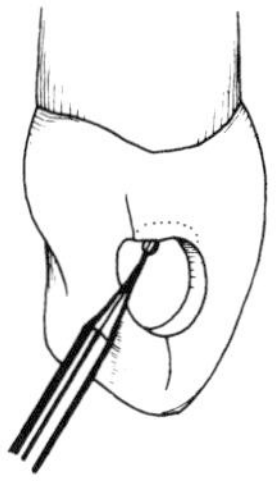 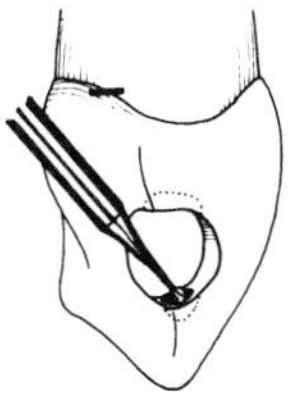	Care must be taken when making an incisal pit because the incisal edge of the tooth may be weakened. **Fig. 10.3e** **Fig. 10.3f**
	Alternatively, and especially in a large cavity with a weak palatal wall, prepare a retentive 'lock' in the palatal surface, using a small flat fissure bur (Fig. 10.3g); this lock should be about 2 mm deep, i.e. just into dentine. Check the enamel margins and smooth if necessary with a chisel or margin trimmer.	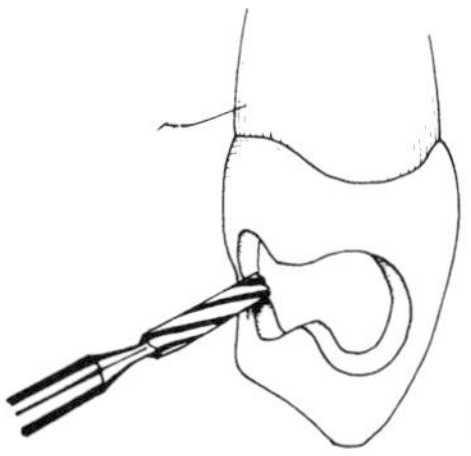 **Fig. 10.3g**	A similar retentive 'lock' may be made in the lingual surface of a mandibular incisor.
5. Wash, dry and assess the cavity preparation	Wash the cavity with water and dry with compressed air. Confirm that the cavity is caries-free and otherwise satisfactory.		
6. Line the cavity	Apply a small amount of quick-setting calcium hydroxide, carried on the end of a fine instrument, to the pulpal wall of the cavity. When it is set, remove any excess from retentive grooves or pits, or from cavity margins, using a small excavator.	The aim is to cover the pulpal wall but not to obliterate retention in the cavity.	
7. Etch the enamel at the margin of the cavity	Apply 30–50% phosphoric acid to the enamel with a cotton wool pledget, sponge pad or small brush. After 1 minute, wash with water and dry thoroughly.	Etching ensures that the composite resin bonds to the enamel to produce a good marginal seal.	The adjacent tooth should be protected from acid by a matrix strip.

Technique: Class III composite resin restoration *(contd)*

Procedure	Method	Rationale	Notes
8. Fit a matrix	Use a cellulose acetate or other suitable matrix strip. Check its fit around the cavity, noting especially its fit at the cervical margin. If possible, wedge it firmly at the cervical margin (Fig. 10.3h), placing the wedge from the labial or lingual side; otherwise hold the strip in place with a finger. 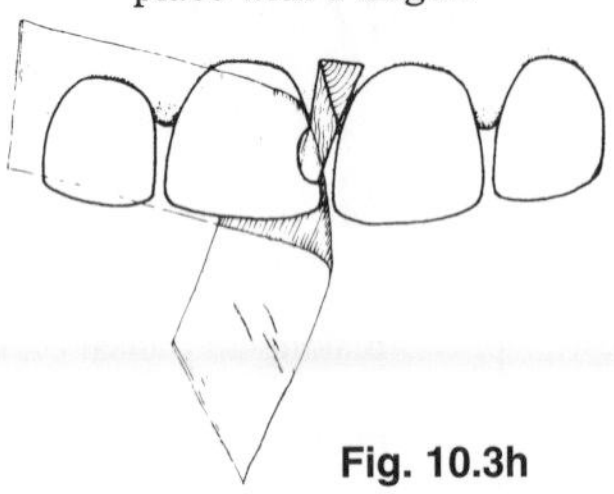	It is often impossible to fit the strip tightly to all margins of the cavity, but fitting to the cervical margin is especially important because it is there that any excess filling material will be most difficult to trim when it is hardened. 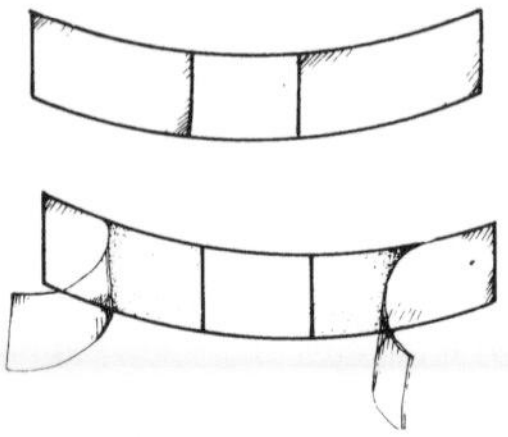	Cellulose acetate matrix strips are most commonly used, but specially-coated soft metal strips are also available for use with autopolymerizing materials. One type of soft metal matrix has adhesive ends which help to maintain it in position around the tooth; when the matrix is positioned, a thin covering film is peeled off and the adhesive end is pressed on to adjacent teeth (Fig. 10.3i).

Fig. 10.3h

Fig. 10.3i

Procedure	Method	Rationale	Notes
9. Fill the cavity	Mix the composite resin according to the manufacturer's instructions (if using an autopolymerizing material). Estimate the amount required to half fill the cavity, carry it to the tooth on a suitable plastic instrument, and work it into the cavity undercuts. Alternatively, use a special syringe to insert composite into the cavity. If using an autopolymerizing resin, fill the cavity within 1 minute. If using a light-sensitive resin, working time is extended. Fold one end of the matrix strip around the palatal surface of the tooth and place an index finger firmly on it, in the palatal concavity. With the other hand, pull the other end of the strip across the labial aspect of the crown and pull it tightly, making sure that it is correctly placed at the cervical margin. Hold the strip in this way, without movement, for the length of time recommended by manufacturer for polymerization to take place.	Moving the strip might disturb the composite resin before it has polymerized, and result in poor adaptation to the cavity margins.	A thin layer of unfilled resin may be applied to the etched enamel before placing the restorative material, but this is not essential. Several types of special syringe are available. Autopolymerizing composite resins harden within about 2 minutes.
10. Finish the restoration	Remove the matrix strip and trim excess beyond the cavity margin with a sharp excavator. If possible, limit any further trimming to the margin of the restoration, using fine diamond or tungsten carbide instruments for accessible parts of the margin, and an abrasive composite finishing strip for the cervical part.	The smoothest surface obtainable on a composite material is that which polymerizes against a smooth matrix strip.	If the bulk of the restoration needs some trimming, zirconium silicate discs leave a smooth surface. Composite polishing paste may also be used.

REFERENCES

Going R E 1984 Sealant effect on incipient caries, enamel maturation, and future caries susceptibility. Journal of Dental Education 48: 35–41

Houpt M, Fuks A, Eidelman E, Shey Z 1988 Composite/sealant restorations: 6 1/2-year result. Pediatric Dentistry 10: 304–306

Raadal M 1978 Follow-up study of sealing and filling with composite resins in the prevention of occlusal caries. Community Dentistry and Oral Epidemiology 6: 176–180

Simonsen R J 1980 Preventive resin restorations: three-year results. Journal of the American Dental Association 100: 535–539

Simonsen R J 1985 Conservation of tooth structure in restorative dentistry. Quintessence International 16: 15–24

Simonsen R J, Stallard R E 1977 Sealant restorations utilising a diluted filled composite resin. Quintessence International, report no. 1514

O'Brien M 1994 Children's dental health in the United Kingdom 1993. Office of Population Censuses and Surveys. Her Majesty's Stationery Office, London, p 25

Welbury R R, Walls A W G, Murray J J, McCabe J F 1990 The management of occlusal caries in permanent molars. A 5-year clinical trial comparing a minimal composite with an amalgam restoration. British Dental Journal 169: 361–366

Treatment of abnormalities of the primary and mixed dentitions

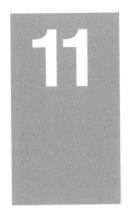

Normal development of occlusion

Table 11.1 Chronology of development of the primary dentition (from Lunt & Law 1974).

Teeth	Calcification begins (months in utero)	Crown complete (months after birth)	Eruption (months)
Incisors	4	$1\frac{1}{2}$–3	6–9
Canines	4–5	9	18–20
First molars	4–5	6	12–15
Second molars	4–6	12	24–36

Root development is complete 1–$1\frac{1}{2}$ years after tooth eruption.

Part Four of this book is concerned with the treatment of abnormalities of the primary and mixed dentitions. However, before considering abnormalities, a short account is given in this chapter of normal development of the occlusion.

11.1 THE PRIMARY DENTITION

Formation of the primary dentition begins after 4–5 months of intrauterine life (Table 11.1). The first teeth usually erupt 6–7 months after birth and all primary teeth have usually erupted by $2\frac{1}{2}$—3 years of age.

Many opinions have been expressed about the features that characterize a normal primary dentition, but three features are seen frequently enough for them to be considered normal:

1. *'Straight' or 'mesial step' second molar relationship.* In most dentitions the primary second molars are in cusp-to-cusp occlusion so that their distal surfaces are in the same vertical plane (Fig. 11.1a). Frequently, however, there is a mesial 'step' in this vertical plane (Fig. 11.1b); this can also be

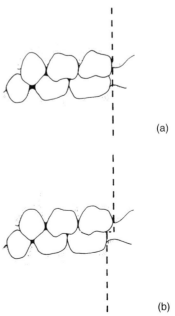

Fig. 11.1 Primary dentition with (a) 'straight' second molar relationship, and (b) 'mesial step' second molar relationship.

129

considered normal (Baume 1950, Ravn 1975).
Distal 'steps' indicate a Class II arch relationship
(Foster & Hamilton 1969).

2. *Incisor spacing.* Spacing between the primary incisors
   is normal, and indicates that the permanent
   successors will probably have adequate space into
   which to erupt. Lack of spacing or imbrication of
   primary incisors are signs that the permanent
   incisors will probably be crowded when they erupt.

3. *Anthropoid (primate) spaces.* The most common sites
   for spaces in the primary dentition are in the canine
   regions (Foster & Hamilton 1969). The 'anthropoid
   spaces' are mesial to the maxillary canines and distal
   to the mandibular canines.

Considerable variations occur in the overbite and
overjet of incisors and it is difficult to define normality
(Foster 1990).

Once the primary dentition is completed, the
dimensions and form of the arches change very little
until permanent teeth begin to erupt; any increases in
width and length that have been reported are small
(Baume 1950, Clinch 1951, Foster et al 1972).
Interdental spaces in spaced dentitions do not increase
in width, nor do spaces develop in unspaced
dentitions. However, two changes may be seen during
this period: attrition of teeth (especially of anterior
teeth), and reduction of overbite and overjet, so that
the incisors may, by the age of 5–6 years, occlude
'edge to edge'.

11.2 ERUPTION OF PERMANENT FIRST MOLARS

The normal or Class I occlusal relationship of permanent first molars is shown when the tip of the mesio-
buccal cusp of the maxillary molar occludes in the
buccal groove of the mandibular molar. Baume (1950)
suggested three ways by which this relationship may be
achieved:

1. In primary dentitions which terminate in marked
   mesial 'steps', the permanent first molars erupt
   directly into Class I occlusion (Fig. 11.2).

2. In spaced primary dentitions with straight terminal
   planes, eruption of permanent first molars pushes
   the mandibular primary molars forward into the
   anthropoid spaces so that mesial-step relationships
   are created. The mandibular permanent first molars
   are then able to erupt into Class I occlusion (Fig.
   11.3).

3. In 'closed' primary dentitions (i.e. those having no
   interdental spaces), mesial movement of the
   mandibular primary molars cannot occur.

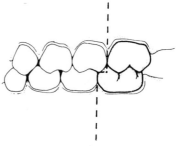

Fig. 11.2 Eruption of permanent first molars directly into Class I relationship.

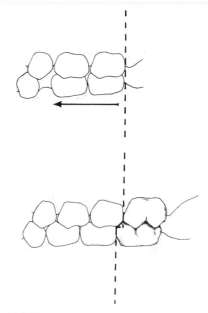

Fig. 11.3 Eruption of permanent first molars into Class I relationship after mesial movement of mandibular primary molars into the anthropoid space.

The permanent molars therefore erupt cusp-to-cusp
(i.e. $\frac{1}{2}$ unit Class II), and normal occlusion is only
achieved when the primary second molars are
replaced by the smaller second premolars (Fig.
11.4a, b). The permanent molars move forward into
the spaces that become available, and since these are
greater in the mandible than in the maxilla (because
mandibular primary second molars are particularly
large teeth), the mandibular permanent molars are
able to move forward more than the maxillary
molars, and establish Class I relationships.

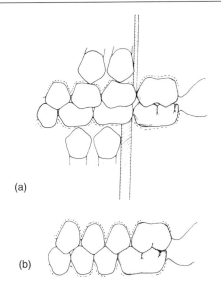

(a)

(b)

Fig. 11.4 (a) Eruption of permanent first molars into cusp-to-cusp (1/2 unit Class II) relationship and (b) establishment of Class I relationship after exfoliation of primary molars.

11.3 ERUPTION OF PERMANENT INCISORS

Spacing between primary incisors is an important factor in allowing the relatively large permanent incisors to be accommodated in the arch. Further

space is provided by labial proclination of permanent incisors, which increases the arch perimeter, and by alveolar bone growth, which increases the intercanine width of the arch. This growth is usually complete when the lateral incisors reach full eruption, so that crowding of incisors at that stage of development does not improve: indeed it may worsen in later years due to pressure from crowded posterior teeth.

Eruption of each tooth pair is usually symmetrical; delay of a few months in the eruption of a tooth after the contralateral tooth has erupted usually indicates an abnormality requiring investigation.

Maxillary incisors often erupt with some distal inclination of their crowns, an appearance sometimes referred to as 'the ugly duckling stage'; usually they straighten gradually with the eruption of lateral incisors and canines (Fig. 11.5).

11.4 ERUPTION OF PREMOLARS AND CANINES

The sum of the mesio-distal dimensions of the primary canine and molars in each quadrant of the dentition always exceeds that of the successional canine and premolars (Fig. 11.6); the excess is accounted for chiefly by the difference in size between the primary second molar and the premolar that replaces it. The excess space, sometimes referred to as the 'leeway

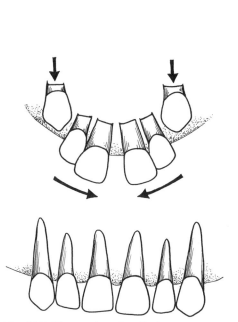

Fig. 11.5 Closure of median diastema.

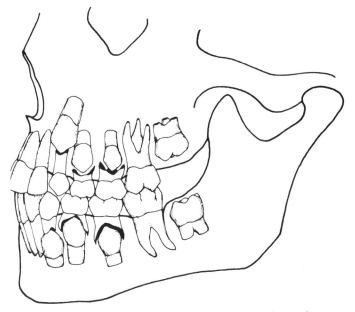

Fig. 11.6 Eruption of permanent canines and premolars. The sum of the mesio-distal dimensions of primary canines and molars is greater than that of their successors.

space', is important in some dentitions for allowing final adjustment of first molar occlusion. Also, it ensures (if the primary teeth are not prematurely removed) that there will be adequate space for the eruption of permanent canines and premolars.

The occlusion does not remain static but undergoes some changes during adolescence. These changes may include a decrease in arch length (mesial movement of premolars and molars) and in intercanine width, and an increase in incisor irregularity. However, it is not possible to predict the changes that will occur in an individual patient (Sinclair & Little 1983).

11.5 CHRONOLOGY OF TOOTH DEVELOPMENT

Knowledge of the chronology of tooth development and eruption is essential to the understanding of the clinical features and aetiology of many of the developmental abnormalities described in the following chapters. The bare facts are given in Tables 11.1 and 11.2 but, since it is not easy to remember all this information, a summary is presented in Table 11.3 in a form that may be easier to assimilate. Because 3–6-month intervals have been used for the primary dentition and 3-year intervals for the permanent dentition, the table only offers a rough guide, but this

Table 11.3 An approximate chronology of tooth development and eruption.

Age	Crown development starts	Crown fully formed	Eruption
	PRIMARY DENTITION		
3–6 months in utero	A B C D E		
3–6 months after birth		A B D	
6–9 months		C	A B
1 year		E	D
1½ years			C
2–3 years			E
	PERMANENT DENTITION		
birth–6 months	[6 1 2*] 3		
3 years	[4 5 7]	[6 1 2]	
6 years		[4 5 7] 3	[6 1 2]
9 years			3†
12 years			[4 5 7] 3‡

* Although included in this group, it must be remembered that *maxillary* lateral incisors start developing later than other incisors (10–12 months)
† mandibular canine
‡ maxillary canine

Table 11.2 Chronology of development of the permanent dentition (from Schour & Massler 1940).

	Calcification begins	Crown complete (years)	Eruption (years)
Central incisors			
mandibular	3–4 months	4–5	6–7
maxillary			7–8
Lateral incisors			
mandibular	3–4 months	4–5	7–8
maxillary	10–12 months		8–9
Canines			
mandibular	4–5 months	6–7	9–10
maxillary			11–12
First premolars	1½–2 years	5–6	10–12
Second premolars	2–2½ years	6–7	10–12
First molars	birth	2½–3	6
Second molars	2½–3 years	7–8	12–13
Third molars	7–10 years	12–16	16–21

Root development is complete 3–4 years after tooth eruption.

is adequate for most clinical applications. It is convenient, as suggested in the table, to think of two distinct groups or 'crops' of permanent teeth, the first comprising the first molars and incisors, and the second the premolars and second molars; canines must be considered separately because crown formation starts with the first group but ends with the second, and the mandibular canines erupt about 3 years before the maxillary canines.

11.6 MONITORING THE DEVELOPING DENTITION

Paediatric dentistry embraces all aspects of the dental care of children, an essential part of which involves monitoring the developing dentition and, when abnormalities are detected, taking interceptive action if appropriate or referring to an orthodontist. This is the field of 'interceptive orthodontics' but it is primarily the province of the dentist responsible for the child's overall dental care, the orthodontist's role being to provide specialist advice and treatment when required.

Dentists should always have an orthodontic opinion about their child patients, and sometimes require an orthodontist's opinion.

Chapters 12 to 22 describe many of the abnormalities that may be detected during the development of the dentition. Points that should be considered routinely when monitoring the developing dentition are summarized in Table 11.4 and reviewed below.

11.6.1 Age 3–6 years

Interdental spacing: A 'normal' ('ideal') primary dentition shows spacing between the anterior teeth (p. 130). Although intercanine arch width increases just before and during eruption of permanent incisors, lack of spacing between primary incisors is a sign that permanent incisors will be crowded when they erupt. This observation makes it all the more important to monitor eruption of permanent incisors because some interceptive action may be indicated to accommodate them in the arch (Ch. 18).

Although various abnormalities may occur in the primary dentition (for example, supernumerary teeth, congenital absence of teeth, double teeth, crossbites), generally no treatment is indicated. Therefore, routine full-mouth examination to detect abnormalities is not justified during this age range—this is better carried out at the age of 8–9 years (see below).

11.6.2 Age 6–8 years

Crowding of erupting permanent incisors: Although lack of spacing in the primary dentition allows a prediction that permanent teeth will be crowded, the first actual sign of crowding is noted when the incisors erupt. An important decision must be taken: either to extract primary canines to provide space for the permanent incisors, or to take no action and reassess the situation when the child is about 10 years of age. This subject is discussed in Chapter 18.

Anterior crossbite: An incipient crossbite of permanent incisors is easily detected, and simple treatment at this age avoids more complicated treatment later (Ch. 19).

Ectopic eruption of permanent first molars: Ectopic eruption of a permanent first molar results in its impaction against the crown or root of the primary second molar. Although the condition may be transient, treatment at this age may be required (Ch. 12).

Open bite and increased overjet: A possible cause of anterior open bite and increased overjet is persistent digit sucking. The child should be gently encouraged to abandon the habit, and a simple appliance may be inserted at about 8–9 years of the age if the child is keen to cooperate (Ch. 21).

11.6.3 Age 8–10 years

Radiographic examination: An important step in monitoring the developing dentition is to establish radiographically that there is a normal number of developing teeth and that there are no abnormalities that might adversely affect the developing dentition. The age of 8–9 years is an appropriate time to do this; the recommended radiographs are outlined on pages 8–9.

Availability of space for unerupted canines and premolars: A normal dentition at the age of 8 years consists of permanent first molars and central and lateral incisors, and primary canines and molars.

If the permanent incisors are in good alignment (showing no imbrication) and all the primary canines and molars are present, it can be said that dental development is progressing normally, and it can be confidently predicted that adequate space exists in the arch to accommodate premolars and permanent canines when they erupt.

If, however, the incisors are imbricated, or premature loss of primary molars has allowed mesial drift of permanent first molars to occur, there will clearly be inadequate space for the canines and premolars to

Table 11.4 Points to consider when monitoring the developing dentition.

Age 3–6 years	Age 6–8 years	Age 8–10 years	Age 10–12 years
Interdental spacing	Crowding of permanent incisors	Radiographic examination	Eruption of premolars and permanent canines
	Anterior crossbite	Availability of space for unerupted canines and premolars	
	Ectopic eruption of permanent first molars	Long-term prognosis of permanent first molars	
	Open bite and increased overjet	Position of maxillary permanent canines	

erupt in good alignment. It is important to assess the degree of space deficiency because this affects further treatment planning decisions during the mixed dentition period: in particular the importance of space maintenance and therefore the importance of conserving the remaining primary teeth. The assessment of the degree of crowding in the mixed dentition is discussed in Chapter 17.

The long-term prognosis of permanent first molars: It is vitally important to make a decision at about this stage of dental development about the long-term prognosis of permanent first molars. The factors that must be considered in making this assessment are outlined in Chapter 22.

It is emphasized that this decision must be made primarily by the dentist who has long-term responsibility for the child's dental care. An orthodontist's opinion may be sought, especially if it is anticipated that the patient will be referred later for orthodontic treatment, but the general practitioner is in a better position to assess all the social and management factors that influence the decision.

The position of maxillary canines: The path of eruption of maxillary permanent canine teeth is longer than that of any other tooth, and it is important to establish, by the age of 10 years, that they are erupting normally.

At about the age of 9 years, maxillary canines that are developing normally become palpable high in the buccal sulcus, above the primary canines; and by the age of 10 years, some mobility of the primary canines should be detectable. If at least one of these signs is not evident by the age of 10 years, radiographs should be taken to determine the position of maxillary canines. Two radiographs are required, taken at different angles to apply the principle of parallax; either

1. two periapicals — directed from mesial and distal to the canine

or 2. two maxillary anterior occlusals — one midline and one oblique

or 3. one off-centre periapical and one midline anterior occlusal.

If the maxillary canine appears to be abnormally placed, a decision must be taken concerning the best course of action. The alternatives are outlined on pages 139–140.

11.6.4 Age 10–12 years

Eruption of premolars and permanent canines: It is important to assess whether there is enough space in the arch for eruption of the premolars and permanent canines in good alignment. If crowding is predicted, or if there are other occlusal irregularities, a full orthodontic assessment must be made. Most orthodontic treatment is commenced between the ages of 10 and 12 years.

REFERENCES

Baume L J 1950 Physiological tooth migration and its significance to the development of occlusion. Journal of Dental Research 29: 132–133, 331–337, 338–348, 440–447

Clinch L M 1951 An analysis of serial models between three and eight years of age. Dental Record 71: 61–72

Foster T D 1990 A textbook of orthodontics, 3rd edn. Oxford, Blackwell, pp 46–47

Foster T D, Hamilton M C 1969 Occlusion in the primary dentition. British Dental Journal 126: 76–79

Foster T D, Grundy M C, Lavelle C L B 1972 Changes in occlusion in the primary dentition between 2 1/2 and 5 1/2 years of age. Transactions of the European Orthodontic Society 1972: 75–84

Lunt R C, Law D B 1974 A review of the chronology of calcification of deciduous teeth. Journal of the American Dental Association 89: 599–606

Ravn J J 1975 Occlusion in the primary dentition in three year old children. Scandinavian Journal of Dental Research 83: 123–130

Schour I, Massler M 1940 Studies in tooth development: the growth pattern of human teeth. Journal of the American Dental Association 27: 1918–1931

Sinclair P M, Little R M 1983 Maturation of untreated normal occlusions. American Journal of Orthodontics 83: 114–123

RECOMMENDED READING

Richardson A 1995 Interceptive orthodontics, 3rd edn. British Dental Association, London, ch 2

Van der Linden P G M 1983 Development of the dentition. Quintessence, Chicago

12 Abnormalities of tooth eruption

12.1 NATAL AND NEONATAL TEETH

Rarely, one or more teeth are erupted at birth or erupt during the first month of life; these teeth are termed natal and neonatal teeth, respectively (Massler & Savara 1950).

The crown of a natal or neonatal tooth may appear normal or it may be a simple shell-like structure; there is little or no root and the crown is loosely attached to the alveolus by soft tissue. At birth most of the crown of a natal tooth may be erupted, or only the incisal edge may be visible, enveloped in soft tissue. Root growth progresses normally and the tooth gradually becomes firmer, but the enamel is often hypomineralized and tends to break away.

Most natal and neonatal teeth are mandibular incisors and are usually of the normal primary dentition, not supernumerary teeth (Bedi & Yan 1990, To 1991).

Treatment

Natal and neonatal teeth should be retained if possible because they are usually part of the normal dentition. However, if most of the crown has erupted and is not therefore supported by soft tissue, the tooth may be so loose that extraction is necessary because it causes discomfort during feeding either to the child or to the mother (if she breast-feeds), or because it might become dislodged and be either swallowed or inhaled.

12.2 'TEETHING'

Eruption of the primary dentition usually begins in the fifth or sixth month of a child's life. The first appearance of normal teeth is eagerly awaited by the parents since it represents an important early milestone in development. In most cases eruption of teeth causes no distress to the child or parents but sometimes the process causes local irritation, which is usually minor but which may be severe enough to interfere with the child's sleep. The small primary incisors usually erupt without difficulty; 'teething' problems are more commonly associated with eruption of the relatively large molars.

The signs of teething may be manifested locally and/or systematically (Seward 1971, 1972a):

Local	Redness or swelling of the gingiva over the erupting tooth.
	Patches of erythema on the cheeks.
Systemic	General irritability, and crying.
	Loss of appetite.
	Sleeplessness.
	Increased salivation and drooling.
	Reduced appetite.
	Increased thirst.
	Circumoral rash.

Treatment

Local

1. *Teething toys.* A baby uses hands and mouth to explore unfamiliar objects. A variety of teething rings,

rattles and keys are available in mothercraft shops. They are designed to satisfy the natural tendency of the child to bite and suck. The baby may obtain relief from soreness by the pressure of biting, and teething toys have a useful function. Parents should be advised to purchase only well-made, smooth toys; rough toys can increase irritation in the mouth, and some cheap products contain high levels of lead.

2. **Teething foods.** Hard rusk or biscuit preparations are used in the same way as teething toys. Teething foods consist mainly of flour and fat. It is important that they should contain no sugar or sweetening, since this might contribute to the development of a 'sweet tooth'.

3. **Topical medicaments.** Various types of ointments and jellies are available for topical application to the gingiva. Common ingredients include salicylates, which combine local counter-irritant and anti-inflammatory properties with systemic analgesic and anti-pyretic effects; antiseptics, which control infection at the site of tooth eruption; and local analgesics, which provide rapid but short-lived pain relief. Some topical preparations for the control of teething problems are listed in Table 12.1. Preparations containing salicylate should not be used very frequently as they may give rise to salicylate poisoning.

Systemic

Treatment by systemic administration of drugs should be considered only if local treatment has been ineffective. Two main types of drugs are used: analgesics (to relieve pain) and hypnotics (to aid sleep).

1. *Analgesics.* Several sugar-free paracetamol preparations are available. 5 ml contains 120 mg of paracetamol.
   Dosage: Up to 1 year—5 ml at bedtime
           1–5 years—10 ml at bedtime

2. *Hypnotics and sedatives.* There is understandable reluctance to prescribe these drugs for very young children. However, a succession of sleepless nights imposes a severe strain on parents and other members of the family, and a short course of a hypnotic drug will help to restore normal rhythms of sleep. It may be necessary to use hypnotics in combination with local and systemic analgesics.
   Chloral Elixir Paediatric BPC. 5 ml contains 200 mg of chloral hydrate.
   Dosage: Up to 1 year—2.5 ml twice daily
           1–5 years—2.5–5 ml three times daily
   Dichloralphenazone Elixir BPC (Welldorm Elixir). 5 ml contains 225 mg of dichloralphenazone.
   Dosage: Up to 1 year—2.5–5 ml at bedtime
           1–5 years—5–10 ml at bedtime

Guidance for the selection of treatment is given below:

Complaint	Treatment
Irritation at site of tooth eruption.	Topical application.
Daytime irritability and fretfulness.	Topical application and systemic analgesic.
Disturbed sleep.	Topical application, systemic analgesic and hypnotic.

12.3 ERUPTION CYSTS

Eruption cysts appear as smooth, bluish swellings of the oral mucosa overlying erupting teeth. They occur most frequently over primary molars, but also over primary anterior teeth and, occasionally, over permanent teeth. Some eruption cysts originate from remnants of reduced enamel epithelium and are true dentigerous cysts, located in soft tissue rather than in bone (Soames & Southam 1993); others are simply an

Table 12.1 Active ingredients in preparations used for the control of teething symptoms.

Name	Local analgesic	Antiseptic	Analgesic/anti-inflammatory agent
Bonjela	none	0.01% cetalkonium chloride 4.6% glycerin 39% alcohol	8.7% choline salicylate 0.05% menthol
Dentinox	0.3% lignocaine hydrochloride	0.1% cetylpyridinium chloride 0.3% polyethoxdodecane 3% alcohol	0.06% menthol 0.08% myrrh tincture
Pyralvex	none	5% anthraquinone glycosides	1% salicylic acid
Teejel	none	0.01% cetalkonium chloride	8.7% choline salicylate

accumulation of tissue fluid and blood in a dilated follicular space around the crown of the erupting tooth and are therefore more correctly termed eruption haematomas (Shafer et al 1983).

Eruption and dentigerous cysts should be considered distinct clinical entities because they differ in several important respects (Seward 1973). For example, eruption cysts are almost always associated with primary teeth and resolve on eruption of the teeth, whereas dentigerous cysts are very rarely associated with primary teeth and do not resolve spontaneously.

Eruption cysts may be painless, but are painful if they become infected or traumatized by opposing teeth.

Treatment

Most eruption cysts are transient and resolve by rupture of the cyst, followed by normal eruption of the tooth. Occasionally the problem persists, causing prolonged crying and loss of sleep. If conservative treatment, as given for teething problems, is ineffective, it may be necessary to excise the cyst.

Simple incision of the cyst with a scalpel under topical or local analgesia may be effective. However, a single incision may heal rapidly and allow recurrence of the cyst; because of this possibility, the more thorough technique advocated by Seward (1972b) may be preferred. A longitudinal incision is made along the side of the swelling and a blade of a pair of 'mosquito' forceps is inserted into the cystic space over the crown of the tooth. The roof of the cyst is then held taut whilst an elliptical portion is cut away.

12.4 INFRAOCCLUSION (SUBMERGENCE)

An infraoccluded tooth is one that has failed to maintain its position relative to adjacent teeth in the developing dentition, and is therefore 'submerged' below the occlusal level. Infraocclusion is usually associated with primary molars but permanent molars are occasionally affected (Oliver et al 1986). Surveys of submerged primary molars in children up to 12 years of age have reported prevalence figures ranging from 1.3% to 8.9% (Andlaw 1977, Kurol 1981).

Mandibular primary molars are affected more commonly than maxillary molars. In most studies the tooth most commonly affected was the primary first molar but in others it was the second molar. The second molar tends to become grossly submerged, perhaps below gingival level, more frequently than does the first molar.

The mechanism of infraocclusion is not properly understood, but appears to be related to ankylosis (Kurol & Magnusson 1984), possibly brought about by excessive bone deposition during the alternating resorption and repair phases that characterize normal root resorption of primary teeth; further occlusal movement of the tooth is retarded or arrested, and it therefore falls below the occlusal level of neighbouring teeth.

Treatment

An infraoccluded primary molar need not always be extracted: many affected primary teeth (especially first molars) exfoliate normally and do not interfere with the eruption of premolars (Brearley & McKibben 1973). However, some form of treatment becomes necessary if there are radiological signs of interference with premolar eruption, or if there is a possibility of adjacent teeth tilting over the submerged tooth, or if there is a danger that the tooth may become submerged below gingival level.

The type of treatment required depends on the degree of infraocclusion (Andlaw 1974):

1. **Minimal infraocclusion (marginal ridge of submerged tooth occlusal to adjacent contact areas)**: Monitor to assess whether the condition worsens. Obtain study models to aid this assessment. Take radiographs every 6–12 months to determine whether premolar eruption is being affected.

2. **Moderate infraocclusion (marginal ridge of submerged tooth just cervical to adjacent contact areas)**: A short period of clinical and radiological observation, as outlined above, may again be appropriate, but in the case of moderate infraocclusion it is more likely that one or more indications for treatment will be present. There are two alternatives:

   a. *Retain the submerged tooth.* If there are no indications of interference with premolar eruption, the submerged tooth may be retained. However, it may be necessary to restore normal contacts with adjacent teeth; this may be achieved by fitting a stainless steel crown (Ch. 8), or by building up the occlusal surface with composite resin (Gorelick 1977).

   b. *Extract the submerged tooth.* It is probable, but not inevitable, that because of ankylosis the tooth will be more difficult to extract than a normal tooth. A surgical approach may be necessary, and appropriate preoperative arrangements for this should be made.

   It is wrong to remove any primary tooth without

considering the effect that the extraction may have on the development of the dentition; the need to balance or compensate the extraction, or to fit a space maintainer, should be considered (Ch. 17).

3. **Severe infraocclusion (marginal ridge at gingival level)**: Extract the submerged molar unless a radiograph shows that resorption of the root is almost complete and that eruption of the successional premolar is imminent. Consideration should again be given to the need to balance the extraction or maintain the space.

Sometimes it is evident that a submerged tooth has never erupted; such teeth inevitably prevent normal eruption of adjacent teeth and therefore must be surgically extracted. A submerged permanent molar should ideally be extracted before it becomes submerged below the gingiva.

12.5 ECTOPIC ERUPTION OF PERMANENT FIRST MOLARS

Ectopic eruption of a permanent first molar results in its impaction against the crown or root of the primary second molar, which may cause resorption of the primary molar root. Usually, further eruption of the permanent tooth is prevented, but occasionally the impaction is temporary (Young 1957). Almost always it is a maxillary molar that is affected.

Although the condition has been associated with crowding and with larger-than-average permanent first molars (Bjerklin & Kurol 1983), affected teeth typically are mesially inclined against the primary second molar, whereas in crowded dentitions permanent molars are distally inclined.

Treatment

The tooth should be disimpacted if possible; if this is unsuccessful it may be necessary to extract the primary second molar.

If the tooth is impacted against the crown rather than the root of the primary molar (Fig. 12.1a) it may be possible to disimpact it using soft brass ligature wire (0.5–0.7 mm diameter), as follows:

1. Anaesthetize the gingiva buccal and palatal to the tooth.
2. Holding the wire in Spencer Wells forceps, pass it under the contact point from buccal to palatal (Fig. 12.1b).
3. Twist the ends together over the contact point; do not overtighten or the wire will snap.
4. Cut off ends, leaving about 5 mm twisted together.

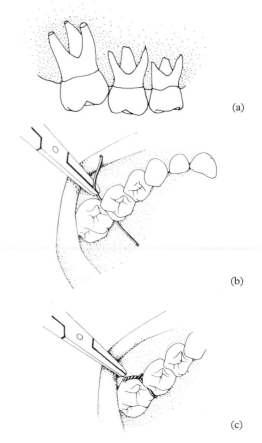

(a)

(b)

(c)

Fig. 12.1 One of the methods of disimpacting an ectopically erupted permanent first molar.

5. Tuck in neatly to avoid traumatizing the cheeks or gingiva (Fig. 12.1c).
6. Review every 2 weeks and retighten.

Although this method is sometimes successful in simple cases, more reliable results are obtained by using an orthodontic appliance. The appliance may be fixed or removable, incorporating a spring engaged either on the mesial surface (if it is accessible) or on an occlusal cuspal incline (Fig. 12.2); a blob of composite

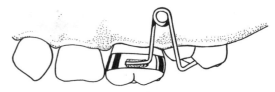

Fig. 12.2 An appliance to disimpact an ectopically erupted permanent first molar.

resin or an orthodontic bracket may be bonded to the occlusal surface against which the spring is to be engaged (Groper 1985).

If treatment to disimpact the first molar is not practicable the primary second molar must be extracted, and consideration should be given to compensating the extraction or to fitting a space maintainer. Balancing extraction is not indicated unless both maxillary permanent first molars are impacted. Cervical traction applied to the first molar with headgear, after extracting the primary second molar, has also been used (Kurol & Bjerklin 1984).

12.6 DELAYED ERUPTION OF PERMANENT TEETH

The data on tooth development given in Table 11.2 conceal the fact that there are considerable normal variations between children. Most cases of apparent delay are in fact within the normal range. Parents should be reassured, and occlusal development reviewed. However, as contralateral teeth usually erupt together, a delay of more than a month or two in the eruption of one of the teeth gives cause for concern.

Localized eruption delay is more common in the permanent dentition than in the primary dentition. Some of the causes are listed below:

Incisors: Delayed resorption of a primary incisor following trauma and death of the pulp. Dilaceration (Ch. 14). Supernumerary teeth (Ch. 15).

Canines: Abnormal eruption path of maxillary permanent canines (see below).

Premolars: Impaction against other teeth due to abnormal angulation or crowding. Retarded resorption of a primary molar. Infraoccluded primary molar (p. 137).

Molars: Impaction against other teeth; especially affecting third molars.

Other conditions, such as dentigerous cyst and regional odontodysplasia, may delay the eruption of any tooth. In addition, very early loss of a primary tooth, followed by bone formation in the socket, may delay eruption of the successor.

Systemic conditions associated with delayed eruption of the teeth include:

> Down's syndrome
> Cleidocranial dysplasia
> Gingival fibromatosis
> Mucopolysaccharidoses
> Congenital hypothyroidism
> Congenital hypopituitarism

12.6.1 Maxillary permanent canines

The path of eruption of maxillary canines is longer than that of other teeth and not uncommonly they deviate from their normal path, usually palatally. Early detection of abnormal eruption is extremely important, and appropriate investigations should form an essential part of examination of all child patients aged 9–10 years (page 134). If by the age of 10 years maxillary primary canines are not mobile and permanent canines are not palpable in the buccal sulcus, radiographs must be taken to determine their position.

Treatment

There are several treatment options (Ferguson 1990):

1. ***Extract maxillary primary canines.*** If abnormal eruption of a maxillary permanent canine is detected before the age of 13 years, extraction of the primary canine frequently results in correction of the path of eruption. Ericson & Kurol (1988) found that 36 of 46 palatally-displaced maxillary permanent canines changed to a normal path of eruption within 1 year of extracting the primary canines; the proportion was even higher in cases in which, on an orthopantomogram, the tip of the canine crown was distal to the midline of the lateral incisor root.

After extracting a primary canine, a radiograph should be taken about 6 months later to determine whether the position of the permanent canine has improved.

2. ***Extract maxillary primary canines and surgically expose the crown of the permanent canine.*** A maxillary permanent canine that might have erupted normally following extraction of its predecessor in a child aged 10–13 years may not erupt in an older patient. Surgical exposure of the crown encourages such a tooth to erupt. The tooth may then be allowed to erupt normally or orthodontic traction may be applied by bonding a bracket to its crown at the time of surgery and attaching a ligature to an orthodontic appliance. Before embarking on this course of treatment the position of the unerupted tooth must be carefully assessed and space must exist or be created in the arch to accommodate it.

3. ***Retain maxillary primary canines and either leave or extract the permanent canine.*** If the position of a maxillary permanent canine is unfavourable, or if its root development has reached an advanced stage, the prognosis is poor for normal eruption or for repositioning following extraction of its predecessor. Retained primary canines may remain functional into adult life, but their appearance later may be considered unacceptable by the patient,

which presents a problem if there is insufficient space for a normal-sized prosthetic replacement, or if orthodontic treatment to open or close the space is not practicable.

Unerupted canines left in situ may cause resorption of lateral incisor roots or, more rarely, may undergo cystic change in the follicular space, in which cases they must be surgically extracted. If they are not extracted, radiographs must be taken at about annual intervals to check for root resorption or cystic change.

4. **Extract maxillary primary canines and transplant the permanent canine.** If the position of the maxillary permanent canine is unfavourable for orthodontic alignment, a possible form of treatment is transplantation of the permanent canine into the primary canine space. Some orthodontic treatment may be required to provide space in the arch, and the transplanted tooth must be splinted, either by attaching the archwire of a fixed orthodontic appliance to a bracket bonded to the buccal surface of the transplanted tooth, or by using one of the methods described on pages 216–218. The management and complications of a transplanted tooth are similar to those of a replanted tooth (p. 219).

Treatment to extract or to bring an unerupted maxillary permanent canine into the arch can be unpleasant for a child. The fact that many such teeth would erupt normally following the relatively simple treatment of extraction of primary canines emphasizes the desirability of diagnosing the condition by the age of 10–11 years, and certainly not later than 13 years.

REFERENCES

Andlaw R J 1974 Submerged deciduous molars: a review with special reference to the rationale of treatment. Journal of the International Association of Dentistry for Children 5: 59–66

Andlaw R J 1977 Submerged deciduous molars: a prevalence survey in Somerset. Journal of the International Association of Dentistry for Children 8: 42–45

Bedi R, Yan S W 1990 The prevalence and clinical management of natal teeth—a study in Hong Kong. Journal of Paediatric Dentistry 6: 85–90

Bjerklin K, Kurol J 1983 Ectopic eruption of the maxillary first permanent molar: etiologic factors. American Journal of Orthodontics 84: 147–155

Brearley L J, McKibben D H 1973 Ankylosis of primary teeth. Journal of Dentistry for Children 40: 54–63

Ericson S, Kurol J 1988 Early treatment of palatally erupting maxillary canines by extraction of the primary canines. European Journal of Orthodontics 10: 283–295

Ferguson J W 1990 Management of the unerupted maxillary canine. British Dental Journal 169: 11–17

Gorelick L 1977 Direct bonding in the management of an ankylosed second deciduous molar. Journal of the American Dental Association 95: 307–309

Groper J N 1985 A simplified treatment for correcting an ectopically erupting maxillary first permanent molar. Journal of Dentistry for Children 52: 374–376

Kurol J 1981 Infraocclusion of primary molars: an epidemiologic and familial study. Community Dentistry and Oral Epidemiology 9: 94–102

Kurol J, Bjerklin K 1984 Treatment of children with ectopic eruption of the maxillary first permanent molar by cervical traction. American Journal of Orthodontics 86: 483–492

Kurol J, Magnusson B C 1984 Infraocclusion of primary molars: a histological study. Scandinavian Journal of Dental Research 92: 564–576

Massler M M, Savara B S 1950 Natal and neonatal teeth. Journal of Pediatrics 36: 349–359

Oliver R G, Richmond S, Hunter B 1986 Submerged permanent molars: four case reports. British Dental Journal 160: 128–130

Seward M H 1971 Local disturbances attributable to eruption of the human primary dentition. British Dental Journal 130: 72

Seward M H 1972a General disturbances attributable to eruption of the human primary dentition. Journal of Dentistry for Children 39: 178–183

Seward M H 1972b Treatment of teething in infants. British Dental Journal 132: 33–36

Seward M H 1973 Eruption cyst: an analysis of its clinical features. Journal of Oral Surgery 31: 31–35

Shafer W G, Hine M K, Levy B M 1983 A textbook of oral pathology, 4th edn. Saunders, Philadelphia, p 261

Soames J V, Southam J C 1993 Oral pathology, 2nd edn. Oxford University Press, Oxford, p 74

To E W H 1991 A study of natal teeth in Hong Kong Chinese. International Journal of Paediatric Dentistry 2: 73–76

Young D 1957 Ectopic eruption of the first permanent molars. Journal of Dentistry for Children 24: 153–162

RECOMMENDED READING

Davis J M, Law D B, Lewis T M 1981 An atlas of pedodontics, 2nd edn. Saunders, Philadelphia, ch 3

Rapp R, Winter G B 1979 A colour atlas of clinical conditions in paedodontics. Wolfe, London

Rock W P, Grundy M C, Shaw L 1988 Diagnostic picture tests in paediatric dentistry. Wolfe, London

Shaw L 1994 Self-assessment picture tests in dentistry. Paediatric Dentistry. Wolfe, London

13 Abnormalities of tooth structure

Dental tissues are formed in two stages: deposition of organic matrix, and mineralization. Disturbance of either stage may cause abnormalities of tooth structure, which are particularly important when enamel is involved. A disturbance of matrix deposition produces hypoplasia, characterized by enamel that is irregular in thickness or deficient in structure; defects may range from small pits or grooves in the enamel surface to gross deficiency. Disturbance during the second stage of development causes hypomineralization; although the enamel is of normal thickness, part of it, at least, is poorly mineralized.

13.1 ENAMEL HYPOPLASIA AND HYPOMINERALIZATION

13.1.1 Local

Developing permanent teeth may be damaged by trauma or by infection associated with their predecessors.

Intrusion or severe displacement of a primary incisor as a result of trauma may affect the developing permanent incisor. The younger the child at the time of injury the greater the chance that the enamel of the permanent tooth will be hypoplastic. If the injury occurs after 4 years of age, hypomineralization rather than hypoplasia is more common, often showing as white or brown patches on the labial surface.

The trauma associated with extraction of a primary molar may damage the developing premolar, especially if the child is under 4–5 years of age, when premolar development is at an early stage.

Similarly, the type of damage that may be caused by infection of a primary tooth depends on the stage of development of the permanent successor.

13.1.2 Systemic

Formation of primary teeth begins in utero (Table 11.1, p. 129). Until birth, the dentition is protected against all but the most severe systemic disturbances; therefore, prenatal enamel usually has a regular, homogeneous structure. There are microscopic differences between pre- and postnatal enamel and sometimes the difference is sufficiently marked to be seen clinically as 'neonatal lines' across the crowns of the teeth that were developing at birth. A well-marked neonatal line, or defective postnatal enamel, is related to systemic upsets at birth or during postnatal development.

The many systemic factors that may affect developing teeth have been reviewed by Pindborg (1982). They include genetically-transmitted factors (e.g. those causing amelogenesis imperfecta), inborn errors of metabolism (e.g. phenylketonuria), neonatal disturbances (e.g. premature birth, hypocalcaemia, haemolytic anaemia), endocrinopathies (e.g. hypoparathyroidism), nephropathies (e.g. nephrotic syndrome), gastrointestinal disease, liver disease and excessive ingestion of fluoride. The common viral infections are often considered to be causes of enamel hypoplasia, but supporting evidence only exists in relation to rubella syndrome.

Enamel hypomineralization or hypoplasia caused by

systemic factors is distributed on the crowns of teeth in a chronological pattern; that is, its distribution is related to the stage of development of the teeth when the disturbance occurred. Thus, if a severe systemic disturbance occurs within the first 6 months of life (which is not uncommon), the following distribution of enamel defects would be expected:

Primary teeth
Molars and canines — cervical–middle $\frac{1}{3}$
Incisors — cervical $\frac{1}{3}$

Permanent teeth
First molars — occlusal $\frac{1}{3}$
Central incisors and mandibular
  lateral incisors — incisal $\frac{1}{3}$
Canines — tips of cusps
[Maxillary lateral incisors would
  not be affected because they
  begin to develop later (p. 132).]

Figure 13.1 illustrates the parts of the crowns of developing permanent teeth that would be expected to be affected by systemic disturbances from birth to 7 years.

When long-term ingestion of excessive fluoride is the cause, the affected enamel can be expected to be distributed all over the crowns of teeth developing during that period.

Although the teeth affected, and the distribution of abnormal enamel, may be predicted from the child's age at which a systemic disturbance occurred (and vice-versa), this prediction is not always exactly reflected by the clinical appearance. For example, one or more of the four first molars (or of the incisors or canines) may show little or no sign of abnormal

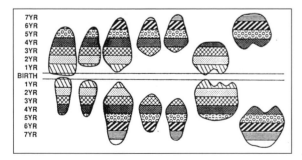

Fig. 13.1 The parts of the crowns of developing permanent teeth that would be expected to be affected by systemic disturbances from birth to 7 years. (Reproduced from R. K. Hall, Pediatric Orofacial Medicine and Pathology, Chapman and Hall 1994, Fig. 11.8, by kind permission of the author and publishers.)

enamel. It seems that a disturbance does not necessarily disrupt all developing teeth to the same degree.

13.1.3 Hereditary (amelogenesis imperfecta)

Amelogenesis imperfecta is a rare hereditary condition in which enamel structure is defective. Fifteen genetically distinct types have been described, classified into four groups: hypoplasia; hypomaturation; hypocalcification and hypomaturation; and hypoplasia with taurodontism (Winter & Brook 1975, Witkop 1988). Most commonly the inheritance pattern is autosomal dominant, but alternatively it can be autosomal recessive, or x-linked dominant or recessive. In almost all cases, both primary and permanent dentitions are affected. The typical appearances of teeth affected by amelogenesis imperfecta are illustrated by Rapp & Winter (1979), Davis et al (1981), and Rock et al (1988).

From the clinical standpoint, two main types need to be considered: hypoplasia and hypomineralization (the latter including the hypomaturation and hypocalcification types). The enamel in hypoplasia types may be thin but otherwise of normal appearance, or it may be pitted, grooved or more grossly deficient in structure. The enamel in hypomineralization types is of normal thickness, and has a smooth surface unless it is chipped and worn away; the areas of hypomineralized enamel vary in size and distribution, and may be opaque white, dull yellow or light brown in colour.

13.1.4 Treatment: general considerations

Hypomineralization and hypoplasia present various clinical problems:

Hypomineralization
Poor appearance of anterior teeth
Chipping of enamel, leaving rough surfaces
Attrition of occlusal enamel
Exposure of dentine — tooth sensitivity
Attrition of exposed dentine

Hypoplasia
Poor appearance of anterior teeth
Food stagnation in hypoplastic areas, predisposing to
  dental caries
Tooth sensitivity if dentine is exposed

The severity of each problem varies greatly. The labial surfaces of anterior teeth may show only very slightly discoloured flecks or minimal surface irregularity, or they may be grossly discoloured or hypoplastic. In some hypomineralization types of amelogenesis imperfecta there is only minimal chipping and wear of enamel: in others there is rapid attrition of enamel and exposure of dentine, causing tooth sensitivity and allowing further attrition. In some hypoplasia cases the deficiency of enamel is limited to minor pitting or grooving: in others there is gross deficiency of tooth structure.

In view of the wide range in the severity of the clinical problems, it is not possible to give precise recommendations for treatment, but a guide is outlined in Table 13.1.

It is important to reassure and encourage the child and parents, who may be demoralized by the appearance of the teeth. They should be advised that treatment is possible, and encouraged to take an active interest in the treatment plan. Without their interest and cooperation it is not practicable to embark on the considerable amount of treatment that would be necessary to conserve the dentition; in severe cases the provision of dentures would be the only alternative.

Table 13.1 suggests that treatment is done only for permanent teeth, starting in the early mixed dentition. However, treatment of primary teeth may be necessary. Stainless steel crowns are ideal restorations for primary molars; conservation of these teeth ensures that the permanent first molars erupt in their normal positions. Anterior primary teeth could be conserved by crowning (Ch. 8), but extraction in severe cases is often justified.

Table 13.1 also indicates that after initial treatment of permanent first molars in the early mixed dentition, a decision must be made either to retain the teeth permanently or to extract them at a time in dental development that will encourage the second molars to occupy their positions. If radiographs show that the unerupted canines and premolars are present, and if it is assessed that there will be sufficient space for their eruption, it may be preferable to extract the permanent first molars when the child is between $8\frac{1}{2}$ and 10 years of age (Ch. 22). This treatment plan is especially indicated if the cause of the defective tooth structure is a systemic disturbance during infancy, because the premolars and second molars will not be affected. If, however, the cause is amelogenesis imperfecta, premolars and second molars will be expected to be similarly affected and there is therefore no advantage to be gained by extracting the first molars; except, perhaps, if extensive restorative treatment is required to maintain the teeth and the child is very uncooperative, when extraction of the first molars under general anaesthesia would allow the restorative treatment to be delayed for a few years.

13.1.5 Treatment of anterior teeth

Small areas of hypomineralized labial enamel may not cause concern to the child or parent and therefore not require treatment. Other cases of localized discoloration or hypoplasia may be treated simply, masking the affected areas with composite resin. Severely hypoplastic teeth, however, require more extensive treatment because the teeth may not only be unsightly but also sensitive as a result of exposed dentine.

Although a porcelain jacket crown may be regarded as the most satisfactory long-term restoration for a severely affected tooth, it is not an appropriate

Table 13.1 Summary of treatment possibilities for hypomineralized or hypoplastic teeth.*

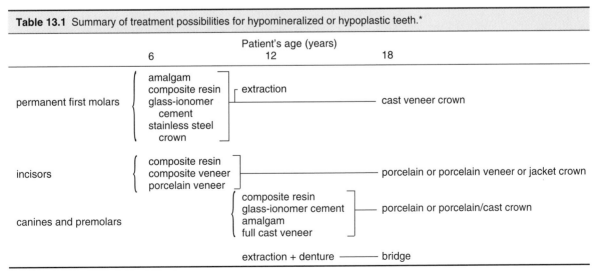

* Refer to text.

restoration for children: it is generally agreed that the amount of tooth reduction necessary to make a porcelain jacket crown places at risk the relatively large pulp of a child's tooth. Therefore, more conservative restorations are preferred: either a composite resin or porcelain veneer.

Composite resin veneer

Composite resin veneers have been considered to offer only temporary treatment for discoloured or hypoplastic anterior teeth (Smith & Pulver 1982, Cooley 1984), but new developments in materials and techniques have raised hopes that they might provide satisfactory long-term alternatives to the porcelain jacket crown (Welbury 1991).

Resins that polymerize when exposed to visible light are generally preferred to autopolymerizing resins because they allow a longer working time; shades may be mixed on the tooth surface until a pleasing result is obtained, and excess may be removed from the margins before initiating polymerization with the light source. The microfilled resins, which contain very small filler particles, have the advantage that they can be polished to a smoother finish than can other types of composite.

The use of composite resin can dramatically improve the appearance of hypomineralized, hypoplastic or discoloured teeth. Unfortunately the surface of composite resin becomes abraded and stained, and therefore the appearance of veneers tends to deteriorate.

Before proceeding with any veneering technique, the decision must be made whether to reduce the thickness of labial enamel before placing the veneer. If enamel thickness is not reduced (the approach often preferred, especially in children) it is inevitable that the labial bulk of the tooth will be increased, which may not be acceptable. On the other hand, the appearance of an instanding or rotated tooth can be improved by the addition of a labial veneer. The decision to reduce the thickness of labial enamel is usually taken when it is considered undesirable to increase the labial bulk of the tooth, and also if the tooth is very discoloured, since additional layers of composite resin may be required to mask severe discolorations.

Composite resin is a translucent material and cannot mask tooth discoloration unless it is used in thick layers, which is usually undesirable. For this reason, colour tints or opaquers are included with products that are marketed specifically as veneering materials.

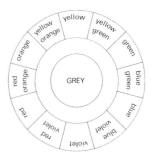

Fig. 13.2 The colour wheel used in selecting colours for colour modification.

A colour tint is used to neutralize the colour of the discoloured tooth to the neutral colour of grey. The colour wheel (Fig. 13.2) indicates which colour must be used to neutralize another. Colours on opposite sides of the wheel neutralize one another; for example, a yellow discoloration is neutralized by the addition of violet.

After the neutral grey colour has been obtained it must be lightened to the desired tooth colour. This can be done by applying one or more thin layers of either a tooth-coloured tint or an opaquer. Opaquers are tooth-coloured and act as reflective screens.

Not all manufacturers provide both colour tints and opaquers, and the recommended methods of using the materials differ. The vehicle for colour tints and opaquers is either the unfilled resin bonding agent, which is applied to etched enamel, or the composite paste that is used to cement the porcelain veneer. It is, of course, essential to follow the manufacturer's instructions carefully, but it is always important to apply layers of colour tint or opaquer very thinly; multiple thin layers may be used if necessary, but thick layers produce a dull, non-translucent appearance.

Porcelain veneer

Porcelain has several advantages over composite as a veneering material. Porcelain veneers are aesthetically superior, are more resistant to abrasion and, being glazed, are less likely to irritate gingival tissues or attract plaque.

Composite resin is used as a lute between the veneer and the tooth, the resin bonding to etched enamel and porcelain. The veneers are thin and fragile but, when bonded to enamel, their strength is more than adequate for veneering purposes (Garber 1989).

Technique: full labial veneer using light-cured composite resin

(If it is decided not to reduce the thickness of labial enamel, proceed to stage 4.)

1. Use a cylindrical or tapered diamond to reduce the thickness of labial enamel by about 0.5 mm. Depressions or grooves 0.5 mm deep may be made first to facilitate this procedure.
2. Finish the preparation 0.5 mm short of the gingival margin (Fig. 13.3a). However, if the cervical part of the tooth crown is hypoplastic or discoloured, finish the preparation subgingivally.
3. Mesially and distally, finish the preparation just labial to the contact points but, if the enamel is hypoplastic or discoloured in those areas, carry the preparation palatal to the contact points.
4. Clean the tooth with a slurry of pumice in water, or with an oil-free prophylaxis paste. Wash the paste away with a water spray and dry the tooth.
5. Isolate the tooth and place a suitable matrix. Use either a conventional straight matrix strip or a shaped strip made specially for the purpose (Fig. 13.3b).
6. Etch, wash and dry the labial enamel as previously described (p. 59).
7. Apply a thin layer of unfilled resin ('bonding agent') to the etched and dried enamel with a fine brush or other

suitable applicator (Fig. 13.3c). Direct the air syringe gently over the surface to remove excess resin. If the enamel is discoloured, a colour neutralizer or an opaquer may be used at this stage. Polymerize the resin.

8. Apply a small amount of filled composite resin of appropriate shade to the central part of the labial surface. Currently available materials vary considerably in their viscosity. The more viscous materials need to be spread with a dental instrument, and may then be smoothed with a small brush; the less viscous materials may be spread easily with the brush. Add further increments of composite resin as required, using different shades if necessary to produce a good colour match with adjacent teeth and to achieve a gradual transition from a relatively dark gingival area to a lighter, more translucent, incisal region.
9. Carefully remove excess material from around the margin before polymerizing the resin (Fig. 13.3d).
10. After the resin has polymerized, remove the matrix, explore the margin carefully and smooth with finishing burs and polishing discs. A scalpel is useful to remove excess at the margin (Fig. 13.3e).

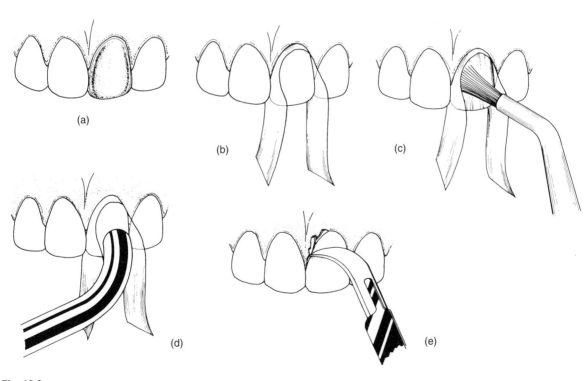

(a)

(b)

(c)

(d)

(e)

Fig. 13.3

Horn (1983), Calamia (1985) and Clyde & Gilmour (1988) reported excellent results with porcelain veneers, but their long-term durability is not yet known. A study evaluating 315 porcelain veneers over periods of up to 63 months found that 53 (17%) developed minor problems and 34 (11%) were failures (Dunne & Millar 1993).

A porcelain veneer may be made to fit a natural tooth surface (Plant & Thomas 1987), but a conservative enamel preparation is generally preferred (Millar 1987).

A further development is a castable glass ceramic material that has physical and mechanical properties similar to those of enamel (McLean 1988). A technique for making labial veneers (and other restorations) has been described (Hobo & Iwata 1985).

Technique: porcelain veneer

1. The enamel preparation is similar to that described for the composite resin veneer. Alternative incisal edge preparations are illustrated in Figure 13.4; the preparations shown at c and d are preferred because they facilitate accurate placement of the veneer on the tooth surface, and also place the porcelain-tooth junction out of sight on the palatal surface of the tooth.
2. Take an impression with a rubber-based impression material. If the incisal edge has been prepared as shown in Fig. 13.4d it may also be necessary to take an impression of the lower arch and a wax registration of the teeth in occlusion.
3. It is not usually necessary to place a temporary restoration but, if it is deemed necessary, flow a layer of acrylic or composite resin on to the labial enamel (which, of course, should not be etched). This usually remains in place if the patient is careful when toothbrushing.
4. Write precise instructions to the laboratory technician. Indicate the shade of tooth to be matched and make a simple drawing to show the area to be covered by the veneer; this is especially important if the veneer is to be placed on an unprepared tooth surface. If facilities are available for clinical photography, a colour print showing the anterior teeth would be helpful to the technician.
5. *The patient's next visit:*
   The veneers must be handled carefully not only because they are small and brittle but also because their fitting surfaces have been etched in the laboratory, and contamination of the etched surfaces must be avoided. Brush a thin layer of silane coupling agent on to the fitting surface of the veneer, and allow it to dry for 5 minutes.
6. Clean the tooth surface with a slurry of pumice in water or with an oil-free prophylaxis paste. Wash the pumice away with water, dry the tooth and then place the veneer in position to confirm that it fits properly.
7. Place a layer of try-in paste (composite resin not containing the light-sensitive catalyst) on the fitting surface of the veneer and try it in again. Check the colour match and invite the patient to comment on it.
8. If colour modification is required, proceed as described on page 144.
9. Remove the try-in paste by placing the veneer in acetone and gently dabbing the paste off with a small sponge pad.
10. Isolate the tooth and place a matrix (Fig. 13.2b).
11. Etch, wash and dry the labial enamel.
12. Apply a thin layer of bonding agent to the etched enamel surface and to the fitting surface of the veneer, and polymerize.
13. Place a layer of composite paste on the veneer (just enough to cover the previously placed bonding agent). Position the veneer on the tooth and gently press it into place.
14. Maintain the veneer in position while removing excess composite with a probe or other convenient dental instrument.
    If the incisal edge of the tooth was reduced, the veneer is firmly located in position but, if not, the veneer may easily be moved out of position while removing excess composite from the margin. To prevent this, use the polymerizing light for 5 seconds; this stabilizes the veneer while still allowing removal of excess composite.
15. When all excess composite has been removed, polymerize fully with the light.
16. Remove the matrix, check all margins carefully with a probe, and trim and polish as necessary with diamond or tungsten carbide finishing burs, and with abrasive discs.
17. A final polish of trimmed margins may be given with composite polishing paste.

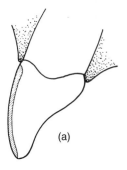
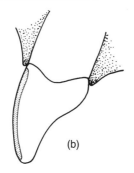
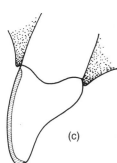
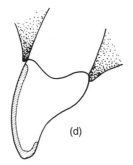

(a)   (b)   (c)   (d)

Fig. 13.4

13.1.6 Treatment of posterior teeth

Small areas of hypoplastic enamel in posterior teeth can be restored with amalgam, composite resin or glass-ionomer cement. However, crowns are required for more severely affected teeth. Stainless steel crowns are ideal semi-permanent restorations for permanent first molars, but are not made in sizes suitable for premolars. Therefore, cast veneers must be made for premolars.

13.2 DENTINOGENESIS IMPERFECTA

Dentinogenesis imperfecta is an hereditary dentinal defect that may occur alone or in association with the skeletal condition of osteogenesis imperfecta (Gage 1985, Witkop 1988). The alternative term 'hereditary opalescent dentine' aptly describes the appearance of the teeth, which vary in colour from grey to brownish blue. Diagnosis is simple because, in addition to their discoloration, the crowns are bulbous, being constricted cervically, and radiographs typically show short, thin roots, and pulp chambers and root canals that are partly or completely obliterated; there may also be periapical areas of radiolucency.

The enamel, which is usually normal, is poorly supported by the defective dentine and therefore tends to flake away. Attrition of exposed dentine occurs, and the teeth may rapidly be reduced to gingival level. Pulp death commonly occurs. All teeth of both dentitions are usually affected, but permanent teeth, especially premolars and second and third molars, are less severely affected.

13.2.1 Treatment

The rationale of treatment is similar to that applied to a severe case of amelogenesis imperfecta of the hypomineralization type: unless teeth (particularly posterior teeth) are crowned they will be worn down by attrition and have to be extracted. Stainless steel crowns are ideal for primary molars and permanent first molars; in the primary dentition it is sometimes sufficient to crown second molars only. However, the teeth may be unsuitable for crowning because they are poorly supported by short, thin roots; an assessment must be made of their suitability for crowning. Much depends on whether the patient is keen to have the considerable amount of treatment that would be required, despite the uncertain prognosis (Mars & Smith 1981, Mendel et al 1981).

If it is decided not to embark on conservative treatment, the teeth should be retained for as long as possible, but the provision of dentures will eventually be necessary, as it is for the patient who first presents with permanent teeth already worn down by attrition. For a young patient it is preferable to make dentures that fit over the tooth remnants, after rounding and smoothing rough edges. This approach ensures the maintenance of the alveolar ridges, but eventually it may become necessary to extract the teeth and provide normal dentures.

REFERENCES

Calamia J R 1985 Etched porcelain veneers: the current state of the art. Quintessence International 16: 5–12

Clyde J S, Gilmour A 1988 Porcelain veneers: a preliminary review. British Dental Journal 164: 9–14

Cooley R O 1984 Status report on enamel bonding of composite, preformed laminate and laboratory fabricated resin veneers. Journal of the American Dental Association 109: 782–784

Davis J M, Law D B, Lewis T M 1981 An atlas of pedodontics. Saunders, Philadelphia

Dunne S M, Millar B J A 1993 A longitudinal study of the clinical performance of porcelain veneers. British Dental Journal 175: 317–321

Gage J P 1985 Dentinogenesis imperfecta: a new perspective. Australian Dental Journal 30: 285–290

Garber D A 1989 Direct composite veneers versus etched porcelain laminate veneers. Dental Clinics of North America 33: 301–304

Hall R K 1994 Pediatric orofacial medicine and pathology. Chapman & Hall, London, ch 11

Hobo S, Iwata T 1985 A new laminate veneer technique using a castable apatite ceramic material. II: practical procedures. Quintessence International 16: 509–517

Horn H 1983 Porcelain laminate veneers bonded to etched enamel. Dental Clinics of North America 27: 672–684

Mars M, Smith B G N 1981 Dentinogenesis imperfecta — an integrated conservative approach to treatment. British Dental Journal 152: 15–18

McLean J W 1988 Ceramics in clinical dentistry. British Dental Journal 164: 187–194

Mendel R W, Shawkat A H, Farman A G 1981 Management of opalescent dentine — report of a long-term follow up. Journal of the American Dental Association 102: 53–55

Millar B J 1987 Porcelain veneers. Dental Update 14: 381–390

Pindborg J J 1982 Aetiology of developmental enamel defects not related to fluorosis. International Dental Journal 32: 123–134

Plant C G, Thomas G D 1987 Porcelain facings: a simple clinical and laboratory method. British Dental Journal 163: 231–234

Rapp R, Winter G B 1979 A colour atlas of clinical conditions in paedodontics. Wolfe, London

Rock W P, Grundy M C, Shaw L 1988 Diagnostic picture tests in paediatric dentistry. Wolfe, London

Smith D C, Pulver F 1982 Aesthetic dental veneering materials. International Dental Journal 32: 223–239

Welbury R R 1991 A clinical study of a microfilled composite resin for labial veneers. International Journal of Paediatric Dentistry 1: 9–15

Winter G B, Brook A H 1975 Enamel hypoplasia and anomalies of the enamel. Dental Clinics of North America (Jan) 3024

Witkop C J 1988 Amelogenesis imperfecta, dentinogenesis imperfecta and dentin dysplasia revisited: problems in classification. Journal of Oral Pathology 17: 547–553

14 Abnormalities of tooth form

14.1 DOUBLE TEETH

Double teeth may be formed either by fusion of two developing tooth germs or by gemination (partial dichotomy) of one tooth germ. If fusion occurs between two teeth of the normal dentition, one of the teeth will appear to be missing from the dentition. If, on the other hand, one element is a supernumerary tooth, the normal number of teeth will be present (including the double tooth). This is also the case when the double tooth is formed by gemination of one tooth germ. Therefore, it is sometimes difficult to decide whether an abnormally large tooth is the result of fusion of a normal and a supernumerary tooth, or of gemination; use of the term 'double tooth' avoids this difficulty (Brook & Winter 1970).

Double teeth are rare: a review of 11 surveys carried out in several countries revealed a prevalence ranging from 0.1% to 1.0% (Brook & Winter 1970). They occur most frequently in the maxillary incisor region, more commonly in the primary than in the permanent dentition, and may be unilateral or bilateral. A large tooth may be identified as a double tooth by notching in its incisal edge, or by a longitudinal groove in its crown, or by partial or complete separation of its roots.

Treatment

No treatment is necessary for primary double teeth, but in the permanent dentition treatment to improve their appearance is usually requested by the patient and parent.

If the pulp chambers and root canals are separate (Fig. 14.1), it is possible to separate the crowns using a fine diamond bur or a guarded diamond disc. To obtain an aesthetic result, it is usually necessary to modify the shapes of the separated parts, which can be done by one of the methods described in Chapter 13. If one part of the double tooth is a supernumerary element, its extraction is usually necessary (Smith 1980, Moore 1984).

Ideally, division of a double tooth should be delayed until the late teenage years to allow some recession of pulp horns to occur, thus reducing the risk of pulp exposure. However, the appearance of the double tooth may be so poor that earlier treatment is demanded. Pulp exposure is then more probable, and may be treated by pulpotomy (Gregg 1985) or pulpectomy (Itkin & Barr 1975). If treatment can be delayed at least until root development is complete

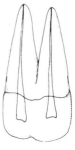

Fig. 14.1 Double tooth with separate pulp chambers.

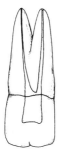

Fig. 14.2 Double tooth with single pulp chamber.

(about 11 years of age), simple root canal treatment may be done before division of the crown (Pearson & Willmot 1995).

If there is a single pulp chamber (Fig. 14.2), division of the crown is not feasible. Some improvement of appearance may sometimes be obtained by accentuating the longitudinal groove in the crown, to simulate two separate teeth.

If conservative treatment is not practicable, extraction becomes necessary, followed usually by provision of a denture or bridge because the space left after extraction of even one double tooth is usually too large to be closed by orthodontic means.

14.2 MALFORMATION OF THE MAXILLARY PERMANENT LATERAL INCISOR

The maxillary permanent lateral incisor is often abnormal in size or shape. The most common abnormalities are a 'peg-shaped' crown and a deep palatal invagination.

Peg-shaped lateral incisors have small, conical crowns and resemble conical supernumerary teeth. They may occur unilaterally (not uncommonly associated with a congenitally absent contralateral tooth) or bilaterally.

Palatal pits occur in many lateral incisors, but sometimes the pit is particularly deep and leads to a chamber formed by invagination of the developing tooth germ; this is known as *dens in dente* or *dens invaginatus*. Caries may begin in the depths of a pit or invagination and quickly involve the pulp.

Treatment

Peg-shaped lateral incisor

If the dental arch is crowded, peg-shaped lateral incisors may be extracted as part of orthodontic treat-

ment. However, this is rarely the treatment of choice because peg-shaped lateral incisors tend to occur in dentitions in which the other teeth are small or in which one or more teeth are congenitally absent.

A normal crown shape can be produced with a porcelain 'thimble' crown. Usually no tooth preparation is required before taking an impression of the tooth. The entire enamel surface of the tooth is acid-etched and the crown is bonded to it with composite resin (as described for porcelain veneer on p. 146).

It is possible but less satisfactory to improve the appearance of a peg-shaped incisor using composite resin in a cellulose acetate crown form or (if using a light-cured resin) by building up in increments. A problem arises in adapting a crown form to the narrow neck of the 'peg' tooth. This may be overcome by making a longitudinal cut in the palatal part of the crown form, overlapping the two sides and sticking with photographic film adhesive (Fig. 14.3).

Deep palatal pits

Ideally, palatal pits should be sealed with composite resin or glass-ionomer cement as soon as the teeth erupt.

If the teeth have erupted and the pits have not been sealed, careful clinical and radiological examination is required to assess whether they are carious.

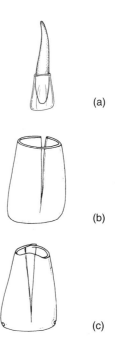

Fig. 14.3 Modifying a cellulose acetate crown form to fit a peg-shaped lateral incisor.

14.3 DENS EVAGINATUS (EVAGINATED ODONTOME)

Dens evaginatus is a tooth in which an evagination of enamel and dentine appears as a tubercle on the occlusal surface. The tubercle is covered with enamel and a fine pulp horn usually extends into the dentine core. The anomaly is most common in people of Mongoloid races but also occurs in Caucasians, and it is found most frequently in premolar teeth but occasionally also in other permanent teeth (Hill & Bellis 1984).

The condition is of clinical significance because the tubercles often become worn or fractured, exposing pulp and leading to pulp necrosis and periapical infection. Since this often occurs within a few years of the tooth's eruption it presents a problem for endodontic treatment.

Treatment

Treatment must be directed at preventing the complications associated with exposure and death of the pulp.

1. If the tubercle causes no occlusal interference, seal the occlusal surface as described in Chapter 5. Use a filled composite resin and flow it around the tubercle and over the adjacent fissures.
2. If the tubercle causes occlusal interference, administer local analgesic and isolate the tooth with rubber dam in readiness for pulp treatment. Reduce the height of the tubercle sufficiently to relieve the occlusal interference and examine it carefully.
   a. If pulp is not exposed, proceed as for 1 above.
   b. If pulp is exposed, perform a conservative partial pulpotomy by removing pulp to a depth of about 2 mm with a small diamond bur, following the technique described on page 213. This creates space to place a calcium hydroxide dressing over the pulp and to seal the cavity with glass-ionomer cement or composite resin. Seal the adjacent fissures with composite resin.

14.4 TALON CUSP

A talon cusp has been defined as 'an additional cusp that prominently projects from the lingual surface of primary or permanent anterior teeth, is morphologically well delineated, and extends at least half the distance from the cemento-enamel junction to the incisal edge' (Davis & Brook 1986). Talon cusps have been reported most frequently on maxillary permanent incisors (Hattab et al 1995), but also on maxillary primary incisors (Hattab & Yassin 1996) and on man-

dibular permanent incisors, and are often associated with other abnormalities (for example, evaginated premolars, peg-shaped maxillary lateral incisors, double teeth, complex odontomes).

A talon cusp may project at an angle from the tooth or lie close to its palatal surface. The junction between cusp and tooth may be smooth or, especially when the cusp lies close to the tooth, it may be grooved or fissured. When the tooth is erupting, before the connection of the cusp and the tooth becomes visible, the cusp may appear to be a supernumerary tooth; it is important not to be hasty and attempt to extract it.

The cusp is composed of enamel and dentine. Pulp projects into it, to a variable degree. Radiography is not usually helpful in determining the outline of the pulp horn.

The main problems presented by talon cusps are caries (associated with plaque retention in the groove or fissure between cusp and tooth) and occlusal interference, which may cause labial displacement of a maxillary tooth as it erupts.

Treatment

1. Soon after the tooth erupts, carefully examine the junction between the cusp and the tooth. If it appears that it might be a site for plaque retention and therefore for caries, seal with composite resin or glass-ionomer cement.
2. If the cusp is causing occlusal interference or has caused tooth displacement, either (a) reduce the cusp gradually over a period of several months, for example by grinding about 1 mm at about monthly intervals (it is hoped that secondary dentine will be formed in response to the grinding and, thus, that pulp exposure will be avoided); or (b) if more immediate improvement is required, administer local analgesic, isolate the tooth with rubber dam in readiness for probable pulp exposure, and remove the amount of cusp necessary to relieve the occlusal interference; place fluoride varnish on exposed dentine. Sometimes considerable reduction of a cusp is possible without exposing pulp. However, if pulp is exposed, perform a conservative partial pulpotomy as described on page 213.

Teeth that have been mildly displaced by the talon cusp will align spontaneously after removal of the occlusal interference.

14.5 DILACERATION

A dilacerated tooth is one that has a distorted crown or root. Dilaceration is most commonly associated with maxillary permanent central incisors. Severe trauma to primary incisors is a common cause of dilaceration, but some cases are not associated with trauma and simply reflect abnormal development of the tooth (Stewart 1978).

Severe injury to a maxillary primary incisor may cause dilaceration of either the crown or the root of the permanent successor, depending on the stage of development of the permanent tooth and its relationship to the root of the primary incisor at the time of injury. Maxillary permanent incisors develop palatal to and very near the root apices of the primary incisors; as they erupt they move over the roots of the primary teeth. Therefore, intrusion or gross displacement of the primary incisor in infancy is most likely to displace the permanent tooth crown palatally. Since further development continues normally, the fully developed tooth has its crown bent palatally; it also has hypoplasia of the enamel in the area of the distortion, as evidence of the traumatic incident (Fig. 14.4a). After about $4\frac{1}{2}$ years of age, when the roots of the permanent incisors are forming and the teeth are moving over the primary incisor roots, the permanent tooth crown and the partially developed root are more likely to be bent labially; the fully-formed tooth then has a bend in its root, but no enamel hypoplasia (Fig. 14.4b).

Dilaceration of the apical third of a permanent incisor root (Fig. 14.4c) is caused by injury to the tooth itself at the age of 8–10 years, after the primary incisors have exfoliated. Intrusion or gross displacement of the tooth are the most likely causes.

Dilacerated teeth that are developmental anomalies not associated with trauma are gently curved from crown to root; the crown is bent labially from the crown–root junction and there is no enamel hypoplasia (Fig. 14.4d).

A dilacerated tooth usually fails to erupt, but may sometimes erupt into an abnormal position and cause displacement of adjacent teeth.

Treatment

Unerupted dilacerated teeth usually must be extracted, but sometimes it is possible to bring a tooth into the arch by a combination of surgery and orthodontics (Howard 1978, Davies & Lewis 1984). Erupted teeth with root dilaceration are also usually extracted if they are in an abnormal position because it is difficult to move them by orthodontic means. Following extraction, the space must either be maintained with a prosthesis (to restore aesthetics and to prevent tilting of adjacent teeth) or closed orthodontically.

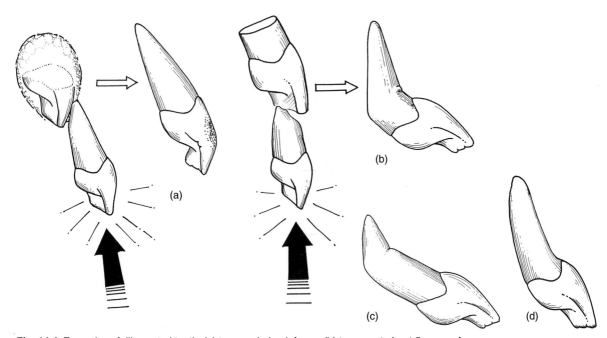

Fig. 14.4 Examples of dilacerated teeth: (a) trauma during infancy; (b) trauma at about 5 years of age; (c) trauma at 8–10 years of age; (d) developmental anomaly.

REFERENCES

Brook A H, Winter G B 1970 Double teeth: a retrospective study of geminated and fused teeth in children. British Dental Journal 129: 123–130

Davies P H J, Lewis D H 1984 Dilaceration: a surgical/orthodontic solution. British Dental Journal 156: 16–18

Davis P J, Brook A H 1986 The presentation of talon cusp: diagnosis, clinical features, associations and possible aetiology. British Dental Journal 160: 84–88

Gregg T A 1985 Surgical division and pulpotomy of a double incisor tooth. British Dental Journal 159: 254 –255

Hattab F N, Yassin O M, Al-Nimri K S 1995 Talon cusp – clinical significance and case management: case reports. Quintessence International 26: 115–120

Hattab F N, Yassin O M 1996 Bilateral talon cusps on primary incisors: a case report. International Journal of Paediatric Dentistry 6: 191–195

Hill F J, Bellis W J 1984 Dens evaginatus and its management. British Dental Journal 156: 400–402

Howard R D 1978 Maxillary anterior displacement and impaction in the mixed dentition. Dental Clinics of North America 22: 635–645

Itkin A B, Barr G S 1975 Comprehensive management of the double tooth: report of a case. Journal of the American Dental Association 90: 1269–1272

Moore K H 1984 A case report of bilateral double teeth. British Journal of Orthodontics 11: 40–41

Pearson A I, Willmot D R 1995 Combined surgical and orthodontic treatment of bilateral double teeth: a case report. International Journal of Paediatric Dentistry 5: 43–48

Smith G A 1980 Double teeth. British Dental Journal 148: 163–164

Stewart D J 1978 Dilacerate unerupted maxillary central incisor. British Dental Journal 145: 229–233

RECOMMENDED READING

Davis J M, Law D B, Lewis T M 1981 An atlas of pedodontics, 2nd edn. Saunders, Philadelphia, ch 3

Rapp R, Winter G B 1979 A colour atlas of clinical conditions in paedodontics. Wolfe, London

Rock W P. Grundy M C, Shaw L 1988 Diagnostic picture tests in paediatric dentistry. Wolfe, London

15 Abnormalities of tooth number

15.1 CONGENITAL ABSENCE OF TEETH

Congenital absence of all teeth (anodontia) is very rare. However, absence of one or of several teeth (hypodontia) is not uncommon.

A review of studies conducted in various countries revealed that the prevalence of hypodontia in the primary dentition ranges from 0.1% to 0.9%, and in the permanent dentition (excluding third molars) from 3.5% to 6.6% (Brook 1974). Hypodontia in the primary dentition is of little clinical significance and usually receives no treatment. However, hypodontia in the permanent dentition demands attention. The permanent teeth most frequently congenitally absent are maxillary lateral incisors and mandibular second premolars, but the results of surveys differ about which of these is the more frequently absent. Absence of a maxillary lateral incisor is often associated with a small peg-shaped contralateral tooth.

The effects of congenital absence of one or more teeth depend largely on the amount of crowding that would have existed had the dentition been complete. Sometimes the absence of a tooth is sufficient to relieve crowding and permit alignment of the remaining teeth; in other cases the missing tooth leaves a space.

Treatment

Treatment planning is influenced primarily by whether the arch is crowded or not; that is, whether there is sufficient space in the arch for the eruption of pre-molars and permanent canines. (The assessment of crowding is discussed in Chapter 17.)

Maxillary permanent lateral incisor

1. *In an uncrowded arch.* Fit a partial denture to replace the missing incisor(s). The denture may be replaced by a bridge in later life. Monitor clinically and radiographically the eruption path of the permanent canine—extract the primary canine if the permanent canine appears to be moving mesial to it.
2. *In a crowded arch.* Either a) fit a prosthesis, as above, and treat the crowding when premolars erupt; or b) allow the canine to erupt into the lateral incisor space, and improve its position if necessary by orthodontic means.

Although it seems a logical approach to allow a canine to use a lateral incisor space in a crowded arch, the final appearance is often disappointing because the canine may be large and bulbous and because the palatal cusp of the first premolar, in contact with the canine, may be visible when the patient smiles. The appearance of a canine may be improved by carefully grinding its tip and greatest bulbosity, or by modifying its shape with etch-retained composite resin.

Mandibular second premolar

1. *In an uncrowded arch.* Treatment depends on the condition of the primary second molar. If it is sound, no action is needed; it may remain functional into adulthood. If, on the other hand, the long-term prognosis of the tooth appears poor, extraction during the mixed dentition period might be followed by some space closure by mesial drift (and tilting) of the permanent first molar. However, in an uncrowded arch, space closure is unlikely to be complete and orthodontic treatment may be needed later to achieve

155

it, or to improve the angulation of the first molar before constructing a bridge.

2. **In a crowded arch.** Absence of a premolar, especially if bilateral, is an advantage in an arch that would otherwise be crowded.

15.2 SUPERNUMERARY TEETH

Supernumerary teeth occur most frequently in the premaxilla and are less common in the primary dentition than in the permanent dentition. In the primary dentition, supernumerary teeth are usually normal or conical in shape; in the permanent dentition they have a greater variety of shapes, and may be classified as follows:

Conical   — small, peg-shaped crown
Tuberculate   — short, barrel-shaped crown
Supplemental — tooth resembling a normal incisor, usually a lateral incisor
Odontome   — varied shape, unsuitable for inclusion in one of the other groups.

The majority of supernumerary teeth are either conical or tuberculate; their characteristic features, which differ in many important respects, are summarized in Table 15.1.

Supernumerary incisor teeth may interfere with the eruption of, or cause displacement or rotation of, adjacent teeth (Gregg & Kinirons 1991).

Multiple supernumerary teeth are a feature of certain syndromes (e.g. cleinocranial dysplasia, Gardner syndrome).

Treatment

Treatment depends on the type and position of the supernumerary tooth and on its actual or potential effect on adjacent teeth.

1. **No treatment.** Supernumerary teeth that are neither interfering with the eruption of teeth, nor causing displacement of erupted teeth, may be allowed to remain; this is often possible with inverted conical types. Periodic radiographic examination is essential to detect any undesirable changes that may occur.

2. **Await eruption and then extract.** Most conical supernumeraries that are not inverted will erupt.

3. **Surgical extraction.** Most tuberculate and inverted conical types, and odontomes, must be extracted. The optimal timing of treatment is controversial: the advantages and disadvantages of early intervention (before the age of 6 years) and of delayed intervention (between the ages of 8 and 10 years) have been discussed by Primosch (1981). Early removal of a supernumerary tooth gives the normal developing tooth the best chance of erupting into its normal position; on the other hand, there is a risk of damaging adjacent developing teeth during surgery. Delaying treatment may result in the normal tooth becoming displaced or rotated, and may allow adjacent teeth to drift into the space as they erupt. The later the supernumerary tooth is removed the less eruption potential the impacted normal tooth will have. Each case must be considered individually, but it has been suggested that the most appropriate time to extract midline supernumeraries is when the lateral incisors are just beginning to erupt (Broadway & Gould 1960).

If there is adequate space in the arch for the unerupted incisor, insert a simple space maintainer. If the space available is inadequate, move adjacent teeth distally with an orthodontic appliance after extracting the primary canines at the same time as the supernumerary tooth. It is important to provide a slight excess of space for the unerupted incisor.

Having removed the supernumerary tooth and provided enough space in the arch, the incisor usually erupts (Mitchell & Bennett 1992). Sometimes, especially if it has previously been displaced by the supernumerary, the incisor does not erupt, and requires further surgery and orthodontic traction to bring it into the arch (Howard 1967).

Table 15.1 Features of conical and tuberculate supernumerary teeth (from Foster & Taylor 1969).

	Conical	Tuberculate
Morphology	Conical, pointed crown Normal root Root development at similar stage to, or ahead of, normal incisor	Barrel-shaped crown with low cusps Little or no root
Position	The majority between central incisors, not necessarily in midline of arch May be inverted	Palatal to incisors Rarely inverted
Eruption	Often erupt with the central incisors Inverted types do not erupt	Rarely erupt
Effect	May cause median diastema Often do not delay eruption of incisors May cause rotation or other displacement of erupted teeth	Usually prevent eruption of incisors

REFERENCES

Broadway R T, Gould D G 1960 Surgical requirements of the orthodontist. British Dental Journal 108: 187–190

Brook A H 1974 Dental anomalies of number, form and size: their prevalence in British schoolchildren. Journal of the International Association of Dentistry for Children 5: 37–53

Foster T D, Taylor G S 1969 Characteristics of supernumerary teeth in the upper central incisor region. Dental Practitioner 20: 8–12

Gregg T A, Kinirons M J 1991 The effect of the position and orientation of unerupted premaxillary supernumerary teeth on eruption and displacement of permanent incisors. International Journal of Paediatric Dentistry 1: 3–7

Howard R D 1967 The unerupted incisor. Dental Practitioner 17: 332–342

Mitchell L, Bennett T G 1992 Supernumerary teeth causing delayed eruption – a retrospective study. British Journal of Orthodontics 19: 41–46

Primosch R E 1981 Anterior supernumerary teeth—assessment and surgical intervention in children. Pediatric Dentistry 3: 204–215

RECOMMENDED READING

Davis J M, Law D B, Lewis T M 1981 An atlas of pedodontics, 2nd edn. Saunders, Philadelphia, ch 3

Rapp R, Winter G B 1979 A colour atlas of clinical conditions in paedodontics. Wolfe, London

Rock W P, Grundy M C, Shaw L 1988 Diagnostic picture tests in paediatric dentistry. Wolfe, London

16 Intrinsic staining of teeth

16.1 CAUSES

There are many causes of intrinsic staining of teeth (Baden 1970, Faunce 1983). Many of the conditions in which intrinsic staining occurs are quite rare, but fairly common is staining of hypomineralized enamel. The discoloration ranges from white to brown, and is either localized or diffuse depending on whether the hypomineralization was caused by local, systemic or hereditary factors (Ch. 13). Similar discoloration is associated with mottled enamel, caused by excessive ingestion of fluoride.

In the past, tooth staining caused by administration of tetracycline drugs during the period of tooth development was not uncommon, but fortunately it has become rare because most physicians are now aware of the undesirable side-effects and do not prescribe tetracycline for children under the age of 7 years, except for rare conditions for which there is no effective alternative. The discoloration ranges from light yellow-orange to dark grey-brown, depending on the type of tetracycline drug and the duration of therapy.

16.2 TREATMENT

Treatment of discoloured teeth is required only to improve their appearance and therefore is limited to anterior teeth, often to maxillary anterior teeth. There are four possible approaches to treatment: etching and abrading; bleaching; veneering; and crowning. Techniques for veneering and crowning are described in Chapter 13, and for bleaching of discoloured non-vital teeth in Chapter 29. The techniques outlined below are for discoloured vital teeth.

16.2.1 Hypomineralized enamel

The white or brown discoloration associated with hypomineralization or with fluorosis is often located in superficial enamel and can therefore be eliminated by careful removal of surface enamel. Techniques involving etching and abrading have proved quite successful (Powell & Craig 1982, Croll & Cavanaugh 1986). The effectiveness of these methods cannot be confidently predicted, but they are simple and, especially with children, worth attempting before embarking on more radical and expensive methods.

Croll and Cavanaugh (1986) illustrated 20 cases in which the technique of etching and abrading had been used; only three were unsuccessful. They emphasized that the acid is extremely caustic and that meticulous care must be taken in handling it. Rubber dam isolation must be effective, the patient's and the dentist's eyes must be protected, the pot containing the acid paste must not be placed where it might be spilled on the patient, and the treatment should only be carried out with a cooperative patient.

It has been estimated that a series of 10 rubbings with pumice–HCl paste removes about a quarter of the thickness of the labial enamel of a maxillary permanent incisor (Waggoner et al 1989). There is no evidence of any effect on the dental pulp.

Powell & Craig (1982) described a similar technique, but used phosphoric acid to etch, and a pumice–water slurry and prophylaxis brush to abrade the tooth surface.

Technique: etching and abrading (Croll & Cavanaugh 1986)

1. Clean the affected tooth surfaces with a pumice–water slurry.
2. Prepare two thick pastes:
   a. pumice powder added to 18% hydrochloric acid
   b. sodium bicarbonate added to water.
3. Isolate the teeth with rubber dam. Copal varnish may be flowed around the gingival margin to improve the seal.
4. Place some of the sodium bicarbonate paste on the rubber dam around the teeth to be treated, to neutralize any acid that may inadvertently be misplaced.
5. Apply the pumice–HCl paste with a wooden tongue blade or cotton wool swab stick (having removed the cotton wool). Spread the paste over the discoloured area and rub it gently over the enamel surface with the wooden applicator. Place a cotton wool roll close to the tooth to absorb any acid that may drip from the tooth. A prophylaxis brush or rubber cup is not used because it would be difficult to avoid splatter and the acid is very caustic.
6. After 5 seconds, thoroughly rinse with water for 10 seconds while using high-volume suction.
7. Apply the pumice–HCl paste for further 5-second periods, rinsing thoroughly after each application. Usually improvement is noted after a few applications; the method is not pursued beyond 12–15 applications.
8. Finally, rinse thoroughly and apply a fluoride gel to the treated surfaces for 3 minutes. Polish with a fluoride prophylaxis paste and finish with a superfine aluminium oxide polishing disc.
9. Neutralize the remaining pumice–HCl paste with the sodium bicarbonate paste before discarding it.

16.2.2 Tetracycline staining

Discoloration caused by tetracycline cannot be polished away because the drug is deposited in both enamel and dentine. Bleaching can be successful in the treatment of yellow discolorations, but is rarely successful for grey discolorations (Reid 1985).

Technique: bleaching (Reid & Newman 1977)

1. Clean the affected surfaces with a pumice–water slurry.
2. Isolate the teeth with rubber dam.
3. Apply 30% hydrogen peroxide on pledgets of cotton wool to the labial and palatal surfaces of the teeth.
4. Activate the hydrogen peroxide. Reid & Newman applied heat with a low-voltage soldering iron, increased the heat to a level that the patient could comfortably tolerate, and maintained it for 30 minutes, keeping the pledgets moist throughout. Light also activates hydrogen peroxide, and a visible light source (of the type used to polymerize composite resins) may be as effective as the application of heat (Howell 1980).

REFERENCES

Baden E 1970 Environmental pathology of the teeth. In: Gorlin R J, Goldman H M (eds) Thoma's oral pathology, 6th edn. Mosby, St Louis, ch 4

Croll T P, Cavanaugh R R 1986 Enamel color modification by controlled hydrochloric acid–pumice abrasion. Quintessence International 17: 81–87 and 157–164

Faunce F 1983 Management of discolored teeth. Dental Clinics of North America 27: 657–670

Howell R A 1980 Bleaching discoloured roof-filled teeth. British Dental Journal 148: 159–162

Powell K R, Craig G G 1982 A simple technique for the aesthetic improvement of fluorotic-like lesions. Journal of Dentistry for Children 49: 112–117

Reid J S 1985 Patient assessment of the value of bleaching tetracycline-stained teeth. Journal of Dentistry for Children 52: 353–355

Reid J S, Newman P 1977 A suggested method of bleaching tetracycline-stained vital teeth. British Dental Journal 142: 261

Waggoner W F, Johnston W M, Schumann S, Schikowski E 1989 Microabrasion of human enamel in vitro using hydrochloric acid and pumice. Pediatric Dentistry 11: 319–322

17 Premature loss of primary teeth

Extraction of a primary incisor detracts from the child's appearance but has little or no effect on the development of the permanent dentition. On the other hand, extraction of a primary canine or molar may result in mesial or distal drift of adjacent teeth into the resulting space and subsequent crowding of permanent teeth.

In the mixed dentition, mesial drift of permanent first molars encroaches on space that is required for the eruption of premolars, and one of the premolars (usually the second) later becomes impacted or deflected out of the arch. When permanent incisors drift distally they encroach on space that is required for the permanent canine in that quadrant; as a result either the canine or a premolar in the quadrant later becomes crowded out of the arch. If distal drift occurs on one side only, following unilateral extraction of a primary tooth, the vertical coincidence of maxillary and mandibular centre lines is lost, that is, there is a 'centre line shift'. A centre line shift is undesirable because it results in asymmetrical crowding, which is more difficult to correct than symmetrical crowding.

17.1 FACTORS INFLUENCING MESIAL AND DISTAL DRIFT

The principal factors that influence the rate and extent of mesial and distal drift of teeth are the degree of crowding in the dental arch, the type of primary tooth that is extracted, and the age of the patient.

17.1.1 Degree of crowding

The rate and extent of mesial or distal drift are directly related to the degree of crowding in the dental arch. In an uncrowded arch there may be little or no movement of teeth following an extraction, but in a crowded arch adjacent teeth quickly move into spaces provided by the extraction of teeth.

17.1.2 Type of tooth extracted

Loss of a primary second molar is especially serious because it allows unimpeded mesial drift of the permanent first molar; however, centre line shift occurs only in very crowded arches. In contrast, extraction of a primary canine allows permanent incisors to drift distally (thus causing a centre line shift), but mesial drift of teeth may be minimal. Extraction of a primary first molar allows some mesial and distal drift to occur.

A summary of the relative amounts of mesial and distal drift that may be expected to follow extraction of different primary teeth is given in Table 17.1. Mesial drift of permanent first molars tends to be greater in the maxilla than in the mandible.

17.1.3 Age of patient

In general, the earlier a primary tooth is extracted the greater the opportunity for drifting of teeth, but over-eruption of opposing teeth may limit movement. If a

Table 17.1 The relative amounts of mesial drift of permanent first molars and distal drift of permanent incisors that may be expected following extraction of a primary tooth.

Primary tooth extracted	Mesial drift	Distal drift
second molar	+++	+
first molar	++	++
canine	+	+++

primary molar is extracted before eruption of the permanent first molar, mesial drift of the latter is inevitable, even in arches that are not crowded. On the other hand, if a primary tooth is extracted shortly before its natural exfoliation, no drift of permanent teeth may occur.

17.2 ASSESSMENT OF CROWDING

Because extraction of a primary tooth can have profound effects on the developing permanent dentition, a tooth should never be extracted before first assessing the likely effects and then planning treatment to prevent or alleviate undesirable effects. Since an important factor that determines drifting of teeth is the degree of crowding in the arch, it is essential to assess this before appropriate treatment can be planned.

During the mixed dentition the degree of crowding in the arch may be assessed by 1) observation of erupting permanent incisors, 2) examination of radiographs, and 3) comparison of the space available in the arch for the eruption of permanent canines and premolars with the estimated size of the unerupted teeth (Mixed Dentition Analysis).

17.2.1 Observation of erupting permanent incisors

The erupting incisors may provide early evidence of crowding. Although minimal imbrication may be relieved by growth, which increases the intercanine arch width up to about 9 years of age, definite over-lapping of contact points indicates that the arch is crowded. Signs of severe crowding are rotation or other displacement of erupting teeth, and resorption of a primary canine root by a permanent lateral incisor.

17.2.2 Radiographic examination

Signs of arch crowding that may be seen on radio-

graphs include distal inclination and 'stacking' of maxillary molars and distal inclination of mandibular molars.

17.2.3 Mixed Dentition Analysis

A quantitative assessment of crowding may be obtained by Mixed Dentition Analysis. The spaces available in each dental arch between the distal surface of the lateral incisors and the mesial surface of the permanent first molars are measured in the mouth or on study models, and the sum of the mesio-distal dimensions of the unerupted canines and premolars is determined in one of the following ways:

1. By using the average mesio-distal dimensions of permanent canines and premolars.
   Mandibular canine and all premolars
   $\qquad$ = 7 mm each (approx.)
   Maxillary canine = 8 mm (approx.)
   Therefore, mandibular canine + two premolars
   $\qquad$ = 21 mm
   Maxillary canine + two premolars
   $\qquad$ = 22 mm
   This method is useful only as a rough guide because the patient may not have teeth of average size.
2. By measuring the mesio-distal dimensions of the four erupted mandibular permanent incisors, and predicting the combined sizes of the unerupted canines and premolars from the correlation that exists between the sizes of the different groups of teeth in an individual.

The latter method is more accurate than that using average values but nevertheless is not very precise; it must therefore be considered as an aid in the assessment of crowding, not as an absolute measurement of crowding. The method is simple and quick to use, and is described on page 163.

The correlation between the sum of mesio-distal widths of mandibular permanent incisors and the sum of widths of canines and premolars was first established by Ballard & Wylie (1947) and followed up by Moyers (1973). In a review of published methods of Mixed Dentition Analysis, Irwin et al (1995) concluded that the method of Hixon & Oldfather (1958), as modified by Staley & Kerber (1980), is the most accurate. However, it is more difficult and time-consuming than the Moyers method because it involves measurement not only of incisors on dental casts but also of premolars on radiographs. It is doubtful whether the marginally greater accuracy of the method is of clinical significance.

Technique: Mixed Dentition Analysis—method based on measurement of mandibular permanent incisors

Procedure	Method	Rationale	Notes
1. Measure the mesio-distal widths of each of the four mandibular incisors	Open a pair of fine-pointed dividers to the greatest mesio-distal width of each incisor in turn (Fig. 17.1a). Mark each width on a straight line (Fig. 17.1b) then measure the combined width (Fig. 17.1c).	Mesio-distal dimension of mandibular incisors is the basis for predicting the sizes of unerupted canines and premolars.	If preferred, measurements may be made on study models of the patient's dentition.
2. Determine the predicted sum of widths of canines and premolars	From a table (Table 17.2) read the predicted sum of widths of the canine and two premolars in each quadrant, based on the sum of widths of mandibular incisors. Alternatively, take half the sum of widths of mandibular incisors. If this is x mm then $x + 10.5$ mm = sum widths mandibular canine and premolars $x + 11.0$ mm = sum widths maxillary canine and premolars.	Correlation between the sizes of the different groups of teeth makes this prediction possible. Similar results are obtained by this method, and tables are not required (Tanaka & Johnston 1974).	Tables are available which give predictions at different levels of probability.
3. Measure the space available in the arch for the unerupted canines and premolars	With dividers, measure from the distal surface of the lateral incisor to the mesial of the permanent first molar in each quadrant (Fig. 17.1d). Make a note of each measurement (in millimetres). If the incisors are imbricated, open the dividers to the combined widths of the central and lateral incisors on one side. Place one point on the centre line and note the position of the other point on the primary canine (or on the gingiva if the canine is absent); measure from this point to the mesial of the permanent first molar (Fig. 17.1e). Repeat for each quadrant.	Measurement of the space available for unerupted canines and premolars must take into account the space required for alignment of crowded incisors.	
4. Estimate the adequacy of space for unerupted canines and premolars	Compare the measurements made in procedures 2 and 3.		

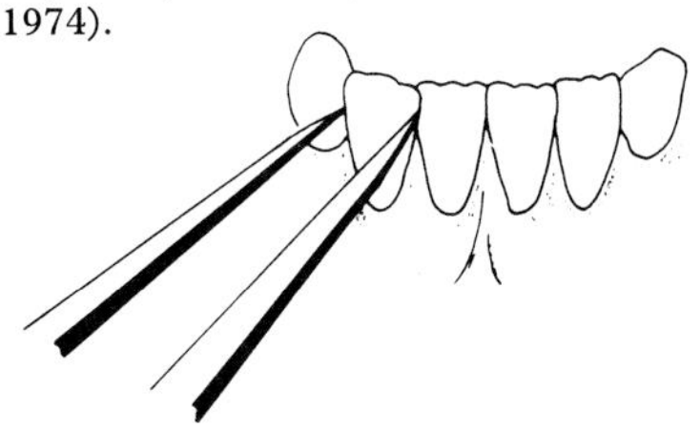

Fig. 17.1a

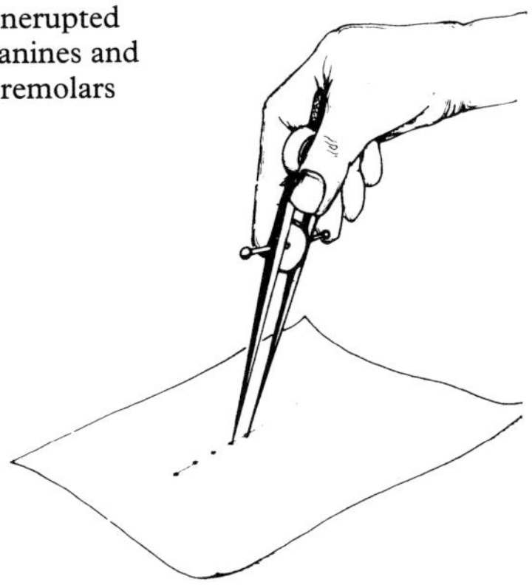

Fig. 17.1b

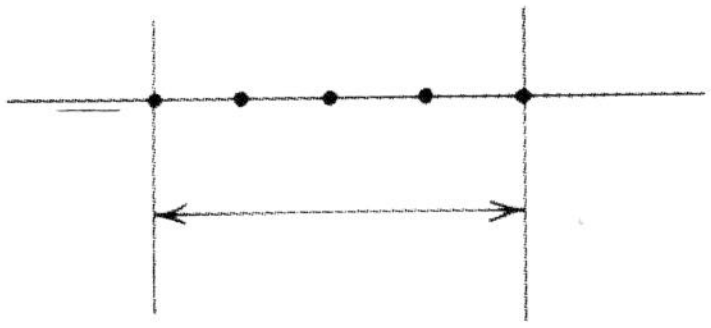

Fig. 17.1c

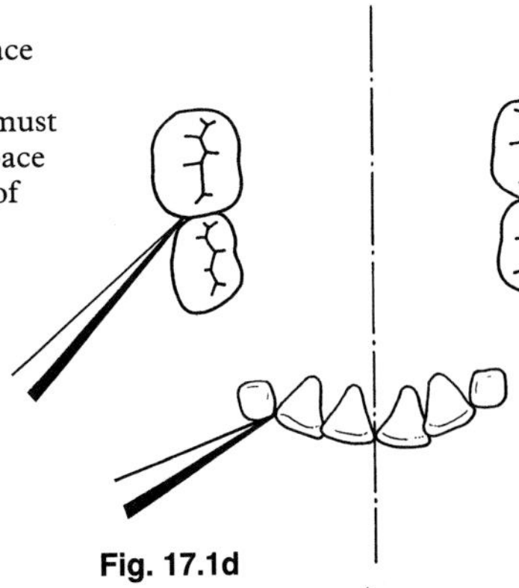

Fig. 17.1d

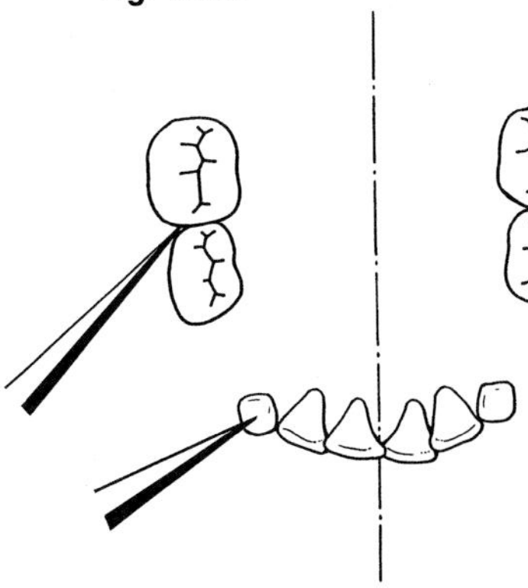

Fig. 17.1e

Table 17.2 Predicted sum of widths of canines and premolars (75% level of probability) based on the sum of widths of mandibular incisors.*

Sum of widths of mandibular incisors (mm)	Predicted sum of widths of canines and premolars in each quadrant (mm)	
	maxilla	mandible
19.5	20.6	20.1
20.0	20.9	20.4
20.5	21.2	20.7
21.0	21.5	21.0
21.5	21.8	21.3
22.0	22.0	21.6
22.5	22.3	21.9
23.0	22.6	22.2
23.5	22.9	22.5
24.0	23.1	22.8
24.5	23.4	23.1
25.0	23.7	23.4

* The data are taken from a much larger table in which the predicted sum of widths of unerupted canines and premolars are given at different levels of probability ranging from 95% to 5% (Moyers 1973). The data in Table 17.2 are those given at the 75% level of probability, which means that there is only a 1 in 4 chance that the actual sum of widths of the unerupted teeth exceeds the predicted sum. This is the level of probability generally used in Mixed Dentition Analysis, but if greater certainty is demanded, 1 mm may be added, which will give predicted sum of widths that will be exceeded in only 1 in 20 cases (95% probability level).

Table 17.3 Example of Mixed Dentition Analysis

	Maxilla		Mandible	
	Right	Left	Right	Left
Sum of widths of mandibular incisors = 22.5 mm				
Predicted sum of widths of canine and premolars	22.3	22.3	21.9	21.9
Space available in quadrant	22.0	22.5	20.5	19.5
Excess or deficiency of space (mm)	−0.3	+0.2	−1.4	−2.4

Having assessed the degree of dental arch crowding by observation of erupting incisors, from radiographs and by Mixed Dentition Analysis (Table 17.3), the dentition may be categorized as one of the following types (Foster 1990):

1. Excess space available for unerupted canines and premolars.
2. Just sufficient space for unerupted canines and premolars.
3. Mild deficiency of space for unerupted canines and premolars.
4. Severe deficiency of space for unerupted canines and premolars.

A summary of the signs of each of these types of dentition is given in Table 17.4.

Table 17.4 Signs of different types of dentition

Type of dentition	Signs
Not crowded —excess space	Spacing between incisors. Radiograph — long axes of maxillary molars vertical. MDA* — space available in arch exceeds that required for eruption of premolars and permanent canines.
Not crowded —just sufficient space	Normal contacts between incisors. Radiograph—long axes of maxillary molars vertical or with slight distal inclination. MDA* — space available in arch equals space required for eruption of premolars and permanent canines.
Mild crowding	Slight overlapping of incisors. Radiograph — distal inclination of maxillary molars. MDA* — space available in arch up to 4 mm less than that required for eruption of premolars and permanent canines.
Severe crowding	Overlapping, rotation or displacement of incisors. Radiograph — marked distal inclination of maxillary molars, with 'stacking'; distal inclination of mandibular molars. MDA* — space available in arch over 4 mm less than that required for eruption of premolars and permanent canines.

*MDA — Mixed Dentition Analysis

17.3 TREATMENT PLANNING

Selection of the most appropriate treatment to accompany the extraction of a primary tooth depends greatly on an assessment of the dentition as outlined above. Alternative forms of treatment, which are summarized in Table 17.5, are to balance the extraction or to fit a space maintainer; only when there is excess space in the arch is neither of these forms of treatment necessary.

Table 17.5 Treatment to accompany extraction of a primary tooth from an intact arch.

Primary tooth to be extracted	Type of dentition	Treatment	Rationale
Canine	Excess space	None	No drifting of teeth is expected.
	Just sufficient space	Usually balance, but a period of close observation may be justified	Centre line shift may or may not occur.
	Mild crowding	Balance. Compensate also if serial extraction is planned (Ch. 18)	Centre line shift is prevented by balancing the extraction.
	Severe crowding	Balance but do not compensate	
First molar	Excess space	None	No drifting of teeth is expected.
	Just sufficient space	Fit space maintainer	A space maintainer ensures that space remains adequate for unerupted canines and premolars.
	Mild crowding	Balance	Balancing prevents centre line shift. Space maintenance is not usually justified because in any case extraction of a permanent tooth from each quadrant is normally required later to relieve crowding.
	Severe crowding	Fit space maintainer	Space maintenance is justified because further space loss might make it necessary to extract more than one tooth from each quadrant to relieve crowding.
Second molar	Excess space	None	No drifting of teeth is expected.
	Just sufficient space	Fit space maintainer	(As for first molar above)
	Mild crowding	Fit space maintainer	Considerable mesial drift of the permanent first molar can be expected if the space is not maintained.
	Severe crowding	Fit space maintainer	Gross mesial drift of the permanent first molar will otherwise occur.

A *balancing extraction* is the removal of a tooth from the opposite side of the same arch to equalize mesial and distal drift of teeth; the tooth extracted is usually, but need not necessarily be, the contralateral tooth. A compensating extraction, which is less frequently justified, is the removal of a tooth from the same side of the opposing arch, to equalize drift in the two arches.

A *space maintainer* is an appliance that is fitted to prevent mesial drift of the permanent first molar. Space maintainers are usually not used to prevent distal drift of permanent incisors because this only occurs if the incisors are crowded; in these cases a balancing extraction is generally preferred to provide space for the incisors to spread out. When space main-tenance is the selected treatment but is impracticable because of unfavourable parental attitudes or poor patient cooperation, balancing extraction should be performed instead, to equalized drift and retain symmetry in the dental arch.

17.4 SPACE MAINTAINERS

It should be emphasized that the best type of space maintainer is the primary tooth itself. If, after assessing the dentition as a whole, it is decided that maintenance of space is important, every effort should be made to conserve the tooth; only if this is impracticable should an artificial space maintainer be considered.

Artificial space maintainers may be fixed or removable. The type of appliance used most commonly to maintain single tooth spaces in the fixed band and loop space maintainer (Fig. 17.2). If the tooth to be banded is very carious, a stainless steel crown is used instead of a band.

To maintain bilateral spaces, a lingual arch is used most commonly in the mandible, and a palatal arch or acrylic removable appliance in the maxilla.

Acrylic removable appliances, which are retained with Adams cribs, are more bulky than fixed appliances, but they are well tolerated by children. However, if space maintenance is required for several years, and if active orthodontic treatment is required subsequently, there is a danger that the child's cooperation may become exhausted before treatment begins. Removable appliances are, therefore, most useful for short-term space maintenance.

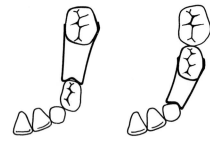

Fig. 17.2 Fixed space maintainers made with stainless steel bands and wire, the bands fitted to a permanent first molar or primary second molar.

Technique: band and loop space maintainer

Procedure	Method	Rationale	Notes
1. Select and fit a band	Select a preformed stainless steel band to fit the tooth distal to the space — either a primary second molar or a permanent first molar. Try the band on the tooth. The correct size band should not seat fully with finger pressure but require the use of a band pusher (Fig. 17.3a). The cervical margin of the band should fit just under the gingival margin. With a band pusher, adapt the margins of the band closely to the tooth.	A tight band is necessary for firm retention of the appliance. If the appliance loosens, demineralization of enamel may occur under the band. If the margin of the band is not subgingival and the patient's oral hygiene is not excellent, cervical caries could occur.	Preformed stainless steel bands are available in a range of sizes. A very secure finger rest is essential when using a band pusher.
2. Take an impression	With the band on the tooth, take an alginate impression of the arch (or of the section of the arch).		Alternatively, before taking the alginate impression, softened impression compound may be moulded over the occlusal surface of the tooth and over the buccal and lingual surfaces of the band; this provides a more positive surface than alginate on which to place the band in procedure 3.
3. Place the band in the impression	Remove the band from the tooth using band-removing pliers, position it accurately in the impression, and secure it with sticky wax.	The band must be carefully placed and secured in the impression to ensure that it is correctly positioned on the model.	

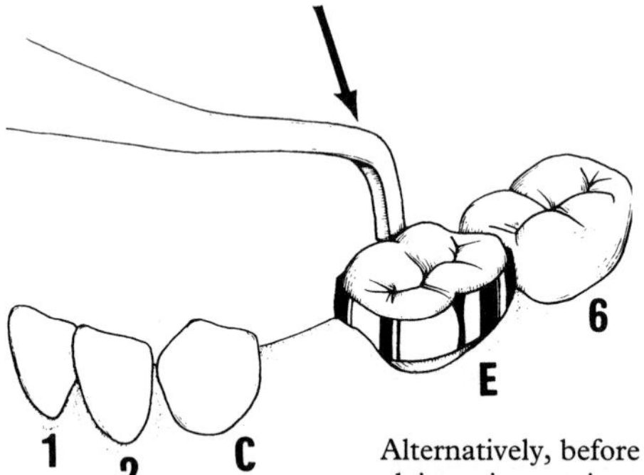

Fig. 17.3a

Technique: band and loop space maintainer *(contd)*

Procedure	Method	Rationale	Notes
4. Cast a stone model	Flow the stone into the impression carefully to avoid dislodging the band. Cut off the tooth that is to be extracted.		Ideally, the space maintainer is made before the tooth is extracted, and fitted as soon as possible after the extraction.
5. Adapt a wire loop	Select a preformed wire loop or bend a loop with 0.7 mm wire. The ends of the loop should rest tightly against the band buccally and lingually; the arms should run on each side of the alveolar ridge close to, or resting gently on, the gingiva; the anterior part should contact the tooth mesial to the space just under its contact area (Fig. 17.3b).	The wire loop should be wide enough to allow partial eruption of the premolar, and must not press on the gingiva.	

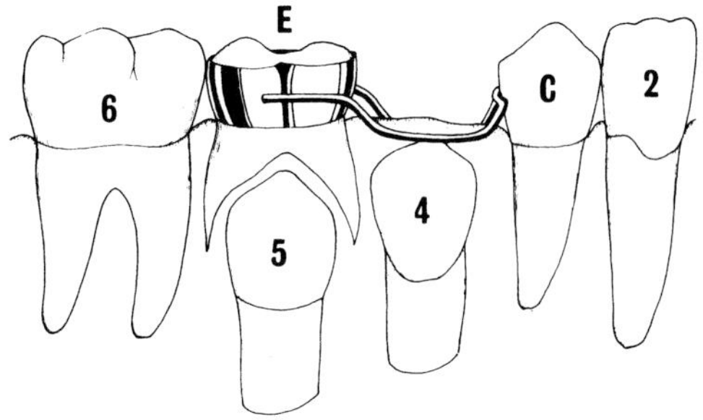

Fig. 17.3b

Procedure	Method	Rationale	Notes
6. Solder the loop to the band	Secure the anterior part of the loop to the model with sticky wax, and cover the wax with plaster. Grind away the stone inside the band on the buccal and lingual sides, that is, inside the parts of the band that are to be soldered to the wire.	Removal of stone inside the band ensures efficient heating of the band, which is essential for soldering.	An alternative method, which makes it unnecessary to grind out stone, is to flow wax into the band on the buccal and lingual sides immediately after placing the band in the impression (procedure 3), that is, before casting the stone model.
	Apply flux to the wire and underlying band, and heat with the soldering flame until the flux dries. Apply silver solder and heat until it flows around the wire.		The surface of the band and wire must be absolutely clean for satisfactory soldering.
7. Smooth and polish the appliance	Smooth the solder with a stone and a rubber wheel. Remove the band from the model for final polishing and to clean the inside of the band.	Smoothing on the model prevents distortion of the appliance.	
8. Try in	Try the appliance in the mouth and check that it fits correctly.		The appliance should be fitted as soon as possible after extraction of the tooth.
9. Cement the band	Clean and dry the tooth. Isolate with cotton rolls and saliva ejector. Apply a creamy mix of polycarboxylate cement to the inside of the band; seat first with finger pressure and then with band pusher and band seater. Remove excess cement when it has set.		

Technique: lingual arch space maintainer

Since most of the procedures in the technique are similar to those used in the band and loop space maintainer, only a few details will be considered here.

1. Fit preformed stainless steel bands to both mandibular permanent first molars. Take an impression, position the bands in the impression and cast a stone model.
2. Bend a lingual arch with 0.9 or 1.0 mm stainless steel wire. The ends of the wire should rest against the middle of the lingual surfaces of the bands. The arch should run mesially on each side level with the crests of the interdental papillae, and contact the lingual surfaces of the mandibular incisors just above the interdental papillae (Fig. 17.4a). If both primary molars on one or both sides are missing, bend the wire down to rest gently on, or just off, the gingiva, on the lingual side of the alveolar ridge. U-loops incorporated into the arch (Fig. 17.4b) permit some adjustment should this be necessary.
3. Check that the arch is passive when placed in position on the model before proceeding to solder.

A lingual arch prevents mesial drift by bracing one first molar against the other. Contact with the mandibular incisors is not essential; indeed, in cases where spontaneous relief of incisor crowding is desired, close contact of the arch against the incisors is undesirable.

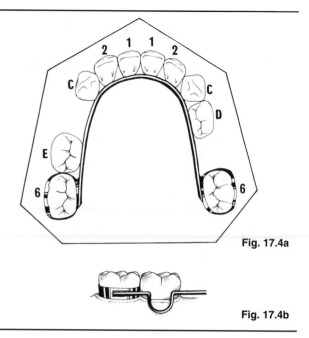

Fig. 17.4a

Fig. 17.4b

REFERENCES

Ballard M L, Wylie W L 1947 Mixed dentition case analysis — estimating size of unerupted permanent teeth. American Journal of Orthodontics and Oral Surgery 33: 754–759

Foster T D 1990 A textbook of orthodontics, 3rd edn. Blackwell, Oxford, p 138

Hixon E G, Oldfather R E 1958 Estimation of the sizes of unerupted cuspid and bicuspid teeth. Angle Orthodontist 28: 236–240

Irwin R D, Herold J S, Richardson A 1995 Mixed dentition analysis: a review of methods and their accuracy. International Journal of Paediatric Dentistry 5: 137–142

Moyers R E 1973 A handbook of orthodontics for the student and the general practitioner. Year Book Medical Publishers, Chicago

Staley R N, Kerber R E 1980 A revision of the Hixon and Oldfather mixed dentition prediction method. American Journal of Orthodontics 78: 296–302

Tanaka M T, Johnston L E 1974 The prediction of the size of unerupted canines and premolars in a contemporary orthodontic population. Journal of the American Dental Association 88: 798–801

18 Crowding of erupting permanent incisors

Crowding of the permanent dentition may be predicted during the primary dentition period if the primary incisors are imbricated, or even if they are well aligned but have no spaces between them (p. 130). The first evidence of crowding of permanent teeth is seen in the incisor regions (usually of the mandible, because mandibular incisors erupt before the maxillary incisors). The central incisors usually erupt normally but there is then inadequate space between these and the primary canines to accommodate the erupting lateral incisors. The lateral incisors either become rotated as they erupt or, in severely crowded cases, resorb the roots of the primary canines, causing their premature loss, or become displaced from the arch (usually lingually).

The eruption of permanent incisors is a milestone in development that excites the interest of every family. When the teeth do not erupt in perfect alignment parents are understandably concerned. Crowding of erupting incisors is, therefore, a common reason for parents to seek a dentist's advice. A fundamental decision must be taken:

1. to postpone treatment and accept the existing incisor crowding, or
2. to extract primary canines, to create space for the permanent lateral incisors. Extraction of primary canines may or may not become part of a serial extraction plan.

18.1 POSTPONEMENT OF TREATMENT

If the incisors are only very mildly crowded, postponement of treatment is easily justified. Some increase in the intercanine width of the arch is expected up to the age of about 9 years (p. 131), which might provide enough space for the lateral incisors. Any crowding that persists is assessed, and orthodontic treatment is considered a few years later, when premolars erupt.

If, however, there is more severe crowding and the incisors are rotated or displaced, postponement of treatment is more difficult to justify to parents because it condemns the child to an ugly appearance for 3 or 4 years, which may be distressing for the child and parents. Nevertheless it may still be considered the best long-term plan.

18.2 EXTRACTION OF PRIMARY CANINES

Extraction of primary canines provides space for lateral incisors to erupt without becoming rotated or displaced or, if they are already erupted, to drift distally and relieve the crowding. However, the incisor crowding is relieved by encroaching on space that should be reserved for the eruption of permanent canines. Thus, extraction of primary canines transfers crowding from the incisor to the canine/premolar region.

18.2.1 Serial extraction

The serial extraction method involves the planned extraction of selected primary and permanent teeth. Classically, the sequence of extraction is as follows (Houston et al 1992, Graber & Vanardsdall 1994):

1. Primary canines—to provide space for the permanent lateral incisors. The canines are extracted

when the maxillary permanent lateral incisors are erupting, at about the age of 8 years.

2. Primary first molars—to encourage early eruption of the first premolars. Primary first molars are extracted about 1 year after extraction of the primary canines.

Since the first premolars are the teeth to be extracted next, it is important to ensure that they erupt before the canines and second premolars. In the maxilla this almost always occurs naturally, but in the mandible the canines and second premolars erupt at about the same time as the first premolars, and extraction of the primary first molars is therefore usually necessary to ensure that the first premolars erupt first.

3. First premolars—to create space for the permanent canines. First premolars are extracted as soon as they erupt.

Serial extraction is a controversial method of treatment that has been described as 'strong in theory but weak in practice' (Ackerman & Proffit 1980). Before embarking on such treatment, a full orthodontic assessment must be made, aided by study models and radiographs. Serial extraction may be considered if: 1) the degree of crowding is mild; 2) the arch relationship is Class I; and 3) all unerupted teeth appear, radiologically, to be in their normal positions and normal in structure.

Serial extraction is complicated if crowding is severe, because considerable mesial drift of permanent first molars can be expected to occur, especially in the maxilla, following extraction of primary first molars and premolars, and this might leave inadequate space for eruption of canines and second premolars. Therefore, if the serial extraction plan is to be pursued in severely crowded cases, space maintenance is essential, ideally by conserving all primary molars but otherwise by fitting artificial space maintainers (p. 165). A disadvantage of using appliances for space maintenance in these cases is that the child would be obliged to wear them for several years: from about the age of 9 years (when primary first molars are extracted) to about 12–13 years (when canines and second premolars erupt), and this might reduce the child's cooperation for further orthodontic treatment should it be required later.

A complication of extracting mandibular primary canines in severely crowded cases is displacement of the developing mandibular permanent canines. By drifting distally and occupying spaces into which the permanent canines should erupt, the lateral incisors often cause distal inclination and buccal displacement of the canines, and this makes their alignment in the

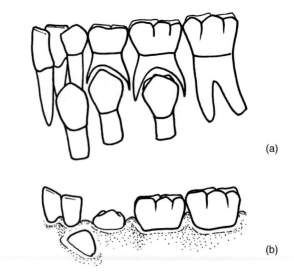

(a)

(b)

Fig. 18.1 (a) Crowded permanent incisors, eruption of mandibular first premolar ahead of canine; (b) canine displaced buccally and inclined distally.

arch more difficult to achieve. This is a particular problem in the mandible because, if eruption of the first premolar is more advanced than that of the canine (which is not uncommon in the mandible), the premolar will also tend to encroach on the canine space in the arch and, by the time it has erupted enough to be extracted, the canine has been displaced buccally (Fig. 18.1). Therefore, if radiographs show mandibular first premolars more advanced in their eruption than the permanent canines, it may be unwise to extract the primary canines.

18.2.2 No serial extraction

The full serial extraction procedure is rarely carried out nowadays, but extraction of primary canines may nevertheless be a useful measure to prevent or alleviate crowding of permanent incisors (Houston et al 1992). If unacceptable crowding is predicted when the lateral incisors are beginning to erupt, extraction of primary canines would prevent rotation or lingual displacement of the lateral incisors and, in the maxilla, possibly a crossbite; if the lateral incisors are already erupted and displaced, spontaneous improvement can be expected.

Before extracting primary canines, however, the developing dentition must be carefully assessed, including the relative stages of eruption of the mandibular canines and first premolars (as indicated above). The malocclusion is reassessed and treated when the premolars erupt.

REFERENCES

Ackerman J L, Proffit W R 1980 Preventive and interceptive orthodontics: a strong theory proves weak in practice. Angle Orthodontist 54: 75–81

Graber T M, Vanardsdall R L 1994 Orthodontics: current principles and techniques, 2nd edn. Mosby, St Louis, p 349–372

Houston W J, Stephens C D, Tulley W J 1992 A textbook of orthodontics, 2nd edn. Butterworth-Heineman, Oxford, p 195

19 Crossbites

dontic treatment plan. Treatment is usually delayed until the child is 10 or 11 years of age, when the occlusion is assessed and a plan made to correct the crossbite in the same course of treatment as any other abnormalities that might exist.

19.1 CROSSBITES IN THE PRIMARY DENTITION

A primary incisor crossbite may be a reflection of a Class III arch relationship, in which case all the maxillary incisors occlude lingual to the mandibular incisors, or it may be caused by a local factor, in which case only one or two incisors may be in crossbite. Unless the crossbite causes a traumatic occlusion no treatment is required; the dentition is reviewed when the permanent incisors erupt.

Primary molar crossbites may be bilateral or unilateral. A bilateral crossbite may be caused by a discrepancy in arch width but a unilateral crossbite is usually caused by a local factor such as premature contact of teeth, usually primary canines, during mouth closure. If abnormal contacts are detected they should be corrected by careful grinding of teeth. Lindner (1989) found that grinding was successful in correcting unilateral crossbites in about 50% of cases. No other treatment is normally considered in the UK for primary molar crossbites, but elsewhere early treatment to expand the maxillary arch is sometimes advocated (Lee 1978, Thilander et al 1984, Lindner 1989).

19.2 PERMANENT FIRST MOLAR CROSSBITE

Crossbite of permanent first molars should not be treated in isolation but as part of an overall ortho-

19.3 PERMANENT INCISOR CROSSBITE

Incisor crossbite may be associated with a skeletal Class III arch relationship. Some children with mild skeletal Class III jaw relationship posture the mandible forwards to achieve a more comfortable occlusion, and this increases the reversed overjet (Foster 1990). More commonly, however, incisor crossbite is caused by local factors. Insufficiency of space in the arch between the primary canines may cause maxillary lateral incisors to be deflected palatally as they erupt, and a primary incisor that is retained because it is non-vital and not being resorbed normally also may deflect its successor palatally.

Anterior crossbites caused by local factors may be prevented by timely removal of the cause. Thus, extraction of maxillary primary canines may allow crowded lateral incisors to erupt in normal alignment, and removal of a retained primary incisor usually allows normal eruption of its permanent successor.

When a maxillary permanent incisor erupts in crossbite, appliance therapy should be started as soon as a small overbite is established; when the crossbite is corrected, the overbite will retain the tooth in its correct position. If there is insufficient space in the arch for the displaced tooth it is, of course, necessary to create space by extracting maxillary primary canines before correcting the crossbite.

Anterior crossbites are most commonly treated with removable appliances such as those illustrated in Figure 19.1. Covering of posterior teeth with acrylic is

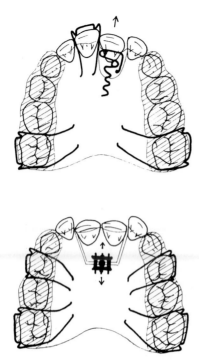

Fig. 19.1 Appliances for the correction of anterior crossbites.

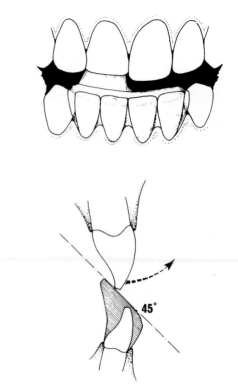

Fig. 19.2 Anterior inclined plane to correct anterior crossbite.

necessary to open the bite sufficiently to allow the maxillary teeth to be moved labially, but as soon as the crossbite has been corrected this 'capping' may be removed and the appliance then worn for a few weeks as a retainer; only a short retention period is needed, provided the overbite is adequate.

If the number of teeth in the maxillary arch is in-sufficient to retain a removable appliance, an inclined plane cemented to mandibular incisors may be used. The appliance may be made of acrylic or cast metal, and should be inclined at about 45° (Fig. 19.2). This appliance is potentially traumatic and should not be used for more than a few weeks.

REFERENCES

Foster T D 1990 A textbook of orthodontics, 3rd edn. Blackwell, Oxford, p 317–320

Lee B D 1978 Correction of crossbites. Dental Clinics of North America 22: 647–668

Lindner A 1989 Longitudinal study of the effect of interceptive treatment in 4-year-old children with unilateral crossbite. Scandinavian Journal of Dental Research 97: 432–438

Thilander B, Wahlund S, Lennartsson B 1984 The effect of early interceptive treatment in children with posterior crossbite. European Journal of Orthodontics 6: 25–34

20 Proclined maxillary permanent incisors

Orthodontic treatment should aim to obtain an acceptable result in the minimum possible time. In most cases this is achieved by delaying the start of treatment until all permanent teeth (other than third molars) have erupted. However, earlier treatment may be considered for a child who has proclined maxillary incisors and an increased incisor overjet, to reduce the risk of trauma to the teeth or to eliminate a source of psychological distress. Boys who participate in contact sports are particularly at risk from trauma, especially if the teeth are inadequately covered by the lips. Girls tend to be more concerned about their appearance and more sensitive to the unkind comments of other children.

Treatment

The essential stages in early treatment of Class II division I malocclusion are as follows (Fulstow 1968, Houston et al 1992):

1. Confirm radiologically that the permanent canines are in satisfactory positions.

2. Start treatment when the crowns of the permanent canines are distal to the roots of the lateral incisors. Extract the maxillary primary canines if the space is required for retraction of incisors.
3. Retract the incisors with a removable appliance (Rock 1990).
4. When the incisors are fully retracted against the mandibular incisors, modify the appliance (or make another appliance) to use for night-time retention for 6 months.
5. Extract maxillary first premolars as soon as they erupt. Sometimes it is advisable to extract primary first molars to accelerate eruption of first premolars. It is hoped that the permanent canines will erupt into premolar spaces, but appliance therapy may be required.

Although conventional treatment of Class II division I malocclusion has fewer potential complications and is usually completed more quickly than the treatment described above, there are important reasons for considering early treatment in certain cases.

REFERENCES

Fulstow E D 1968 The early treatment of Angle's Class II division I malocclusion. Dental Practitioner 19: 137–144
Houston W J B, Stephens C D, Tulley W J 1992 A textbook of orthodontics, 2nd edn. Butterworth-Heineman, Oxford, p 230

Rock W P 1990 Treatment of Class II malocclusions with removal appliances. Part 2—Class II division I treatment. British Dental Journal 168: 206–209

21 Persistent digit sucking

Digit sucking occurs so commonly in young children that it must be regarded as normal behaviour. The effects on the dentition vary according to the way in which the thumb or fingers are sucked, but include anterior open bite (usually asymmetrical), proclination of maxillary incisors, and retroclination of mandibular incisors. Most children give up the habit by the age of 4–5 years.

Treatment

Parents must be reassured that the dental effects of digit sucking are usually reversible when the habit stops: overbite and overjet return to normal unless prevented by the action of the lips and tongue.

The dentist must try to achieve rapport with the child by an understanding and sympathetic approach, so that cessation of the habit becomes a matter of mutual concern. If the habit has not ceased by the age of 8–9 years, a simple passive removable appliance may be fitted, mainly to act as a reminder to the child. With or without an appliance, the habit is usually abandoned by about 10 years of age, when children begin to take greater interest in their teeth and in their appearance generally. If the habit persists, insertion of an appliance as part of orthodontic treatment finally breaks the habit.

In the USA, fixed appliances which incorporate wire 'cribs' that prevent thumb or fingers from being placed in the mouth are sometimes used in the early mixed dentition (Gellin 1978).

REFERENCES

Gellin M E 1978 Digital sucking and tongue thrusting in children. Dental Clinics of North America 22: 603–619

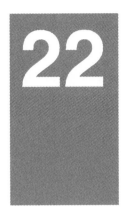

22 Permanent first molars with poor long-term prognosis

Permanent first molars are very important teeth in the dentition and every effort should be made to conserve them by fissure sealing or by prompt treatment of early lesions. Fortunately the prevalence of caries in these teeth in children of all age groups in the UK has declined considerably in recent years, as shown by the results of the national surveys in 1983 and 1993 (Todd & Dodd 1985, O'Brien 1994). For example, 56% of 9-year-old children in 1983 had permanent first molars that were decayed or that had been filled or extracted, compared with 26% in 1993, and for 12-year-olds the figures were 79% in 1983 and 50% in 1993. Permanent first molars may also be hypomineralized or hypoplastic, associated with amelogenesis imperfecta or with a systemic disturbance during infancy (pages 141–142).

If permanent first molars are so severely affected by caries, hypomineralization or hypoplasia that their long-term prognosis is assessed to be poor, extraction may be the most appropriate treatment option. Undesirable effects on the occlusion may be minimized by balancing and compensating extractions and, if possible, by extracting the teeth at the most appropriate time in the development of the dentition, which is usually between the ages of $8\frac{1}{2}$ and 10 years; the developing second molars then have the best chance of erupting into the first molar spaces and a satisfactory occlusion may be established without appliance therapy.

22.1 ASSESSMENT OF LONG-TERM PROGNOSIS

It is an important responsibility of children's dentists to assess the long-term prognosis of permanent first molars in child patients by the age of 8 or 9 years, so that a decision can be made on whether to conserve or extract the teeth. Signs that indicate a poor prognosis include the following:

1. Large amalgam restorations already present.
2. Recurrent caries in teeth already restored.
3. Lingual demineralization or caries in mandibular molars, and buccal demineralization or caries in maxillary molars, especially around existing restorations.
4. Abnormal enamel structure (e.g. hypoplasia).
5. Unfavourable attitudes of the child and parent regarding dental care.
6. Poor oral hygiene.
7. Poor patient cooperation.

22.2 TREATMENT PLANNING

22.2.1 General factors

When the permanent first molars are assessed to have a poor prognosis, the following factors must be considered before a decision is made to extract them.

1. Congenital absence of teeth

Clearly, plans to extract first molars become complicated if other teeth are found to be congenitally absent. However, the absence of third molars has only a marginal effect on the decision. Indeed the germs of the third molars may not have begun to calcify at the age of $8\frac{1}{2}$–10 years, which is the ideal age at which to extract first molars (see below). Therefore the decision to extract first molars must often be made without knowledge of the development of third molars.

2. Hypoplasia of premolars

One or more unerupted permanent teeth may be hypoplastic due to infection of the primary predecessor or to trauma during extraction of the primary tooth; second premolars are most commonly affected. It may be possible to detect severe hypoplasia on a radiograph and to decide that the prognosis of the hypoplastic tooth is worse than that of the first molar.

3. Occlusal relationship and degree of crowding

In general, the most favourable conditions for extraction of first molars are a Class 1 occlusal relationship and mild buccal segment crowding (i.e. insufficiency of space for eruption of canines and premolars). The desired mesial movement of mandibular second molars is encouraged if the developing dentition is crowded; maxillary molars move mesially even in the absence of crowding.

4. Stage of dental development

Extractions must be timed to maximize bodily mesial movement of the developing second molars, and to minimize mesial tilting. The ideal time to extract mandibular first molars is when root formation of the second molars is just beginning (as shown on a radiograph), which is usually between the ages of $8\frac{1}{2}$ and 10 years; this gives the second molars every opportunity to move forward bodily (Fig. 22.1). Earlier

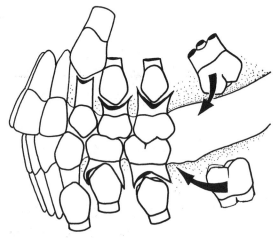

Fig. 22.1 Ideal stage of dental development for extraction of permanent first molars.

extraction is generally undesirable because mandibular second premolars have a tendency to drift distally, and very early extraction of first molars encourages this tendency. On the other hand, if extractions are delayed until after 10 years of age, the second molars will show less bodily movement and more tilting. Thus, extraction of mandibular first molars at the age of $8\frac{1}{2}$–10 years is a compromise between the need to extract early to encourage mesial drift of second molars, and the need to delay to discourage distal drift of second premolars.

In the maxilla, unerupted second molars tend to be distally inclined, especially in a crowded arch, and they readily drift mesially by moving into more upright positions. Therefore, extraction of maxillary molars can often be delayed until about 11 or 12 years of age without affecting the final occlusion.

22.2.2 Ideal conditions for extraction

Having considered the factors outlined above, the ideal conditions for extracting first molars that have a poor long-term prognosis are:

1. Unerupted canines, premolars and second molars are visible on a radiograph and show no evidence of abnormality.
2. The occlusal relationship is Class I.
3. There is mild buccal segment crowding, i.e. there is insufficient space in the arch for the eruption of canines and premolars.
4. The patient is between $8\frac{1}{2}$ and 10 years of age.

Under these conditions, extraction of the four first molars is fully justified, and often results in a satisfactory occlusion with acceptable contacts between second premolars and second molars; sometimes, final orthodontic adjustment may be required later. This outcome is preferable to that resulting from extraction of first molars several years later, following repeated repair and enlargement of restorations.

If, however, all the conditions outlined above are not satisfied, it would be prudent to consult an orthodontist before proceeding with treatment. For example, if the patient has severe incisor crowding or a Class II malocclusion with increased overjet, it may be preferable to delay (if possible) the extraction of maxillary first molars until the maxillary second molars erupt, and then to fit an appliance to hold the second molars in position after the first molars are extracted, thus preserving space for retraction of premolars and correction of incisor crowding or overjet (Crabb & Rock 1971). However, this treatment would have to be delayed until the second molars are erupted sufficiently to be banded, which might not be until the child is over 13 years old, at which age children tend to become less willing to undergo lengthy orthodontic treatment. The alternative approach is to extract the maxillary first molars at the same time as the mandibular molars, which encourages the maxillary second molars to erupt earlier, usually by 12 years of age. Treatment can then proceed either by retracting the second molars and premolars, using headgear, and then the anterior teeth; or by extracting a premolar unit and retracting the anterior teeth. The latter course ensures that treatment is completed quickly, but sacrifices a second tooth unit in the dentition. The choice of treatment plan partly depends on an assessment of the patient's interest and cooperation.

22.2.3 Balancing and compensating extractions

When only one or two of the four permanent first molars need to be extracted or are assessed as having poor long-term prognosis, it is necessary to consider the need to balance or compensate the extraction(s) (i.e. to extract the contralateral or opposing tooth/teeth, respectively). In addition to the general factors outlined above, two main factors must be considered:

1. The occlusal relationship of the teeth
2. The adequacy of space in the dental arches for eruption in good alignment of premolars and permanent canines.

The guidelines summarized in Table 22.1 are based on three different clinical situations.

Clinical situation 1

— occlusal relationship Class I
— inadequate space for premolars and canines

   Compensation. Extraction of one or both mandibular first molars from a dentition in Class I occlusion should be accompanied by compensating extraction(s) of maxillary molar(s) because otherwise the latter would over-erupt and prevent the desired mesial movement of mandibular second molars (Fig. 22.2). If the maxillary molars are sound this treatment plan may

seem rather extreme, and it requires careful explanation to parents, but it is the correct plan in this situation. Maxillary second molars readily move forward to occupy the first molar positions.

On the other hand, extraction of one or both maxillary first molars need not be compensated by extraction of the mandibular molar(s) because the latter do not over-erupt significantly and therefore do not impede mesial movement of the maxillary second molars (Fig. 22.3).

   Balancing. Extraction of a maxillary or mandibular first molar from a dentition having inadequate space for erupting premolars and canines is usually balanced by extraction of the first molar(s) on the other side. However, if the latter are sound teeth, an alternative plan to relieve crowding on that side might be based on extraction of first or second premolars or, possibly, second molars.

Clinical situation 2

— occlusal relationship Class I
— adequate space for premolars and canines

   Compensation. The same guidelines apply as for clinical situation 1. However, because there is no inherent crowding in the dental arches there is little tendency for mesial movement of mandibular second molars. Even in uncrowded arches, unerupted maxillary second molars readily move forward after extraction of maxillary first molars but, if the long-term prognosis of mandibular first molars is considered to be poor, they should be extracted early (age 8 would be preferable to age 10) to give the second molars the maximum time to move forward as they erupt.

   Balancing. Balancing extractions are not required because crowding of premolars and canines is not predicted.

Clinical situation 3

— occlusal relationship Class II (requiring orthodontic treatment)
— inadequate space for premolars and canines

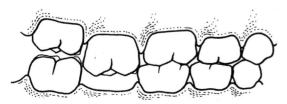

Fig. 22.2 Over-eruption of a maxillary permanent first molar following extraction of the mandibular first molar.

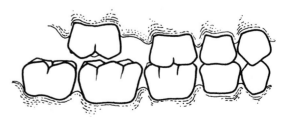

Fig. 22.3 No over-eruption of the mandibular permanent first molar following extraction of the maxillary first molar.

Table 22.1 A summary of guidelines for compensating or balancing extractions of permanent first molars (assuming extractions between the ages of $8\frac{1}{2}$ and 10 years, and all unerupted canines, premolars and second molars confirmed radiographically as present and not hypoplastic).* (Adapted from Mackie et al 1989.)

Permanent first molar(s) to be extracted	Clinical situation		
	1 Class I inadequate space for canines/premolars	2 Class I adequate space for canines/premolars	3 Class II inadequate space for canines/premolars
Mandibular			
one	compensate possibly balance	compensate do not balance	compensate? possibly balance
both	compensate	compensate	compensate?
Maxillary			
one	do not compensate possibly balance	do not compensate or balance	do not compensate possibly balance
both	do not compensate	do not compensate	do not compensate

* Refer to text

Compensation. As pointed out on pages 180-181, there are differing views about whether compensating extraction of a maxillary molar in a Class II case is better carried out at the same time as the enforced extraction of the mandibular molar or delayed (if practicable) until maxillary second molars erupt. It is therefore sensible for general dental practitioners to know the views of the orthodontist to whom they refer their patients.

If maxillary first molars are sound, an alternative plan to correct a Class II malocclusion might be to retain the maxillary molars and make space for retraction of maxillary anterior teeth by extracting maxillary first or second premolars. However, over-eruption of the maxillary molars may present a problem, unless they occlude with mandibular primary second molars (which they might in a Class II case).

If a maxillary molar must be extracted, there is no need for compensating extraction of the mandibular molar, for the same reasons as given under clinical situation 1.

Balancing. Since space must be provided for eruption of premolars and canines and for retraction of maxillary anterior teeth, balancing extractions usually are indicated. If, however, the first molars on the 'balancing' side are sound, orthodontic treatment might be based on the extraction of a maxillary and a mandibular premolar.

Not included in Table 22.1 is the relatively uncommon Class III case. Treatment of Class III malocclusions is complex and referral to an orthodontist is indicated, but an important aim must be to conserve maxillary teeth. If a maxillary molar must be extracted, balancing extraction of the contralateral tooth should not be carried out unless this tooth also cannot be restored, and compensating extractions should not be carried out unless the mandibular molars have a poor prognosis and there is inadequate space for eruption of premolars and canines.

Also not included in Table 22.1 are the cases in which three, or two diagonally opposite, first molars need to be extracted. In each case the appropriate treatment is, almost invariably, to extract the other one or two first molars, provided the child is between $8\frac{1}{2}$ and 10 years old, and that all unerupted canines, premolars and second molars have been confirmed radiographically as present and not hypoplastic.

REFERENCES

Crabb J J, Rock W P 1971 Treatment planning in relation to the first permanent molar. British Dental Journal 131: 396–401

Mackie I C, Blinkhorn A S, Davies P H J 1989 The extraction of permanent first molars during the mixed-dentition period—a guide to treatment planning. Journal of Paediatric Dentistry 5: 85–92

O'Brien M 1994 Children's dental health in the United Kingdom 1993. Office of Population Censuses and Surveys. Her Majesty's Stationery Office, London, p 28

Todd J E, Dodd T 1985 Children's dental health in the United Kingdom 1983. Her Majesty's Stationery Office, London, p 31

23 Tooth wear and erosion

Tooth wear may be caused by attrition, abrasion or erosion, or by any combination of the three processes. Attrition is caused by tooth-to-tooth contact; abrasion by object-to-tooth contact (e.g. toothbrushing); and erosion by a chemical process not directly associated either with mechanical or chemical traumatic factors, or with dental caries.

23.1 DENTAL EROSION

The prevalence of dental erosion was measured for the first time on a national scale in a survey of children's dental health in the United Kingdom in 1993 (O'Brien 1994). Over 50% of 5- and 6-year-old children were reported to have eroded surfaces on one or more primary incisors, and in almost a quarter of these children erosion had progressed into dentine or pulp. Erosion generally involved two-thirds or more of the affected surfaces. Erosion was also found in the permanent dentition, 51% of 14-year-old children being affected. These findings, however, should be considered with caution, because it was stated that the dentists who examined the children had difficulty in agreeing whether or not erosion was present, and in differentiating between erosion and attrition. Since attrition of primary teeth is normal in the late primary dentition (page 130), it is possible that a proportion of the lesions reported as erosion were in fact attrition.

Dental erosion may be caused by extrinsic or intrinsic factors. Extrinsic factors include acidic foods and drinks, especially fruit drinks and carbonated beverages (Millward et al 1994), the consumption of which has increased dramatically since the 1950s. A high proportion of soft drinks consumed in the UK is consumed by young children, 42% being drunk by those aged below 9 years (Rugg-Gunn et al 1987). Excessive consumption of acidic foods and drinks is especially hazardous in the primary dentition because the enamel and dentine are thinner than in the permanent dentition. Intrinsic causes of dental erosion include recurrent vomiting resulting from an abnormality of the gastrointestinal tract or from psychological disorders such as anorexia or bulimia nervosa (Milosevic & Slade 1989).

Treatment

Vigilance is needed to detect early subtle changes in the enamel that are indicative of erosion, so that appropriate intervention can be made.

1. Take a careful social, dental and medical history, and ask the parent to complete a 3-day diet record (page 38).
2. If dietary factors are identified, give appropriate advice: to reduce the frequency of intake of erosive food and drink, to confine drinks to mealtimes, and to drink acidic beverages through a straw to reduce the erosive effect on anterior teeth, which are usually the most severely affected.
3. Give oral hygiene instruction. Ensure that an appropriate toothbrush and a correct technique are used. Advise against brushing immediately after consuming an acidic food or drink as this is likely to accelerate loss of enamel by abrasion (Davis & Winter 1980).
4. If gastric regurgitation is a problem the patient should be under the care of a physician. Advise the use of an alkaline mouthwash, to be used

immediately after regurgitation to neutralize the gastric acid. Alternatively, make a mouthguard (page 204), to be worn at times of high risk, which can be loaded with an alkali such as magnesium hydroxide or sodium bicarbonate. At other times the mouthguard can be used for self-application of fluoride gel.

5. If tooth sensitivity is a problem, advise use of a fluoride mouthrinse (page 48) and a toothpaste containing strontium chloride and fluoride, and apply topical fluoride varnish (page 44).

6. The arrest or progress of erosion can be monitored using standardized photographs and study models cast from silicone impressions.

7. Only when it is certain that the cause has been identified and removed should consideration be given to restoring the affected teeth, otherwise erosion will merely continue around the restorations. Restoration of anterior teeth usually involves the use of veneers, either composite resin or porcelain. However, if buccal and lingual surfaces of teeth are affected full coverage crowns may be indicated.

REFERENCES

Davis W B, Winter P B 1980 The effect of abrasion on enamel and dentine after exposure to dietary acid. British Dental Journal 148: 253–256

Millward A, Shaw L, Smith A J, Rippin J W, Harrington E 1994 The distribution and severity of tooth wear and the relationship between erosion and dietary constituents in a group of children. International Journal of Paediatric Dentistry 4: 151–157

Milosevic A, Slade P D 1989 The orodental status of anorexics and bulimics. British Dental Journal 167: 66–70

O'Brien M 1994 Children's dental health in the United Kingdom 1993. Her Majesty's Stationery Office, London, p 74

Rugg-Gunn A J, Lennon M A, Brown J G 1987 Sugar consumption in the United Kingdom. British Dental Journal 167: 339–364

RECOMMENDED READING

Eccles J D 1978 The treatment of dental erosion. Journal of Dentistry 6: 217–221

Kleier D J, Aragon S B, Averbach R E 1984 Dental management of the chronic vomiting patient. Journal of the American Dental Association 108: 618–621

Treatment of periodontal and oral soft tissue lesions

Part 5

24 Periodontal disease

24.1 CHRONIC MARGINAL GINGIVITIS

Chronic marginal gingivitis is widespread in children. A survey in 1993 of child dental health in the UK (O'Brien 1994) showed that the condition was present in 26% of 5-year-old children, 53% of 7-year-olds, 63% of 11-year-olds and 52% of 15-year-olds.

Gingivitis is relatively uncommon in healthy preschool children, but occurs around primary teeth as they loosen and resolves after the teeth are shed. The prevalence increases between the ages of 6 and 8 years as the first permanent teeth erupt, and again at about 10–13 years as canines, premolars and second molars erupt, associated with the presence of plaque around the erupting teeth and an increased susceptibility of the gingival tissues to bacterial irritation (Matsson 1993). Other common local irritants include rough edges of carious cavities and overhanging margins of restorations. The prevalence of gingivitis also increases during puberty, associated with commencement of sex hormone secretion.

Treatment

1. Remove local irritating factors by carrying out a prophylaxis, restoring carious cavities, and replacing or smoothing unsatisfactory restorations.
2. Give oral hygiene instruction and dietary advice (Ch. 3).

24.2 GINGIVITIS ARTEFACTA

Gingivitis artefacta is a self-inflicted lesion, most commonly on a gingival margin or papilla, and often inflicted with a finger nail. If the child is asked to indicate the site of discomfort, the offending finger may be placed precisely on the lesion, clearly indicating its cause. However, a pencil or other sharp object may sometimes be the cause. The lesion may be an ulcer or a localized stripping of the gingival margin from the tooth, which may expose the root surface.

This type of behaviour by a child is usually initiated by minor gingival irritation, for example by an inflamed papilla or an exfoliating tooth, but sometimes psychological factors are involved and the injuries are more serious (Stewart & Kernohan 1972).

Treatment

1. Examine closely to detect any possible source of local irritation, and treat as necessary.
2. Identify the cause (finger nail or other sharp object). Gain the child's and the parent's cooperation in breaking the habit. If a finger nail is the cause, placing a piece of adhesive bandage on it serves as a reminder.
3. Patients with psychological disturbances may need to be referred for treatment before any improvement in their gingival condition can be achieved.

24.3 LOCALIZED GINGIVAL RECESSION

Localized gingival recession in children is seen most frequently on the labial surface of a mandibular permanent incisor (Fig. 24.1); the condition is sometimes referred to as a 'Stillman's cleft'.

The affected tooth is often positioned more labial in the arch than the other incisors and therefore has little or no supporting labial bone. Occlusal trauma may also be a factor, often associated with an anterior crossbite or deep overbite.

Another complicating factor may be a labial frenum that is attached high into the free gingival margin, and which may pull the gingival margin away from the tooth during normal movements of the lips. The high frenal attachment may also make it difficult for the child to keep the gingival margin clean with a toothbrush. The situation may be further complicated by a very shallow labial sulcus, with little or no attached gingiva over the root of the tooth.

Minor degrees of gingival recession may have no clinical significance because recession often decreases spontaneously if good oral hygiene is maintained (Andlin-Sobocki et al 1991). If it is severe, however, and exposes the root surface ('true' gingival recession), action is required to correct it.

Treatment

1. Give oral hygiene instruction. Encourage the child to pull the lower lip downwards to improve access to the site.
2. For future reference, take a clinical photograph or impressions for study models to record the existing degree of recession.

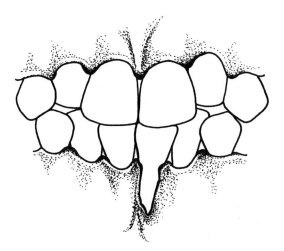

Fig. 24.1 Localized gingival recession.

3. If there is no true gingival recession, monitor the situation at 6-month or annual intervals; the condition sometimes resolves with normal growth and increased alveolar height.
4. If there is true gingival recession and if the child is unable to clean the site satisfactorily because of a shallow sulcus or high frenal attachment, periodontal surgery is generally required.
5. If the tooth is labially positioned in the arch or in traumatic occlusion, orthodontic treatment may be advisable. Either (a) align the tooth after creating space by extraction of one or more teeth in the arch, or (b) extract the tooth (if its labial displacement is so severe that the alveolar bone labial to it is very thin), and align the other incisors. A fixed appliance is required to close the space and achieve satisfactory tooth angulations.

24.4 GINGIVAL ENLARGEMENT

Gingival enlargement may be caused by inflammatory hyperplasia of gingival tissues associated with chronic irritation or with systemic diseases such as leukaemia or an endocrine imbalance. The affected gingiva is soft, tender, hyperaemic and bleeds easily.

Gingival enlargement may also be caused by fibrous hyperplasia, which may be a local reaction to chronic irritation and present as a fibrous epulis (page 197). The aetiology of more generalized forms may be uncertain, but some cases are associated with drug therapy and others are hereditary (e.g. gingival fibromatosis).

24.4.1 Gingival enlargement associated with drug therapy

Gingival enlargement is often seen in children suffering from epilepsy and receiving the drug phenytoin; the prevalence has been reported to be between 36% and 67% (Livingston & Livingston 1969) and its severity varies considerably. Gingival enlargement is also a side-effect of the immunosuppressive drug cyclosporin, which is used to prevent rejection following transplantation of tissue or an organ. Such operations are becoming increasingly common.

Neither phenytoin nor cyclosporin is directly responsible for the hyperplastic reaction but they appear to increase the sensitivity of gingival tissues to irritants from the dental plaque.

Treatment

1. Give the child and the parents detailed instructions

and every possible assistance in establishing and maintaining efficient plaque control.

2. Advise the use of chlorhexidine, as mouthwash or toothpaste. The mouthwash solution may be applied with a toothbrush, since handicapped patients may not be capable of mouthrinsing.

3. If the condition is severe, hyperplastic tissue may be removed by surgery, but this will recur unless plaque control is excellent.

4. Consult the child's physician. Although phenytoin is a safe and effective drug for the control of epilepsy, it is sometimes possible to change to another drug that does not cause gingival hyperplasia. On the other hand cyclosporin is a unique and life-saving drug; corticosteroids may be an alternative but they cause serious side-effects in children.

24.4.2 Gingival fibromatosis

Gingival fibromatosis is an hereditary (autosomal dominant) condition in which there is usually generalized but sometimes local fibrous enlargement of the gingival tissues. The condition usually appears in young children but if it is not too severe it may remain unnoticed until adolescence or adulthood. Gross enlargement may interfere with the occlusion of teeth, and if it is in the anterior part of the mouth it is unsightly.

Treatment

Excision of excess tissue, but it tends to recur.

24.5 PERIODONTITIS

Periodontitis is much less common than gingivitis in children. However, periodontal bone destruction, sometimes severe, may occur not only in children suffering from severe systemic disease but also in apparently healthy children.

24.5.1 Early chronic periodontitis

Evidence of early chronic periodontitis may be found in children by careful probing for loss of connective tissue attachment. A survey of a group of 15-year-old English children showed that 46% had loss of attachment of at least 1 mm, and 11% of at least 2 mm (Lennon & Davies 1974). Generally only a few sites are involved. A horizontal pattern of bone loss is most common and the degree of bone loss is related to oral hygiene. Signs of periodontitis in a child indicate a poor prognosis for periodontal health in adulthood.

Treatment

1. Remove subgingival plaque and any calculus from the affected sites and carry out thorough prophylaxis.

2. Instruct and motivate the child to maintain excellent oral hygiene, paying particular attention to flossing in the affected sites.

3. Review regularly and repeat scaling and prophylaxis as necessary.

24.5.2 Prepubertal periodontitis

Prepubertal periodontitis affects the primary teeth of very young children. Localized and generalized forms were described by Page et al (1983).

The localized form usually presents by the age of 4 years in apparently healthy children and affects only a few teeth. Plaque deposits may be minimal and gingival inflammation mild, but deep pockets are detected on probing and seen radiologically, and periodontal bone destruction is rapid. Affected children may also suffer from otitis media and upper respiratory tract infections.

Generalized prepubertal periodontitis begins earlier (at about the time of tooth eruption) and affects all the primary teeth. Both the marginal and attached gingiva are acutely inflamed and, because of this, toothbrushing may be abandoned and the teeth become covered by heavy plaque deposits. Periodontal bone destruction is even more rapid than in the localized form of the disease. The children may also suffer from otitis media.

The generalized form of prepubertal periodontitis described by Page et al (1983) is now believed to be the oral manifestation of leucocyte adhesion deficiency disease (Watanabe 1990). Similar periodontal problems may present in children suffering from systemic conditions such as neutropenia, agranulocytosis, blood dyscrasias, hypophosphatasia and Papillon Lefevre syndrome (Glenwright & Rock 1990) but, strictly speaking, these should not be defined as generalized prepubertal periodontitis.

Treatment

Refer the patient to a specialist for blood tests and other investigations, to rule out the possibility of underlying systemic disease.

Treatment is difficult because of the rapid progress of the disease and the young age of the patients. However, it is possible to control the localized form of the disease.

1. Thoroughly scale affected roots (general anaesthesia facilities may be required).

2. Prescribe a course of antibiotics. Penicillin has been used (Page et al 1983) but other broad-spectrum antibiotics may be preferred, for example co-amoxiclav (Augmentin) which is available as a suspension for children. Tetracyclines should not be used for patients of this age, to avoid the risk of causing discoloration of developing teeth.
3. Emphasize to the parents the importance of efficient plaque removal, for which they must be responsible. Demonstrate an efficient technique for brushing and flossing the child's teeth (Ch. 3).
4. See the child at least every 3 months, perform prophylaxis or scaling as required and emphasize the importance of meticulous oral hygiene.

The generalized form of the disease cannot be controlled and extraction of teeth will be necessary.

24.5.3 Juvenile periodontitis

Juvenile periodontitis is an uncommon disease characterized by severe destruction of alveolar bone around one or more permanent teeth. The disease is most frequently seen in adolescents but children as young as 10–11 years may be affected. The prevalence of the disease varies in different racial groups but is most prevalent in the Negroid race. A survey of a group of 14–19-year-old children in England reported a prevalence of 0.1% (Saxby 1984). A familial pattern has been noted; a patient's siblings should be examined. Several types of bacteria are probably involved in the aetiology of the condition, but *Actinobacillus actinomycetemcomitans* is especially implicated.

Localized and generalized forms of juvenile periodontitis have been described (Lindhe 1989) but there is disagreement on whether these represent different manifestations of the same disease or two different entities.

Localized juvenile periodontitis affects incisors and first molars. The characteristic vertical pattern of bone resorption results in early involvement of the root furcation of first molars. Characteristically, plaque deposits are minimal and the gingiva appears normal, but the deep periodontal pockets bleed on gentle probing. Severely affected teeth are mobile and anterior teeth may drift. In the generalized form the pattern of bone loss may be vertical or horizontal, and usually involves most teeth in the dentition.

Treatment

The disease can be controlled but tends to recur (Lindhe & Liljenberg 1984).

1. Prescribe tetracycline: 250 mg to be taken four times daily for 2 weeks; or co-amoxiclav (Augmentin junior suspension): 5 ml to be taken three times daily for 2 weeks.
2. A non-surgical approach may be attempted first: thorough sub-gingival scaling (several treatment sessions may be required), and oral hygiene instruction, with particular emphasis on flossing in the affected sites.

   A surgical approach may be required: raising mucoperiosteal flaps greatly improves access to the affected sites. Prescribe chlorhexidine mouthwash (0.2% chlorhexidine gluconate solution) to be used several times a day for 2 weeks following surgery.
3. Review regularly to monitor the effect of treatment and to assess the patient's oral hygiene. Give encouragement and further advice on oral hygiene, and perform further scaling, as necessary.

Irrigation of the periodontal pockets with antimicrobial solutions during surgery, and later by the patient at home (using an oral irrigation device) has also been recommended (Rams et al 1985)

If conservative treatment is unsuccessful, or is not undertaken because the patient is uninterested or uncooperative, extraction and prosthetic replacement of badly affected teeth is the only alternative treatment.

REFERENCES

Andlin-Sobocki A, Marcusson A, Persson M 1991 Three-year observations on gingival recession in mandibular incisors in children. Journal of Clinical Periodontology 18: 155–159

Glenwright H D, Rock W P 1990 Papillon Lefevre syndrome. A discussion of aetiology and a case report. British Dental Journal 168: 27–29

Lennon M A, Davies R M 1974 Prevalence and distribution of alveolar bone loss in a population of 15-year-old schoolchildren. Journal of Clinical Periodontology 1: 175–182

Lindhe J 1989 Textbook of clinical periodontology, 2nd edn. Munksgaard, Copenhagen, ch 6

Lindhe J, Liljenberg B 1984 Treatment of localized juvenile periodontitis: results after 5 years. Journal of Clinical Periodontology 11: 399–410

Livingston S, Livingston H L 1969 Diphenylhydantoin gingival hyperplasia. American Journal of Diseases of Children 117: 265–270

Matsson L 1993 Factors influencing the susceptibility to gingivitis during childhood — a review. International Journal of Paediatric Dentistry 3: 119–127

Page R C, Bowen T, Altman L et al 1983 Prepubertal periodontitis. 1. Definition of a clinical disease entity. Journal of Periodontology 54: 257–271

O'Brien M 1994 Children's dental health in the United

Kingdom 1993. Office of Population Censuses and Surveys. Her Majesty's Stationery Office, London, p 64

Rams T E, Keyes P H, Wright W E 1985 Treatment of juvenile periodontitis with microbiologically modulated periodontal therapy (Keyes technique). Pediatric Dentistry 7: 259–270

Saxby M 1984 Prevalence of juvenile periodontitis in a British school population. Community Dentistry and Oral Epidemiology 12: 185–187

Stewart D J, Kernohan D C 1972 Self-inflicted gingival injuries: gingivitis artefacta, factitial gingivitis. Dental Practitioner 22: 418–426

Watanabe K 1990 Prepubertal periodontitis: a review of diagnostic criteria, pathogenesis, and differential diagnosis. Journal of Periodontal Research 25: 31–48

RECOMMENDED READING

Jenkins W M M, Allan C J 1994 Guide to periodontics, 3rd edn. Butterworth-Heinemann, Oxford, chs 14, 15

Manson J D, Eley B M 1995 Outline of periodontics, 3rd edn. Butterworth-Heinemann, Oxford, chs 18, 20

25 Viral, bacterial and mycotic infections affecting the oral soft tissues

25.1 VIRAL INFECTIONS

25.1.1 Acute herpetic gingivostomatitis

Acute herpetic gingivostomatitis is caused by the herpes simplex virus, which is the most common cause of acute gingival inflammation in children. Acute herpetic gingivostomatitis occurs most frequently in infants between the ages of 1 and 3 years, but adults may also be affected. The child becomes unwell and refuses to eat. Within about 24 hours, the mouth is very sore, the temperature is raised, and cervical lymph nodes are enlarged and tender. Vesicles about 3 or 4 mm in diameter form on the gingiva and oral mucosa, particularly on the dorsum of the tongue and on the hard and soft palate; the vesicles soon burst and leave shallow, painful ulcers. The gingiva is diffusely inflamed. The lesions heal spontaneously within about 10 days.

Treatment

1. Reassure the parent that the disease is self-limiting. Recommend a soft diet of cold rather than hot foods, and a high fluid intake.

2. Although no further treatment is essential, one or more of the following methods may be used:
   a. *Systemic anti-viral drugs*
      Acyclovir (Zovirax): one 200 mg tablet or 5 ml elixir to be taken five times a day for 5 days. This drug is used especially for the treatment of herpes simplex infections in immunosuppressed patients.
   b. *Topical application to the ulcer*
      (i) Carboxymethylcellulose Gelatin Paste (Orabase): A paste that adheres to mucous membranes and, by covering the ulcers, provides some relief from pain.
      (ii) Choline Salicylate Dental Paste (Bonjela, Teejel): Contains an anti-inflammatory and analgesic substance in a base that adheres to the oral mucosa.
      (iii) Chlorhexidine Gel (Corsodyl Gel): Contains 1% chlorhexidine gluconate.
      These preparations must be applied carefully with a cotton applicator several times a day; in practice many parents find this very difficult or impossible.
   c. *Mouthwash*
      (i) Tetracycline Mouth-bath (Tetracycline Mixture): Contains 125 mg tetracycline hydrochloride in 5 ml.
      (ii) Chlorhexidine Mouthwash (Corsodyl Mouthwash): Contains 0.2% chlorhexidine gluconate. Mouthwash solutions rinsed around the mouth for 2–3 minutes several times a day would help limit secondary infection; unfortunately infants and young children are not able to rinse in this way.

3. If the child cannot sleep, prescribe a hypnotic drug (Ch. 12).

25.1.2 Recurrent herpes infection – herpes labialis

Following primary herpetic infection, a balance is

established in the body between the virus and the immune response. If the balance is upset by a disturbance such as the common cold, a fever or other factors, secondary lesions appear which take the form of small clusters of vesicles around the vermilion borders of the lips. The vesicles enlarge, coalesce, become covered by scabs and heal without scarring within about 10 days.

Treatment

Prescribe Zovirax cream (5% w/w acyclovir). If the cream is applied as soon as redness or a prickly sensation indicates the onset of a lesion, the appearance of vesicles may be prevented; if applied when the vesicles start to form, the healing period may be halved (Fiddian et al 1983).

25.1.3 Herpangina

Herpangina is caused by a Coxsackie group A virus. The disease affects infants and young children and is heralded by fever and sore throat. The child is ill for 3–5 days.

Vesicles similar to those of primary herpes infection appear in the throat and on the soft palate, and break down into small ulcers. However, their distribution differs from that in primary herpes: they are mainly confined to the throat, and the gingiva is not affected. Healing occurs rapidly, within 3 or 4 days.

Treatment

No treatment is necessary, other than reassuring the parents and recommending a soft diet with adequate fluids, but analgesics and antipyretics may be prescribed.

25.1.4 Hand, foot and mouth disease

Hand, foot and mouth disease is caused by a strain of Coxsackie group A virus, and generally affects children of school age. However, the child may not feel unwell, as there is little, if any, fever; the chief complaint is a rash on the hands and feet. In the mouth there are small ulcers scattered on the oral mucosa, but there are no vesicles; the gingiva is not affected. The rash and oral ulcers disappear within about 1 week.

Treatment

No treatment is required, but if the oral ulcers are painful they may be treated with Carboxymethyl-cellulose Gelatin Paste or Choline Salicylate Dental Paste (p. 193).

25.1.5 Other viral infections

Mouth lesions may be associated with several other viral infections, including chickenpox, glandular fever, mumps and measles. The oral lesions of chickenpox usually accompany the skin lesions and take the form of vesicles which burst and leave small ulcers. Glandular fever is accompanied by acute gingivitis and stomatitis. Inflammation of the mucosa at the openings of the parotid ducts is common in mumps. Koplik's spots are characteristic of measles; they appear mainly on the buccal mucosa as small, irregularly-shaped blue-white specks surrounded by a bright red margin, several days before the appearance of skin lesions.

Treatment

If the mouth lesions are painful, recommend a soft diet, with cold rather than hot food, and the use of Orabase or Bonjela as described above.

25.2 BACTERIAL INFECTIONS

25.2.1 Acute necrotising ulcerative gingivitis (Vincent's infection)

Acute necrotising ulcerative gingivitis (ANUG) is associated with the organisms *Fusobacterium nucleatum* and *Borellia vincentii*. The disease is rare in healthy children under 16 years of age in the UK. ANUG is most common in young adults, and a number of predisposing factors have been noted, which include mental stress and local irritation from plaque, calculus deposits, or smoking.

The disease is characterized by rapid destruction of interdental papillae and the formation of grey, punched-out ulcers. The condition may be localized to a single papilla, but in severe cases extensive areas of both the free and attached gingiva may be affected. There may be marked halitosis, which is characteristic of the condition.

Treatment

1. If it is possible without causing intolerable pain, remove gross calculus and debris from the gingival margins by gentle scaling and by irrigation with hydrogen peroxide solution (20 vols).
2. Prescribe Metronidazole Tablets, one 200 mg tablet to be taken three times a day for 3 days. Metronidazole acts specifically against obligate anaerobes and does not otherwise disturb the normal oral flora.
3. After about 1 week, when the acute phase has subsided, carry out more thorough scaling; an

ultrasonic scaler provides a rapid and efficient method of doing this.

4. Give detailed oral hygiene instruction. An adequate standard of oral hygiene is necessary to avoid recurrence.

25.3 MYCOTIC INFECTIONS

25.3.1 Candidiasis (candidosis)

Candidiasis is caused by the fungus *Candida albicans*, which is commonly present in the mouth as a yeast-like saprophyte. Under certain conditions the fungus grows rapidly and the yeast-like forms are replaced by pathogenic mycelial forms which grow in the epithelium of the oral mucosa and produce characteristic lesions. Candidiasis is the most common oral manifestation of HIV infection.

Two main types of candidiasis are seen in children: acute pseudomembranous candidiasis (thrush) and chronic atrophic candidiasis (denture stomatitis).

Acute pseudomembranous candidiasis (thrush)

Thrush is not uncommon in the newborn and in weak, undernourished infants, but it may also occur in apparently healthy children. A baby may become infected at birth by direct contact with *Candida* infection of the mother's vagina, which is not uncommon in pregnant women. Thrush may also result from prolonged use of antibiotics or steroids; *Candida albicans* is resistant to most of the commonly used antibiotics and may multiply when other microorganisms are suppressed.

The oral lesions are soft, elevated, creamy-white patches that cover small or large areas of the oral mucosa; the patches can be rubbed off, and leave raw, bleeding surfaces.

Treatment:

1. Prescribe an antifungal drug. The alternatives are:
   a. Topical
   Miconazole (Daktarin Oral Gel): Contains 25 mg miconazole per ml in a sugar-free gel. Gel should be smeared over the affected area with a clean finger.
   b. Systemic
   Either
   (i) Miconazole (Daktarin Tablets): Each tablet contains 250 mg miconazole. One tablet should be sucked slowly four times daily for 10 days.
   For young children who will not suck the tablets, the oral gel (see above) may be used

systemically. Child under 2 years: 2.5 ml twice daily; 2–6 years: 5 ml twice daily; over 6 years: 5 ml four times daily.

or (ii) Fluconazole (Diflucan capsules): Capsules contain 50 mg fluconazole. One tablet daily for 7–14 days. Alternatively, Diflucan Powder for Oral Suspension, 50 mg fluconazole in 5 ml.

or (iii) Nystatin (Nystan Oral Suspension): Contains 100 000 units per ml. 1 ml to be given after food, three to four times daily.

or (iv) Nystatin (Nystan Pastilles): each pastille contains 100 000 units nystatin. One pastille should be sucked slowly four times daily for 7–14 days. The pastilles are more palatable than other nystatin preparations but they contain sugar.

2. Advise the parent to wash the infant's feeding utensils carefully after each meal and to store them in an antiseptic solution (e.g. Milton).

Chronic atrophic candidiasis ('denture stomatitis')

This type of candidiasis affects the palatal mucosa under a denture or removable orthodontic appliance. The mucosa underlying the appliance becomes inflamed, appearing bright red and spongy. Springs or screws on the appliance may become buried in the inflamed tissue.

Clearly, conditions under the appliance of the affected patient must be favourable for the multiplication of *Candida albicans*, but local irritation from rough or ill-fitting appliances, or from poor oral hygiene, may also be a factor.

Treatment:

1. Prescribe Daktarin Oral Gel, as for thrush (above). Advise the child to apply the gel not only to the affected area but also to the fitting surface of the appliance; *Candida* grows on the surface of acrylic dentures as well as on the oral mucosa (Davenport 1970). Alternatively, prescribe Dumicoat denture lacquer, which contains miconazole 50 mg/g, to be applied to the fitting surface of the appliance three times at weekly intervals.

2. Inspect the fitting surface of the appliance and smooth any sharp edges.

3. Give detailed instructions in oral hygiene and in the care of the appliance. The appliance must be rinsed after meals and, when at home, brushed with a toothbrush.

4. Ideally, the appliance should not be worn until healing has occurred, but this would allow relapse of any orthodontic tooth movement previously

achieved. Therefore, instruct the patient to wear the appliance for 2 or 3 weeks at night only (this prevents relapse and allows time for the mucosa to heal) and to keep the appliance in an antiseptic solution.

REFERENCES

Davenport J C 1970 Oral distribution of Candida in denture stomatitis. British Dental Journal 129: 151–156

Fiddian A P, Yeo J M, Stubbings R, Dean D 1983 Successful treatment of herpes labialis with topical acyclovir. British Medical Journal 286: 1699–1701

26 Miscellaneous soft tissue lesions

26.1 EPULIS

The term 'epulis' is used to describe localized tumours of the gingiva. Three types of epulis occur in children: fibrous epulis, pyogenic granuloma and giant cell epulis. They are the result of local irritation which causes minor injury to the gingiva; this permits infection by oral bacteria, which is followed by chronic inflammation and proliferation of granulation tissue. The epulis remains covered by oral epithelium. Most epulides are found on a gingival margin or papilla in the anterior part of the mouth.

26.1.1 Fibrous epulis

In the fibrous epulis, which is the most common type, granulation tissue is largely replaced by fibrous tissue. It has a smooth surface, which has the colour of normal oral mucosa.

26.1.2 Pyogenic granuloma

The pyogenic granuloma contains dilated blood vessels and its colour ranges from dark red or purple to pale red. A pyogenic granuloma may, in time, change its character to that of a fibrous epulis.

26.1.3 Giant cell epulis

This type of epulis contains large multinucleated osteoclasts ('giant cells') in proliferating granulation tissue. The epulis is soft, maroon or purple in colour, and bleeds easily. It remains localized in the gingiva but occasionally causes superficial resorption of the underlying bone.

Treatment

1. Excise the epulis and a small area of normal tissue at its base. The epulis must be removed down to bone, and the bone curetted to minimize the chance of recurrence. Dress the wound with a pressure dressing until it is completely epithelialized (after about 2 weeks). Send the tissue for histological examination to confirm the diagnosis.
2. Examine the area closely to detect any possible sources of gingival irritation that may have initiated the lesion.
3. Check oral hygiene and local plaque retention factors.

26.2 ENDOSTEAL GIANT CELL GRANULOMA

The endosteal giant cell granuloma is similar histologically to a giant cell epulis but originates within the bone. It is rare and is seen on the gingiva only if it erodes through the bone; it then appears as a purplish nodule on the gingiva. It is more common in the mandible than in the maxilla and is diagnosed radiologically.

Treatment

The granuloma must be surgically removed.

26.3 PAPILLOMA

A papilloma is a small epithelial tumour consisting of a core of connective tissue covered by stratified squamous epithelium. The surface has a rough, warty appearance. A papilloma may be up to 1 cm in diameter, is pedunculated, and appears most frequently on the soft palate near the uvula, on the gingiva and on the tongue. It may be either soft and red, or firm and white, depending on the degree of keratinisation of the epithelium.

Treatment

Excise the papilloma as described for an epulis.

26.4 GEOGRAPHIC TONGUE (ERYTHEMA MIGRANS)

Geographic tongue is a benign lesion of unknown aetiology that occurs on the dorsum of the tongue, and which may be seen in young infants. The lesions are usually erythematous and have a white or yellow border, and they occur in patches that vary in size, shape and distribution. They are symptomless.

Treatment

No treatment is required, other than reassuring the patient and parent that the condition is harmless.

26.5 APHTHOUS ULCERS

Aphthous ulcers occur commonly in adults and children, but rarely in infants. There are three types: minor, major and herpetiform (Field et al 1992). The minor type is the most common. The ulcers are shallow, oval or round in outline (about 2–6 mm in diameter) and appear, often several at a time, mainly on the buccal mucosa and tongue. They may be painful, or only painful when traumatized. They heal within 7–14 days without scarring, but tend to recur.

Major aphthous ulcers are much larger, often more than 1 cm in diameter, and are much more painful. They may appear anywhere on the oral mucosa but are found most frequently on lips, soft palate and pillars of the fauces. They may take up to 2 months to heal, leaving scars. Herpetiform ulcers are very small (less than 1 mm in diameter) and painful. They may appear in large numbers and are found especially on the lateral and ventral surfaces of the tongue and on the floor of the mouth. They may coalesce to form a large ulcer. Healing may take several weeks, the larger ulcers leaving scars.

The aetiology of aphthous ulceration is unknown but it has been associated with an alpha-haemolytic streptococcus (*Strep. sanguis*) and with various immunological abnormalities. Predisposing factors include psychological stress, allergies, trauma and, occasionally, deficiencies in haematinics (e.g. iron, folate or vitamin B_{12}) which may be caused by disorders such as coeliac disease.

Treatment

If the ulcers are not very painful and systemic factors have been excluded, no treatment is required other than reassurance that the condition is self-limiting. However, in more severe cases some form of treatment should be given. Many methods have been tried, which reflects the uncertain aetiology of the condition.

a. Mouthwashes
  (i) Benzydamine hydrochloride (Difflam Oral Rinse or Difflam Spray): Contains 0.15% w/v benzydamine hydrochloride. Spray delivers 150 µl per puff.
       Rinse to be used every $1\frac{1}{2}$–3 hours.
       Spray — child 6–12 years: 4 puffs every $1\frac{1}{2}$–3 hours.
            — child over 12 years: 4–8 puffs every $1\frac{1}{2}$–3 hours.
  (ii) Chlorhexidine gluconate solution (Corsodyl mouthwash): Contains 0.2% w/v chlorhexidine gluconate, to be used three or four times a day.
  (iii) Tetracycline Mixture BPC: Contains 125 mg tetracycline hydrochloride in 5 ml, to be used three times a day.
b. Topical application to the ulcers
  (i) Carboxymethylcellulose Gelatin Paste (Orabase):
       The paste adheres to the oral mucosa; covering the ulcers makes them less painful.
  (ii) Choline Salicylate Dental Paste (Bonjela, Teejel):
       An anti-inflammatory and analgesic agent in a base that adheres to the mucosa.

(iii) Triamcinolone Dental Paste BPC (Adcortyl in Orabase):
A corticosteroid in carboxymethylcellulose gelatin paste.

These preparations must be applied several times a day by a parent, using a cotton applicator. This is only feasible if the child is reasonably cooperative, if there are not too many ulcers present and if the ulcers are near the front of the mouth.

c. Lozenges to dissolve in the mouth
Hydrocortisone Lozenges BPC (Corlan Pellets): Contain 2.5 mg hydrocortisone, to be used two to four times a day, starting as soon as the patient senses that ulcers are developing.

26.6 MUCOCELE

There are two types of mucocele: the mucous extravasation cyst, and the mucous retention cyst. They occur most commonly on the lower lip (Fig. 26.1).

Extravasation cysts are much more common than retention cysts and they occur as a result of trauma to a small duct or a minor salivary gland, for example by biting the lip or tongue. Saliva escapes into the tissues and appears as a bluish blister up to 1 cm in diameter.

Treatment

Excise the mucocele together with the underlying mucous gland tissue.

26.7 GINGIVAL CYSTS OF THE NEWBORN

Gingival cysts are extremely common in newborn babies; Fromm (1967) found them in 1028 (76%) of 1367 babies examined, and Cataldo & Berkman

(1968) in 167 (80%) of 209 newborns. The cysts are white or creamy in colour, 0.5–3 mm in diameter, and appear singly, in clusters of five or six or sometimes in large numbers. They are of no clinical significance because they disappear within a few months.

Three types of gingival cyst are recognized: Epstein's pearls, Bohn's nodules and dental lamina cysts. Epstein's pearls are the most common and are found along the mid-palatine raphe; they are derived from epithelial rests trapped within the mid-palatine suture. Bohn's nodules occur on the buccal and lingual aspects of the alveolar ridges and on the palate away from the midline, and originate from epithelial remnants of developing mucous glands. Dental lamina cysts occur only on the crests of the alveolar ridges and are formed from remnants of dental lamina.

Treatment

No treatment is required, other than to reassure the parents.

26.8 ABNORMAL FRENA

26.8.1 Persistent upper labial frenum

In infancy the labial frenum has a low attachment near to the crest of the alveolus. As the alveolus grows down and the permanent incisors begin to erupt the attachment of the frenum normally moves higher on the alveolus so that it does not obstruct the eruption of the central incisors. Sometimes, however, the frenum remains attached to the crest of the alveolus after the permanent central incisors have erupted. Such a persistent frenum may be unsightly and may also be the apparent cause of a median diastema. However, it is unwise to assume that a persistent frenum is the sole or even a contributory cause of a diastema because it is normal for a diastema to be present between the permanent maxillary central incisors when these teeth first erupt. This appearance is known as the 'ugly duckling' stage of occlusal development and is usually resolved when the permanent maxillary canines erupt (p. 131). Some median diastemas have a familial background, especially in children of the Negroid race, and often the space is a localized manifestation of a low tooth:tissue ratio.

Treatment

1. Take a maxillary anterior occlusal radiograph – the median diastema may be associated with congenitally missing lateral incisors or with a midline supernumerary tooth.

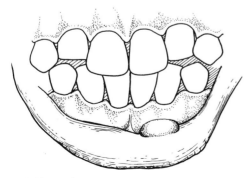

Fig. 26.1 Mucocele.

2. If an unacceptable median diastema persists after the eruption of permanent canines, a frenectomy may be indicated, followed by orthodontic treatment to close the space.

26.8.2 Short lingual frenum

In infants the lingual frenum is short and attached near the tip of the tongue. Normally the attachment progressively retreats as the tongue lengthens but sometimes the frenum remains attached close to the tip. In such cases movement of the tongue is restricted and the condition is referred to as 'tongue tie'.

Speech difficulties may be caused by the inability of the tip of the tongue to reach or to exert enough pressure on the palate and maxillary incisors. However, this diagnosis should only be made after consulting a speech therapist.

Treatment

1. The condition may resolve spontaneously, so no treatment should be considered before the age of 3 years.
2. If it is confirmed that the frenum is causing speech problems, frenectomy must be considered.

REFERENCES

Cataldo E, Berkman M D 1968 Cysts of the oral mucosa in newborns. American Journal of Diseases of Children 116: 44–48

Field E A, Brookes V, Tyldesley W R 1992 Recurrent aphthous ulceration in children: a review. International Journal of Paediatric Dentistry 2: 1–10

Fromm A 1967 Epstein's pearls, Bohn's nodules and inclusion cysts of the oral cavity. Journal of Dentistry for Children 34: 275–287

Treatment of traumatic injuries to teeth

Part 6

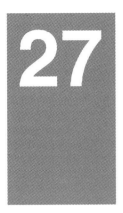

27 Prevention of trauma to teeth

Trauma to children's teeth occurs quite commonly. Permanent incisors showed signs of having been traumatized in 6% of 8-year-old children and in 17% of 12-year-old children examined in the UK in 1993 (O'Brien 1994a). At all ages, the prevalence was higher in boys than in girls; for example, among 12-year-old children, 25% of boys and 9% of girls showed evidence of trauma. Predisposing factors are Class II Division I malocclusion, increased incisor overjet and inadequate lip coverage of maxillary incisors (O'Mullane 1973, O'Brien 1994b).

27.1 MOUTHPROTECTORS

Mouthprotectors are used most commonly by young adults who participate in contact sports. Because less than 10% of injuries to the anterior teeth of children under 15 years of age are associated with contact sports (Winter & Kernohan 1966, O'Mullane 1973), there is little justification for recommending mouthprotectors for all these children. However, mouthprotectors can be strongly recommended for certain children who are particularly at risk during contact sports; for example, those with increased incisor overjet and incompetent lips. In addition, because some sports (e.g. rugby football) become progressively rougher during the teenage years, the use of mouthprotectors by these children should be encouraged; their value in protecting children playing American football has been shown (American Dental Association 1973).

Three types of mouthprotector are available (Turner 1977, Welbury & Murray 1990):

1. *The stock protector.* Made of latex rubber and commonly used by boxers, this type of protector is not recommended for children because it is poorly retained in the mouth, being held in position only by the opposing teeth; a near-fatal accident has been reported in which a protector of this type occluded the airway of an injured rugby player.

2. *The protector made in the mouth.* These are of two types:
   a. A firm outer 'shell' shaped in the form of a dental arch which is filled with a special type of acrylic resin and placed in the mouth; the resin sets in the mouth but remains resilient at mouth temperatures (Coe Dental Guard).
   b. A 'blank' of polyvinyl acetate-polyethylene or polyvinyl chloride material which is softened by inserting into hot water (75°C), placed in the mouth, and moulded with the tongue and fingers (Coe Rediguard).

   Both these types of protector are satisfactory if they are accurately fitted in the mouth; to ensure this, professional supervision is required. However, neither is as satisfactory as the type described below.

3. *The professionally-made protector.* This type of mouthprotector is most highly recommended because it is made on an accurate model of the patient's maxillary arch; however, since it is made professionally, it is the most expensive. Various materials are available, but ethylvinylacetate (Drufosoft, Dreve, Germany) is commonly used, in sheets 3–6 mm thick.

Technique: mouthprotector

Procedure	Method	Rationale	Notes
1. Take an alginate impression	Take an upper alginate impression and cast a stone or plaster/stone model.	The mouthprotector will be made on the model.	
2. Outline the periphery of the mouth-protector	Draw a pencil line on the model (Fig. 27.1a) a. buccally and labially—about 3 mm from the muco-buccal fold, avoiding the frena; b. palatally—about 10 mm from the molar gingival margins and behind the rugae; c. distally—about 3 mm behind the most distal tooth in the arch. OPTIONAL—Scribe a shallow groove along the pencil line.	The pencil line defines the outline to which the vinyl material will later be cut. This amount of coverage provides adequate support, sufficient retention and optimum comfort. The groove will be reproduced as a ridge on the vinyl and be an aid when trimming to shape.	

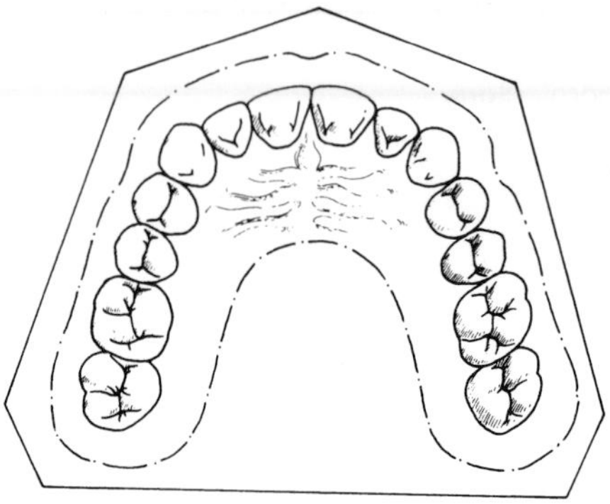

Fig. 27.1a

3. Mould the vinyl material to the model	Place a sheet of ethylvinylacetate material (at least 3 mm thick) on the model. Ideally, use a mechanical apparatus which heats the material and uses either vacuum, pressure, or both, to adapt it over the model. If the apparatus is not available, heat the vinyl sheet either in hot water (75°C) or with a bunsen flame, and mould it by hand.	The mechanical apparatus moulds the vinyl material quickly and efficiently.	If additional protection is considered desirable, the thickness of material over the posterior teeth can be increased, as described by Chandler et al (see text).
4. Trim	After allowing the material to cool, remove it from the model and trim with scissors to the previously marked outline (Fig. 27.1b).	Rough edges would traumatize the soft tissues.	
5. Smooth the cut margin	Smooth the cut margin by passing it lightly over a flame. Replace the mouthprotector on the model and ensure that it has not become distorted during trimming and smoothing.		
6. Try in the mouth and adjust if necessary	Try the mouthprotector in the mouth and further trim the margin if necessary to ensure the patient's comfort. If the occlusion of the opposing teeth on the mouthprotector is uneven, place it again on the model and soften the area(s) of premature contact by heating with a flame. Replace it in the mouth (after checking that it is not too hot) and ask the patient to close firmly.		

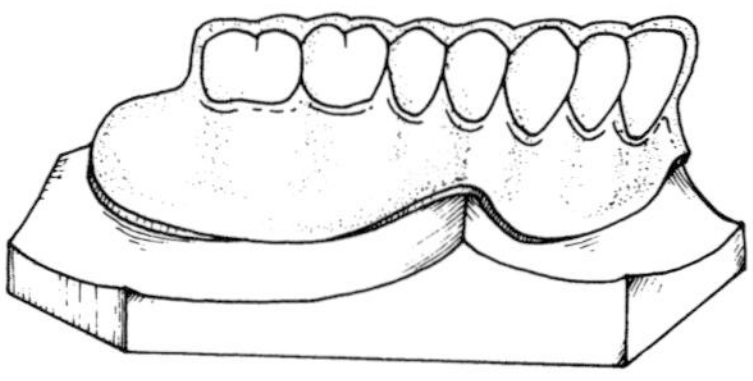

Fig. 27.1b

The type of mouthprotector described on page 204 offers protection to maxillary anterior teeth. However, during strenuous exercise, the mouth is held open to allow mouthbreathing, and there is then a risk of injury to the base of the skull from a blow to the lower jaw. For this reason Chandler et al (1987) suggested that mouthprotectors should open the bite and support the mandible in the 'position of heavy breathing'. To achieve this they cut strips of 1.5 mm and 3 mm ethyl-vinylacetate material to cover the occlusal surfaces of the maxillary posterior teeth on the stone model (extending posteriorly from distal of the canines), heated the strips in a flame and adapted them to form a 4.5 mm thickness of material over the occlusal surfaces (this was found to be the optimum thickness).

Finally they moulded a sheet of the same material at least 3 mm thick over this as described above. They stated that this type of mouthprotector was well accepted by athletes.

27.2 EARLY TREATMENT OF PROCLINED MAXILLARY INCISORS

A child with a gross Class II Division I malocclusion is particularly at risk from trauma to anterior teeth. If, in addition, the child participates in contact sports or has already suffered trauma, there is a strong case for early correction of the malocclusion. This treatment is discussed in Chapter 19.

REFERENCES

American Dental Association 1973 Mouth protectors: 11 years later. Report of Bureau of Dental Health Education, Council on Dental Materials and Devices. Journal of the American Dental Association 86: 1365–1367

Chandler N P, Wilson N H F, Daber B S 1987 A modified maxillary mouthguard. British Journal of Sports Medicine 21: 27–28

O'Brien M 1994 Children's dental health in the United Kingdom 1993. Office of Population Censuses and Surveys. Her Majesty's Stationery Office, London, (a) p 79, (b) p 81

O'Mullane D M 1973 Some factors predisposing to injuries of permanent incisors in school children. British Dental Journal 134: 328–332

Turner C H 1977 Mouth protectors. British Dental Journal 143: 82–86

Welbury R R, Murray J J 1990 Prevention of trauma to teeth. Dental Update 17: 117–121

Winter G B, Kernohan D C 1966 The importance of mouthguards. British Dental Journal 120: 564–565

RECOMMENDED READING

Scheer B 1994 Prevention of dental and oral injuries. In: Andreasen J O, Andreasen F M (eds) Textbook and color atlas of traumatic injuries to the teeth, 3rd edn. Munksgaard, Copenhagen

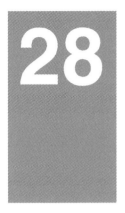

28 Assessment and immediate treatment of traumatized permanent anterior teeth

28.2 TREATMENT OF CROWN FRACTURES

28.2.1 Pulp protection

A traumatized tooth that is not fractured, or fractured through enamel only, requires no immediate treatment other than smoothing of rough edges, unless the tooth is loose, in which case splinting may be necessary (p. 216). As in all cases of trauma, pulp vitality should be reviewed for at least 2 years; first after about 1 month, and then at 3- to 6-month intervals.

A tooth that is fractured through dentine requires immediate treatment. The pulp must be protected against the irritation it would suffer from thermal stimuli passing through the exposed dentine, and from bacteria that might invade the pulp through the dentinal tubules. It is also important to stabilize the position of the tooth by restoring crown shape.

The pulp is protected by covering exposed dentine with a suitable insulating material, usually calcium hydroxide, which must in turn be protected if it is to remain in place and fulfil its function. Usually this is achieved with composite resin, but occasionally this is not feasible and a stainless steel crown may be used. If the fractured tooth fragment is available it may be possible to reattach it to the tooth.

28.1 ASSESSMENT

A child whose teeth have been injured can be expected to be upset and anxious when attending for treatment. It is essential to allay this anxiety while assessing the child and the nature of the injury. A suggested outline for history-taking and examination is given below:

History and examination

Information sought	Rationale
History	
Social	Questioning a child and parent as suggested on page 5 helps to establish rapport and to allay anxiety. With a child who has suffered an injury, however, and especially if the child is in pain, the social history should be abbreviated, although not ignored.
Dental	
How did the injury occur? Direct or indirect trauma to the teeth?	Indirect trauma, e.g. a blow on the chin, is more likely to cause jaw fracture than is a direct blow on a tooth.

History and examination (contd)

Information sought	Rationale
Where did the injury occur?	If the wound is contaminated with soil, a tetanus toxoid injection may be indicated (see below).
When did the injury occur?	If the crown is fractured (especially through the pulp), the longer the interval between injury and treatment the poorer the prognosis.
Is a tooth fractured? If so, where is the fractured piece?	If the fractured piece cannot be accounted for, a chest radiograph should be obtained to exclude the possibility of its inhalation. If the fragment is available it may be possible to reattach it to the tooth (p. 212).
Is the child in pain? If so, from a tooth or elsewhere?	Pain suggests the site of injury; however, many fractured teeth are not painful immediately after injury, and pain is an unreliable indication of the degree of injury.
Was the child concussed, or has he/she suffered from headache, vomiting or amnesia since the injury?	The possibility of brain damage must be excluded. If any suggestive symptoms are reported, the patient should be referred to a hospital for further investigation and the family doctor informed.
Has the child received dental care in the past?	Regular attenders are more likely to be interested and cooperative in receiving treatment to save injured teeth.
Medical	
Is the child in good general health? Congenital heart defect or history of rheumatic fever?	If the child has a congenital heart defect, endodontic treatment may be justified only if the tooth is vital, and should be carried out under antibiotic cover to avoid the risk of bacteraemia causing bacterial endocarditis.
	If the tooth has a necrotic pulp, infected tissue would remain in lateral canals even after endodontic treatment, and be a possible source of bacteraemia in the future.
	However, all congenital heart defects do not carry the same risks of bacterial endocarditis. Therefore, the child's paediatrician should be consulted before a decision about endodontic treatment is made.
Bleeding disorders?	Bleeding disorders are relevant if soft tissues are lacerated, or if teeth are to be extracted.
Allergies?	If antibiotics are to be given, penicillin should be avoided if there is a history of allergy.
Tetanus immunization status?	If the wound is contaminated with soil and the child has not had a 'booster' injection within the last 5 years, the child should be referred to a hospital or to the family doctor for a tetanus toxoid injection.

Examination

Extra-oral
During history-taking, observe the following:

1. Facial swelling, bruising or lacerations?	Lacerations of the face may require suturing.
2. Limitation of mandibular movement, or mandibular deviation on opening or closing the mouth?	These are signs that the jaw may be fractured.
3. Are wounds clean or contaminated?	Antibiotics and/or tetanus toxoid may be required if wounds are contaminated.

Carefully palpate the face and jaws and note any painful areas.

Intra-oral

If a tooth is fractured, note whether the fracture is through enamel only, or whether it also involves dentine or pulp. Note any tooth displacement.	Treatment will differ according to the extent of fracture.
Palpate teeth and alveolus to detect any mobility. If soft tissues are lacerated, examine carefully to detect any embedded tooth fragments.	Displaced teeth will need to be repositioned, and mobile teeth may require splinting. Lacerations of the lips or tongue require suturing, but those of the oral mucosa heal quickly and usually do not need suturing.

Radiographic

Take periapical radiographs of traumatized teeth; take two radiographs from different angles (Fig. 28.1).	Periapical views show root fractures and the stage of root development. Two radiographs are essential because a root fracture may not be detectable if the fracture line runs at a large angle from the X-ray beam (as in 2 in Fig. 28.1).

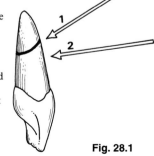

Fig. 28.1

History and examination *(contd)*

Information sought	*Rationale*

If the lips are lacerated, take radiographs to determine whether tooth fragments are embedded:

lower lip — occlusal view using 'occlusal' film held between the teeth (Fig. 28.2)

upper lip — lateral view: either using 'occlusal' film held by the patient at the side of the mouth, or a lateral skull view.

If there is a suspicion of jaw fracture, other radiographs will be required, e.g.
— lateral oblique
— panoramic
— lateral skull
— anterior-posterior skull.

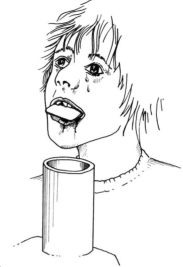

Fig. 28.2

Pulp vitality tests are often misleading at this stage because the teeth may be concussed. However, a positive response to pulp testing indicates a good long-term prognosis for pulp vitality (Rock et al 1974). During history-taking and examinations, signs that might suggest child abuse should not be overlooked (Ch. 31).

Composite resin

As an emergency measure, unfilled or filled composite resin may simply be applied as a bandage over the calcium hydroxide dressing, retained on acid-etched labial and palatal enamel; the technique is described on page 210. Thus, restoration of the tooth is postponed until a subsequent visit. However, restoration of the crown with composite resin (p. 224) may be carried out at the initial visit if the tooth has not suffered any other injuries and if the child is not too upset by the traumatic experience.

Stainless steel crown

In the past, before the advent of the acid-etch technique, stainless steel crowns were frequently used to retain a protective dressing on fractured dentine. They are rarely used nowadays, but are still occasionally useful if the nature of the fracture is such that insufficient enamel is available for retention of resin, because they are retained primarily by a tight fit around the gingival margin of the tooth. Stainless steel crowns require no tooth preparation (unless the tooth is in contact with adjacent teeth) and are fairly easy to fit; the technique is described on page 211. Their only disadvantage is their poor appearance, but this is rarely a problem with

a child patient if it is explained that pulp protection is the essential treatment at this stage and that an aesthetic restoration will be made as soon as possible.

Re-attachment of the crown fragment

If the crown fragment is recovered after the accident, it may be possible to reattach it to the tooth; this method has become feasible with the advent of dentine-bonding agents. No long-term studies on the longevity of this type of restoration have yet been published, although Andreasen & Andreasen (1994) have quoted preliminary studies that indicate 50% loss within 5 years. Therefore this type of restoration can at present only be considered semi-permanent.

If the fracture line through dentine is assessed as being not very close to the pulp, the fragment may be reattached immediately. If, however, the fracture runs close to the pulp, a calcium hydroxide dressing should be placed over the exposed enamel and dentine and retained with composite resin (or a stainless steel crown) for at least 1 month, the fragment being stored in sterile saline; it is advisable to cover enamel as well as dentine with calcium hydroxide, so as to keep the enamel free of composite resin and thus retain a fresh enamel surface for bonding of the crown fragment.

Technique: composite resin bandage

Procedure	Method	Rationale	Notes
1. Polish the labial and palatal enamel surfaces	Use a slurry of pumice and water or an oil-free prophylaxis paste to polish labial and palatal surfaces of the fractured tooth. Wash off the pumice with a water spray.	Polishing removes plaque and pellicle that might interfere with subsequent acid etching. Pumice is preferred to commercial prophylaxis pastes because the latter may contain fluoride and/or oily constituents that reduce the effectiveness of acid etching.	This stage is not essential and may be omitted, especially if the tooth is sensitive to pressure.
2. Isolate the tooth	Isolate the tooth by placing a cotton roll in the labial sulcus, and use a saliva ejector.	For the treatment to be successful it is essential that the tooth is kept isolated from saliva.	Although ideal isolation is obtained by placing a rubber dam, this is often not practicable in the emergency treatment of a fractured tooth.
3. Etch labial and palatal enamel	After drying the tooth, apply a proprietary acid etchant in gel form with a small cotton wool pledget or fine brush. Apply the gel to labial and palatal enamel, extending about 4 mm from the fractured edge along the full mesio-distal width of the tooth. Do not apply gel to the fractured incisal surface. It is not necessary to etch the mesial or distal surfaces. Keep the gel in contact with labial and palatal enamel for 1 minute.	Using a gel avoids the risk of acid flowing on to the fractured surface. Etching about 4 mm from the fractured edge provides sufficient area for bonding of the composite resin. Although the fractured dentine has been protected with calcium hydroxide, it is prudent to avoid the possibility of acid seeping beneath it. Approximal surfaces need not be etched because crown restoration is not the aim of this treatment.	Some gels are coloured to aid accurate placement. If time is available and it is decided to restore the crown at the same session, mesial and distal surface enamel must also be etched. A 1-minute application has been normal practice for many years but 30 seconds is now considered adequate.
4. Wash and dry the enamel surface	With an assistant holding the tip of a high-volume aspirator suction tube close to the tooth, wash the gel off with a stream of water directed at each surface for at least 15 seconds. Do not allow the patient to rinse. Holding the lip away from the tooth, remove the wet cotton roll from the sulcus and replace with a dry one. Dry the etched enamel thoroughly by directing oil-free compressed air to each surface for 30 seconds.	Simultaneous washing and aspiration prevents acid from entering the mouth and causing an unpleasant taste. Inadequate washing, or contamination of the etched surface by saliva, reduces the subsequent bond strength of resin to enamel. Inadequate drying, or contamination by oil, also reduces the subsequent bond strength.	
5. Apply the bandage	Apply the composite resin to the etched enamel and over the calcium hydroxide dressing previously placed over the incisal surface (Fig. 28. 3). Allow the material to polymerize and smooth if necessary with a fine stone or abrasive disc.		

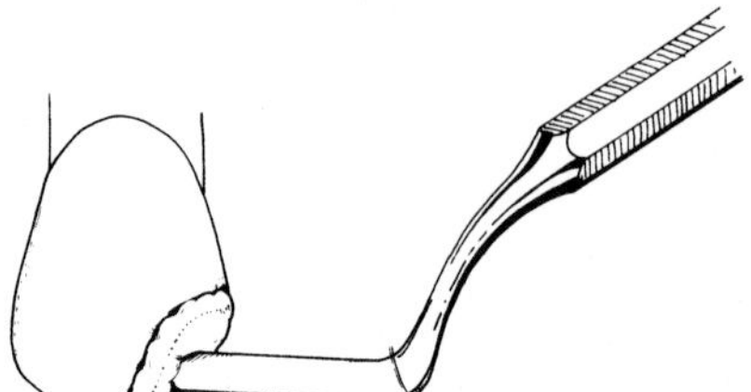

Fig. 28.3

Arrange to see the patient within 3 or 4 weeks to test pulp vitality and to restore the crown (p. 223). Crown restoration is important not only for aesthetic reasons but also to prevent: (1) movement of adjacent teeth into the space, (2) over-eruption of the opposing tooth, and (3) labial drift of the fractured tooth (if the incisal edge is no longer under the control of the lower lip).

Technique: stainless steel crown

Procedure	Method	Rationale	Notes
1. Select a crown	Measure the mesio-distal width of the fractured tooth at the gingival margin using dividers or a gauge. Select a crown of the same size, or slightly larger. Check the fit by placing it on the tooth.	If a crown of the exact size is not available, a slightly larger size should be used; later the edge can be turned in with a contouring plier to produce a tight fit.	
2. Trim the crown	Place the beaks of the dividers at the incisal edge and gingival margin of the tooth, in the centre of the labial aspect (Fig. 28.4a). Transfer this measurement to the stainless steel crown and mark the position of the gingival edge with a dental instrument or bur. Similarly, mark the position of the gingival margin on the mesial, distal and palatal aspects. With a pair of strong crown scissors, join the marks; this will approximate the gingival contour.	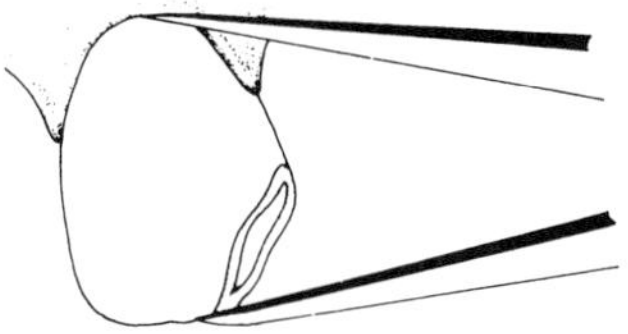 **Fig. 28.4a**	
3. Try the crown on the tooth	After smoothing the cut edge of the steel crown with a stone, try it on the tooth. If necessary, reduce the crown further by cutting or stoning the edge.	A rough edge would traumatize the gingiva when trying the crown in place. The margin of the crown should be placed just within the gingival crevice.	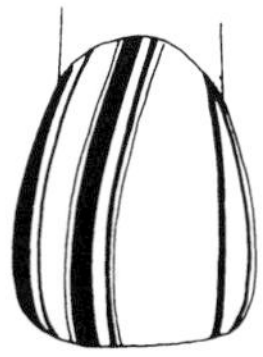
4. Contour the margin of the crown	Use a contouring plier to contour the margin of the crown so that it is a tight fit (Fig. 28.4b).	Contouring is necessary to produce a good fit at the gingival margin; this is essential to ensure good retention and to avoid gingival irritation.	**Fig. 28.4b**
5. Cut 'window' in the labial face of the steel crown	With a diamond bur make a hole in the labial face of the crown in a position that will be located on the enamel surface (Fig. 28.4c). OPTIONAL—enlarge this 'window' to uncover as much enamel as possible (Fig. 28.4d, e).	Exposing labial enamel permits subsequent vitality testing without removing the crown. Exposing a larger area of enamel improves the appearance of the crown.	An alternative method is to cut a V-shaped notch extending from the palatal gingival margin of the crown—but pulp testing near the gingival margin may give false positive results.
6. Smooth the margin of the crown	Smooth the cut margin of the crown with a stone and finally with a rubber wheel.		
7. Cement the crown	Cover the dentine on the fractured surface with calcium hydroxide (if this has not previously been done). Cement the crown with quick-setting zinc oxide-eugenol or polycarboxylate cement. If the entire labial surface of the steel crown has been cut away (as in Fig. 28.4e), add composite resin to replace the fractured portion of crown.	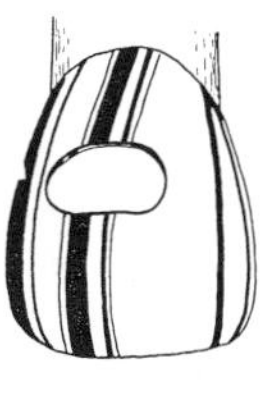 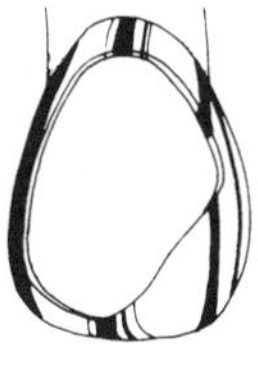	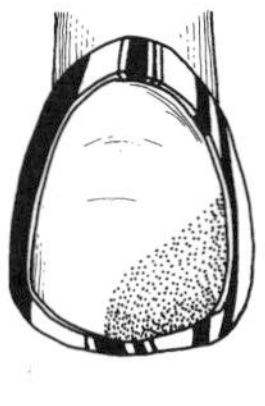

Fig. 28.4c   Fig. 28.4d   Fig. 28.4e

Technique: reattachment of crown fragment

Procedure	Method	Rationale	Notes
1. Check the fit of the fragment to the tooth		The fragment must be a close fit (Fig. 28.5a), although small deficiencies are acceptable—they will be restored with composite resin.	

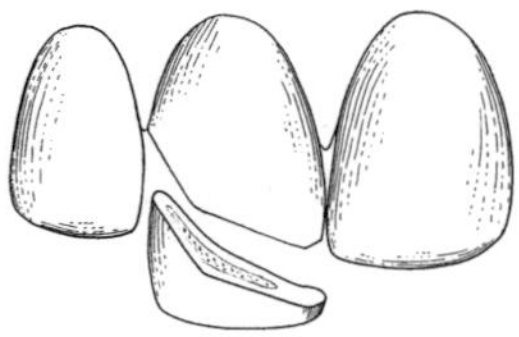

Fig. 28.5a

Procedure	Method	Rationale	Notes
2. Clean the fracture surfaces and adjacent enamel	Use a pumice–water slurry to clean the opposing fracture surfaces and also the adjacent enamel on the tooth and fragment to at least 2 mm from the edges of the fracture.	The surfaces must be cleaned in preparation for etching of enamel and conditioning of dentine.	
3. Etch enamel, wash and dry	Isolate the tooth. Apply etchant (ideally a coloured gel preparation) to the enamel on both fracture surfaces (keeping it off the dentine), and also the enamel all around the tooth and fragment, extending about 2 mm from the edges of the fracture. Wash with water for 15 seconds and dry for 30 seconds.	Using a coloured gel etchant makes it easier to localize on the enamel and to avoid contact with dentine.	
4. Condition the dentine	Apply dentine-bonding agent to the dentine, following the manufacturer's directions.		
5. Reattach the crown fragment	Use a mixture of filled and unfilled composite resin. Place resin on both fracture surfaces and carefully position the fragment on the tooth. Remove excess resin and polymerize.	It is important for the resin to flow satisfactorily so that close contact of the fragment to the tooth can be achieved.	If the fragment is very small, a piece of sticky wax or gutta percha attached to its incisal edge makes it easier to handle.
6. Strengthen the attachment	With a small round diamond bur reduce enamel thickness by about 0.5 mm labially and palatally, extending about 2 mm from the fracture line on the tooth and fragment sides, finishing in a chamfer. On the labial side make the finishing line irregular in outline (Fig. 28.5b). Etch the newly exposed enamel, wash, dry, apply filled composite resin, and smooth.	An enamel-composite junction is less perceptible if its outline is irregular.	Another technique has been described (Burke 1991) in which the only tooth preparation was to bevel the enamel edge of both the tooth and the fragment, before etching and reattaching the fragment.

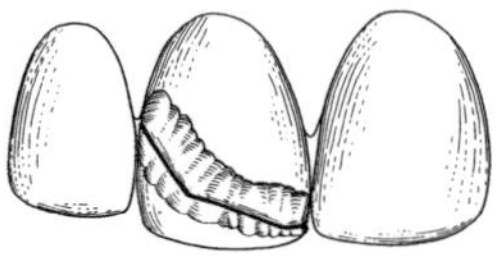

Fig. 28.5b

28.2.2 Pulp capping

When a tooth is fractured through dentine, it is necessary merely to protect the pulp against chemical or thermal injury. However, when the fracture involves pulp, some form of pulp treatment becomes necessary. Sometimes the pulp is not actually exposed but can be seen as a reddish shadow beneath a thin layer of dentine; such cases should be treated as if the pulp were exposed, because inevitably the pulp will have become infected before treatment is started.

Pulp capping with calcium hydroxide may be justified if the child presents within a few hours of injury, if the pulp exposure is pin-point in size, and if the root apex is open (Ravn 1982). However, pulp capping has been found to be less successful than pulpotomy (Fuks et al 1982), presumably because the pulp often becomes contaminated before treatment is carried out.

It may be argued that pulp capping is justified only for teeth with completed root development because, should the pulp die, root canal treatment is an uncomplicated procedure. In contrast, if the pulp dies in a tooth with immature root development, the problems in treatment are much greater (Ch. 29); for this reason pulpotomy or partial pulpotomy is the treatment of choice for such teeth.

Even when partial or full pulpotomy is the planned treatment, pulp capping may sometimes be done as an emergency measure. Time may not be available to complete a pulpotomy at the emergency visit and, moreover, the child may be upset and uncooperative as a result of the injuries. However, the child should be seen again as soon as possible (ideally within 24 hours) for the pulpotomy to be done.

Before pulp capping, the exposed pulp and surrounding dentine should be cleaned gently with a cotton wool pledget moistened in sterile saline or sterile water, and then dried with a cotton wool pledget; water or compressed air from a 'triplespray' should not be used as these would cause pain. A quick-setting type of calcium hydroxide is usually used, and it must be protected by one of the methods described on pages 210–211.

28.2.3 Vital pulpotomy and partial pulpotomy

Pulpotomy implies removal of all coronal pulp. The aims of pulpotomy of a vital tooth are to remove infected pulp tissue and to preserve healthy radicular pulp. In an immature tooth, root development will continue if the radicular pulp remains healthy, but if it dies the root apex will remain open and present a problem in endodontic treatment. Assessed radiologically, root development of maxillary incisors appears complete by the age of about 10 or 11 years, but it has been shown that further closure of the apex occurs up to 14 or 15 years of age (Friend 1966).

Vital pulpotomy has long been established as the treatment for an immature tooth that has sustained a fracture involving pulp, and has been shown to be highly effective (Jackson et al 1990). However, a partial pulpotomy technique first described by Cvek in 1978, and supported by Fuks et al (1987), has now become accepted as the treatment of choice. The technique is more conservative than pulpotomy, not only in the amount of pulp removed but also in the amount of tooth substance destroyed. The size of pulp exposure and the time elapsed before treatment do not appear to be critical for the success of treatment.

However, a critical factor in deciding whether full pulpotomy is necessary is the appearance of the amputated pulp surface when the partial pulpotomy is performed; if its colour and the extent of bleeding suggest that the underlying coronal pulp is inflamed or necrotic, partial pulpotomy will not be the appropriate treatment. Both techniques are described below.

Technique: vital partial pulpotomy

1. Administer local analgesic and place rubber dam. The maintenance of a sterile operating field is essential. If rubber dam cannot be placed, cotton wool rolls and a saliva ejector must be used and carefully maintained in position throughout the treatment.
2. With a sterile cylindrical or pear-shaped diamond bur enter the pulp at the site of the pulp exposure (Fig. 28.5a). Running the handpiece at high speed, make a cavity about 2 mm deep while washing and cooling with a constant stream of sterile water or saline from a syringe (Fig. 28.5b); this technique causes minimal irritation to the underlying pulp. Carefully examine the amputated pulp; if it does not

have a normal red colour and is not bleeding normally, the partial pulpotomy should be carried to a deeper level or a full pulpotomy carried out.
3. After controlling bleeding with sterile cotton wool pledgets, place a layer of calcium hydroxide over the pulp surface (either paste or powder or a hard-setting product) and seal the cavity with glass-ionomer cement.

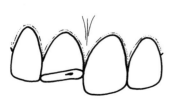

Fig. 28.6a

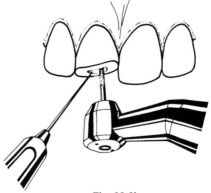

Fig. 28.6b

Technique: vital pulpotomy

1. As stage 1 partial pulpotomy.
2. Use a diamond or tungsten carbide bur at high speed to outline the access cavity in the palatal surface of the tooth. Prepare this cavity in dentine but do not extend into the pulp (Fig. 28.7a). Make the cavity triangular in shape and large enough to give good access to the pulp chamber and pulp horns (Fig. 28.7b).
3. Wipe the cavity and the surrounding area with a cotton wool pledget soaked in a disinfectant solution and use only sterile instruments and materials (ideally from a sterile pre-packed tray) from this stage to the end of treatment. Deepen the cavity until the pulp is exposed (Fig. 28.7c) and, with a fissure bur, remove the entire root of the pulp chamber.
4. With a round bur revolving slowly, or with a sharp excavator, amputate the pulp at the floor of the pulp chamber. Remove amputated pulp, including pulp horns, with an excavator (Fig. 28.7d) and wash the pulp chamber

with sterile water or saline from a syringe; do not use water or compressed air from a 'triplespray' because the water is not sterile and the air pressure would irritate the pulp. Dry and control haemorrhage with sterile cotton wool pledgets, avoiding pressure.

5. When haemorrhage has ceased, place calcium hydroxide paste or powder in the floor of the pulp chamber (Fig. 28.7e). Paste is best applied fairly thickly on the end of a small instrument; powder is insufflated through a 'Jiffy' tube. Do not exert pressure on the radicular pulp.
6. Place a layer of quick-setting calcium hydroxide over the paste before sealing the cavity with glass-ionomer cement (Fig. 28.7f).
7. Arrange to see the patient within a few weeks to test pulp vitality and to restore the crown (Ch. 29). Part of the pulp chamber can be used to contribute to the retention of the composite resin restoration.

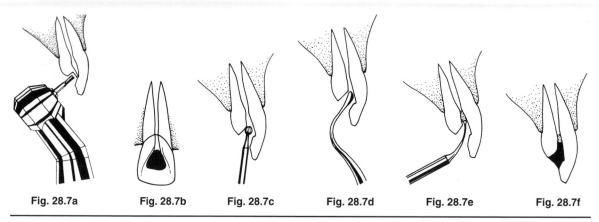

| Fig. 28.7a | Fig. 28.7b | Fig. 28.7c | Fig. 28.7d | Fig. 28.7e | Fig. 28.7f |

28.2.4 Pulpectomy

Pulpectomy (removal of coronal and radicular pulp) is the usual treatment when a tooth with a fully developed root becomes fractured through the pulp. If the pulp exposure is pinpoint in size and the patient presents within a few hours of injury, pulp capping may be adequate treatment. It is, however, essential to monitor pulp vitality during the next 2 years and to intervene with pulpectomy and root canal filling if there is evidence of pulp death.

The technique of pulpectomy and root canal treatment will not be described here; the reader is referred to textbooks of endodontics.

28.3 TREATMENT OF ROOT FRACTURES

The main decision that must be taken concerning the immediate treatment of a root-fractured tooth is whe-

ther to splint the tooth, and this decision depends on the position of the fracture. The main purpose of splinting is to encourage repair of the fracture (p. 215), but repair is only important if the long-term stability of the tooth depends on it. If the fracture is through the apical $\frac{1}{3}$ of the root (Fig. 28.8a) there is sufficient length of root coronal to the fracture line to provide adequate periodontal support for the tooth without repair of the fracture; there is therefore no need to splint (unless the tooth has been loosened by breakdown of the periodontal attachment). Thus, an apical $\frac{1}{3}$ root fracture does not per se cause loosening of the tooth, and no treatment is required other than to review pulp vitality and to carry out endodontic treatment if required (Ch. 29).

If, however, the fracture is through the middle $\frac{1}{3}$ or cervical $\frac{1}{3}$ of the root (Fig. 28.8b, c) repair of the fracture is essential to stabilize the tooth; splinting is therefore required if the tooth is to be retained. Splinting methods are discussed in the next section.

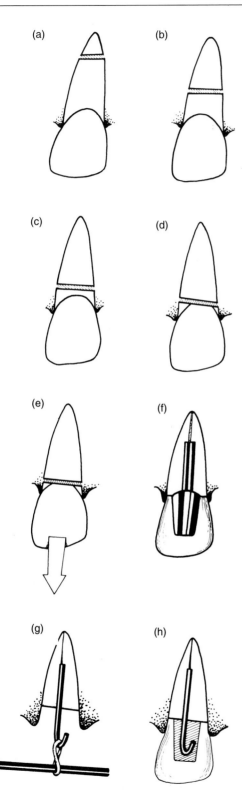

The prognosis for most root-fractured teeth is good (Zachrisson & Jacobsen 1975). However, when a fracture is close to the gingival crevice (Fig. 28.8d) the prognosis is poor and splinting is not recommended; in these cases a decision must be made either to extract the coronal portion and retain the root for construction of a post crown (Fig. 28.8e, f), or to extract the two fragments and make a prosthetic replacement.

When the decision is made to extract the coronal portion only, immediate treatment must also include removal of pulp and the placement of a temporary dressing in the remaining root portion. However, this treatment (extraction and pulpectomy) may be postponed, and the coronal fragment temporarily splinted in position; this course of action might be indicated if the child is upset and uncooperative.

After a coronal fragment is extracted, it may be found that the face of the root lies too far subgingival to permit adequate access for its preparation and for taking an impression. This problem may be resolved by either surgical or orthodontic means; the latter approach is preferred. A piece of steel wire, bent into a hook at one end, may be cemented into the root canal (after pulp extirpation), and traction applied by an orthodontic elastic band attached to a labial arch wire (Fig. 28.8g). Alternatively, a composite resin core or even a crown may be made over the wire hook (Fig. 28.8h) and an orthodontic bracket bonded to its labial surface. When the root has been extruded sufficiently, root canal treatment can be completed and a post crown made.

28.4 SPLINTING

Trauma may loosen a tooth either by breaking the periodontal attachment to the alveolar bone or by fracturing the root. Splinting may be required to stabilize a loosened tooth until healing of the periodontal ligament occurs or until repair of a root fracture takes place.

28.4.1 Loosened (subluxated) teeth

Splinting is not an essential prerequisite for periodontal healing; indeed, prolonged splinting delays healing and encourages root resorption. However, it is often desirable to splint the tooth to protect it from further trauma during the healing period. The decision on whether to make a splint depends principally on the degree of tooth mobility; grossly mobile teeth should be splinted, but less mobile teeth may be left unsplinted if the child is sensible enough

Fig. 28.8

to follow instructions and to take obvious pre-cautions.

The splinting period is kept as short as possible. Even for the severest cases, for example a replanted tooth, the splint can be removed after about a week; but it would not be unreasonable to prolong this to 2 weeks, and it should be extended to 3–4 weeks if alveolar bone is fractured.

28.4.2 Displaced (luxated) teeth

Teeth that have been displaced must be repositioned before they are splinted. Those that have been displaced labially or palatally, or that have been extruded, may be repositioned by digital pressure. Avulsed teeth may be replanted (p. 219).

Teeth that have been intruded do not need to be splinted because they are supported by alveolar bone, but they present special problems because intrusion usually results in rapid pulp death and external root resorption. These complications have been found to occur especially when intruded teeth are surgically repositioned by the use of forceps; for this reason more gentle extrusion by orthodontic means is recommended (Spalding et al 1985). To do this, an orthodontic bracket is bonded with composite resin to the labial surface of the tooth (if the tooth is completely intruded it must be pulled down gently with forceps just far enough to allow a bracket to be attached).

Although intruded teeth with incompletely formed roots sometimes re-erupt spontaneously, early orthodontic treatment is recommended for these as well as for mature teeth (which do not re-erupt). Pulp death may occur and root resorption may begin within 2–3 weeks and it is important that the teeth are extruded sufficiently to allow access to the pulp chamber for endodontic treatment. Orthodontic treatment may be delayed only when an immature tooth has suffered a minor degree of intrusion and access to the pulp chamber has not been compromised; the tooth may then be given the opportunity to re-erupt spontaneously.

Endodontic treatment of mature intruded teeth should be carried out as soon as possible because pulp death is inevitable. After pulpectomy, the root canal should be filled with calcium hydroxide paste (p. 231) which inhibits external root resorption. However, this treatment can be delayed for immature teeth because it is possible that the pulp will survive; close observation is essential, and radiographs should be taken every 2–3 months to check for the earliest signs of external root resorption. The rationale of endodontic treatment of intruded teeth is similar to that of replanted teeth.

28.4.3 Teeth with root fractures

A longer splinting period, 2–3 months, is recommended for the treatment of root fractures when the aim is to promote repair of the fractured root.

Ideally a hard tissue repair occurs and the fragments become firmly united, but a connective tissue repair may be satisfactory. Sometimes, however, little or no repair takes place, the fracture site becomes filled with inflamed granulation tissue, and the tooth remains loose.

28.4.4 Types of splint

Fixed splints

Convenient materials for making splints are acrylic or composite resins that are produced for making temporary crowns and bridges. The material can be either applied across the labial surfaces of the teeth (Fig. 28.9) or used to bond an arch wire to the teeth (Fig. 28.10).

The tooth to be splinted must be supported while the splint is being made, and this is usually done with a finger placed over its incisal edge. An alternative method utilizes impression compound (Croll & Johnson 1982). A piece of softened compound is placed on the incisal edges of the mandibular incisors (assuming the traumatized tooth is a maxillary incisor), the patient is asked to close the teeth together and the compound is moulded over the palatal surfaces and incisal edges of the maxillary incisors (but kept away from the labial surfaces). The traumatized tooth is supported in this way while the splint is made.

The splint is retained by bonding the material to acid-etched labial enamel. However, it is an advantage

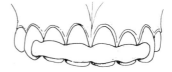

Fig. 28.9 Resin splint.

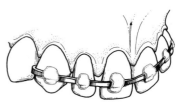

Fig. 28.10 Arch wire and resin splint.

Technique: acrylic or composite resin splint

1. The teeth to be splinted should include at least one tooth mesial and at least one distal to the loose tooth. Clean the labial surfaces of the teeth with a pumice–water slurry or an oil-free prophylaxis paste. The traumatized tooth must be cleaned very gently while supporting it firmly as described above; if, despite these precautions, the tooth is painful, cleaning may be limited to gentle rubbing with a moist cotton wool roll.
2. Isolate and dry the teeth.
3. Etch the incisal third of the labial surfaces of the teeth for $\frac{1}{2}$ –1 minute with 30–50% phosphoric acid. A gel form of etchant is preferable if control of gingival bleeding is incomplete because gel is less easily displaced from the tooth surface than solution.
4. Wash and dry the etched surfaces.
5. Mix the resin according to the manufacturer's instructions and flow it across the teeth, over the etched areas (Fig. 28.9).
6. When the resin begins to harden, remove excess and, when it is set, smooth any rough edges.

Technique: wire and resin splint

1. Use either round or rectangular wire (about 0.020" diameter or about 0.018" x 0.025"). Multistrand wire (0.018" diameter) is recommended because it is easily bent and its slightly rough surface aids adhesion of the composite resin. If suitable orthodontic wire is not readily available, a paper clip may be used.
2. Bend the wire to fit the incisal third of the labial surface of the teeth to be splinted; it should fit closely, but not necessarily very accurately. It is helpful to bend a short tag to fit around the distal surface of the tooth that will be at one end of the splint; this helps to relocate the wire in exactly the same position after making adjustments to its shape.
3. Clean the labial surfaces of the teeth to be splinted, isolate and dry the teeth, and etch the labial enamel.
4. Place a small amount of resin on the etched areas, position the wire over the teeth and add more resin until the parts of the wire lying over the labial surfaces are covered (Fig. 28.10).

if the splint can be easily removed at the end of the splinting period, and for this reason acrylic resin may be preferred to composite resin for all except root-fractured teeth. Acrylic resin is retained satisfactorily on etched enamel for the short (1–2 week) splinting period that is usually required (Awang et al 1985), but composite resin may be preferred for root-fractured teeth because the stronger bond of composite resin to etched enamel may be necessary to retain the splint for the 2–3 month period that is required.

The two types of splint described, and illustrated in Figures 28.9 and 28.10 fulfil most of the requirements of an ideal splint: they are easy to make and are retained reliably; they do not impinge on the gingiva; and they allow access for pulp testing, and for endodontic treatment should this be required. The only disadvantage is that the progress of periodontal reattachment cannot be assessed without first removing the splint. Although the general guidelines regarding splinting periods are usually satisfactory, some teeth may remain splinted longer than is necessary and others may require further splinting, which would involve the inconvenience of making a new splint. Removable splints have an advantage in this respect because they allow simple assessment of periodontal reattachment.

Removable splints

A removable splint can be used at any time in preference to those described above, but is particularly useful if several adjacent teeth have been loosened or if there are no teeth present on either side of the traumatized tooth. For example, a 7- or 8-year-old child with traumatized maxillary central incisors may not have lateral incisors sufficiently erupted to provide support, and the primary canines may be absent or carious. One of the removable splints described below would offer a solution to this problem.

The splints are made on plaster-stone casts of the dentition. Alginate is a suitable impression material, but precautions must be taken to avoid displacing, or even extracting, the loose tooth. Moderately loose teeth need only be covered with petroleum jelly (Vaseline), but a very loose tooth, for example a replanted tooth, should be supported while the impression is taken. An old dental instrument adapted to the labial surface of the tooth and bent over its incisal edge provides adequate support (Fig. 28.11). Alternatively, the tooth can be covered with thin casting wax or metal foil (Fig. 28.12) which is adapted closely to the labial and palatal surfaces of the teeth, but not pressed between the teeth, so that it comes away in the impression.

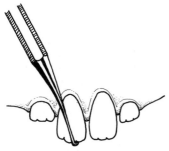

Fig. 28.11 Stabilizing a very mobile tooth with a dental instrument while taking an impression.

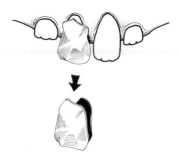

Fig. 28.12 The use of thin metal foil to facilitate taking an impression of a very loose tooth.

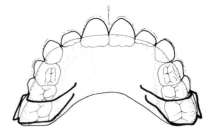

Fig. 28.13 Removable acrylic splint, showing occlusal coverage and Adams cribs (the cribs are not essential).

The splint should be made in the laboratory immediately or with minimal delay, thus avoiding the need for a temporary splint.

1. Removable acrylic splint. This type of splint has been extensively used in Northern Ireland. When first described (Stewart 1963) the splint incorporated Adams cribs on permanent first molars (Fig. 28.13), but further experience has shown that cribs are not required; the splint is retained satisfactorily without them (Saunders 1991).

The acrylic is extended over the incisal edges of the anterior teeth and 2–3 mm on to their labial surfaces (Fig. 28.13). It is usually necessary to cover occlusal surfaces of posterior teeth because, if this is not done, the only occlusal contact would be between mandibular incisors and palatal acrylic; the slight opening of the bite produced by occlusal coverage is easily tolerated by child patients. However, if the patient has an incomplete overbite there might be sufficient clearance for palatal acrylic, making it unnecessary to cover posterior teeth.

The patient is instructed to remove the splint for cleaning after meals and before retiring to bed.

2. Removable thermoplastic vinyl splint. Various thermoplastic materials are available which may be used for making splints. A suitable material is ethylvinylacetate (Drufosoft, Dreve, Germany), which is used for making mouthprotectors (Skyberg 1978). The splint is made in the same way as a mouthprotector; the technique is described in Chapter 27. The splint is removable and the patient is given the same instructions as those outlined for a removable acrylic splint.

The fact that a removable splint can be removed by the patient may be considered to be a disadvantage. However, the experience of those who use removable splints is that they are not removed because patients feel more comfortable and secure wearing them. If the patient's sense of responsibility is in doubt a removable splint should not be used. The main disadvantages of using a removable splint are the laboratory time and expense involved in its construction. On the other hand, an advantage of using a removable splint is the ease with which the progress of periodontal reattachment can be assessed, which ensures that the splint is discarded at the optimal time. It is possible that a removable splint, by allowing the tooth slight movement, encourages more rapid periodontal reorganization and reattachment. Such movement is, however, undesirable for the repair of a root fracture, for which a fixed splint is preferred.

28.5 REPLANTATION (REIMPLANTATION)

Replantation is the replacement in its socket of a tooth that has been avulsed. The tooth usually becomes firm within a few weeks, but its long-term prognosis is dependent on many factors. The prognosis is most favourable if the tooth is replanted within half an hour of avulsion and if, before replantation, the periodontal tissues attached to the root are kept moist and not disturbed.

Under ideal conditions, normal healing occurs and the tooth remains healthy. Unfortunately, the majority of replanted teeth show progressive root resorption: either inflammatory resorption, or replacement resorption and ankylosis. The rate of progress of resorption varies greatly; the tooth may be lost within a few months or it may survive for several years.

After replanting the tooth, it must be stabilized by splinting, but only for 1–2 weeks; a longer splinting period encourages root resorption. Root canal treatment will almost certainly be required if the replanted tooth has a fully developed root, but may not be necessary if the root apex is open and the tooth was replanted immediately after avulsion. Root resorption may sometimes be arrested by root canal treatment and filling with calcium hydroxide.

Despite its uncertain prognosis, replantation of an avulsed permanent tooth is usually justified, especially in children (Mackie 1992). One of the factors determining the prognosis is the length of time that the tooth remains out of the mouth. Therefore, if a parent or guardian telephones to report the accident, he or she should be encouraged to replant the tooth (assuming there is no unfavourable medical history). The following instructions should be given:

1. Hold the tooth by its crown, not by its root.
2. Remove any particles of dirt that may be present on the root surface by rinsing with cold water (for a few seconds only) or by dabbing very gently with a wet tissue (wetted preferably with saliva rather than with water).
3. Replant the tooth carefully in its socket (ensure that the parent can differentiate the labial from the palatal surface of the tooth).

4. Ask the child to keep it in place by biting on a handkerchief.
5. Report to the surgery as quickly as possible.

If the parent is unwilling or unable to carry out these instructions, directions must be given on how to transport the tooth to the surgery. This is a crucial factor influencing the prognosis, because it is essential to maintain the vitality of the periodontal tissues attached to the root surface. The ideal method is for the tooth to be placed in the child's mouth (or even the parent's mouth); the lower labial sulcus may be recommended as a safe place. If they are unwilling to do this they should be advised to place the tooth in milk, which has been shown to be a satisfactory medium for maintaining the vitality of the periodontal tissues (Blomhof & Otteskog 1980); water is a poor medium. If milk is not available, the tooth should be placed in a clean tissue or handkerchief moistened with the child's or the parent's saliva.

When the patient reaches the surgery, the tooth should immediately be placed in saline so that it can be examined and cleaned. A dental and medical history is taken and the extra-oral and intra-oral injuries are examined. If it is decided to replant the tooth, this should be done without further delay; the taking of radiographs may be postponed until after the tooth has been replanted (except when there is a suspicion of alveolar fracture that would complicate replantation).

If a parent reports that a tooth was avulsed but not recovered, it is essential to obtain a chest radiograph to exclude the possibility that it was inhaled.

Technique: replantation

Procedure	Method	Rationale	Notes
1. Prepare the patient	Inform the patient and parent of the need to splint the tooth for 1–2 weeks, of the probable need for root canal treatment, and of the uncertain prognosis.	Unless the tooth is replanted under ideal conditions, root resorption and eventual loss of the tooth is inevitable. If the patient is not keen to receive the necessary treatment, prosthetic replacement may be preferable.	If the patient has severe incisor crowding and/or an increased overjet, orthodontic treatment involving closure of the space may be considered to be preferable to replantation.
2. Prepare the tooth	When the patient brings the avulsed tooth to the surgery, place it immediately in a dish containing sterile saline. Hold the tooth by its crown and gently wash or dab away any mud or dirt (Fig. 28.14a). Do not remove or damage adherent periodontal tissues.	Preservation of undamaged periodontal tissues greatly improves the prognosis of replantation.	It is possible to remove the pulp and fill the root canal while holding the tooth by its crown, but the available evidence strongly indicates that it is preferable to replant the tooth immediately and to defer root canal treatment for a few weeks until the tooth is firm again after splinting.

Technique: replantation *(contd)*

Procedure	Method	Rationale	Notes
3. Prepare the tooth socket	Anaesthetize the area. Inspect the socket and surrounding tissues and clean if necessary with sterile saline or water. Do not disturb the blood clot in the socket.		Local analgesic may not be required if the tooth was avulsed less than about 2 hours previously. If a firm blood clot has already formed, it is necessary to break it up gently with a sterile instrument.
4. Replant the tooth	Replace the tooth carefully in its socket (Fig. 28.14b), without using force.		
5. Make a splint	Splint the tooth by one of the methods described on pages 216–217.		
6. Prescribe antibiotic	Prescribe a course of oral penicillin.	The tissues will certainly have become infected.	If the patient is allergic to penicillin, or has received penicillin during the previous 3 months, an alternative should be prescribed (Appendix 2).
7. Check tetanus immunization status	Arrange for tetanus toxoid injection if necessary (p. 208).		

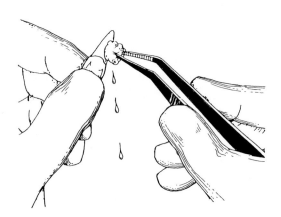

Fig. 28.14a

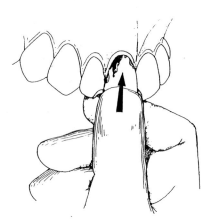

Fig. 28.14b

Follow-up

1–2 weeks after replantation:
1. Remove the splint carefully. The tooth will not yet be firm, but will soon become so, and a longer splinting period encourages root resorption.
2. Take a periapical radiograph of the tooth to serve as a baseline for subsequent assessment of root resorption and of periapical involvement.

3–4 weeks after replantation:
1. The tooth should now be firm enough for endodontic treatment to be carried out. For a tooth with a fully-developed root, pulpectomy and root canal filling with calcium hydroxide should be carried out without further delay. An immature tooth may remain vital if it was replanted under ideal conditions and may therefore be monitored for a longer period; if it remains vital, it may be expected to give a vital response to pulp testing after about 1–2 months.
2. Test the vitality of adjacent teeth that might also have been traumatized.
3. If the patient wishes to participate in contact sports, make a mouthprotector (Ch. 27).

Technique: replantation *(contd)*

At about 3–4 week intervals:
1. Take further radiographs of replanted immature teeth that have not been root-filled. At the first sign of root resorption, carry out root canal treatment and fill the canal with calcium hydroxide.
2. Test pulp vitality of replanted immature teeth and of adjacent teeth.

At about 3-month intervals:
Take radiographs of replanted teeth that have been root-filled with calcium hydroxide; replace the calcium hydroxide dressing if there are signs of active root resorption.

REFERENCES

Andreasen J O, Andreasen F M 1994 Textbook and color atlas of traumatic injuries to the teeth, 3rd edn. Munksgaard, Copenhagen

Awang H, Hill F J, Davies E H 1985 An investigation of three polymeric materials for acid-etch splint construction. Journal of Paediatric Dentistry 1: 55–60

Blomhof L, Otteskog P 1980 Viability of human periodontal ligament cells after storage in milk or saliva. Scandinavian Journal of Dental Research 88: 436–440

Burke F J T 1991 Reattachment of a fractured central incisor tooth fragment. British Dental Journal 170: 223–225

Croll T P, Johnson R 1982 Stabilisation of a traumatised tooth for application of a splint. Journal of Dentistry for Children 49: 357–358

Cvek M 1978 A clinical report on partial pulpotomy and capping with calcium hydroxide in permanent incisors with complicated crown fracture. Journal of Endodontics 4: 232–237

Friend L A 1966 The root treatment of teeth with open apices. Proceedings of the Royal Society of Medicine 59: 1035–1036

Fuks A B, Bielak S, Chosak A 1982 Clinical and radiographic assessment of direct pulp capping and pulpotomy in young permanent teeth. Pediatric Dentistry 4: 240–244

Fuks A B, Chosack A, Klein H, Eidelman E 1987 Partial pulpotomy as a treatment alternative for exposed pulps in crown-fractured permanent incisors. Endodontics and Dental Traumatology 3: 100–102

Jackson K, Rock W P, Potts A J C 1990 Vital pulpotomy of fractured immature incisors—a retrospective study. Journal of Paediatric Dentistry 6: 103–108

Mackie I C 1992 An investigation of replantation of traumatically avulsed permanent incisor teeth. British Dental Journal 172: 17–20

Ravn J J 1982 Follow-up study of permanent incisors with complicated crown fractures after acute trauma. Scandinavian Journal of Dental Research 90: 363–372

Rock W P, Gordon P H, Friend L A, Grundy M C 1974 The relationship between trauma and pulp death in incisor teeth. British Dental Journal 136: 236–239

Saunders I D F 1991 Personal communication

Skyberg R L 1978 Stabilisation of avulsed teeth in children with the flexible mouthguard splint. Journal of the American Dental Association 96: 797–800

Spalding P M, Fields H W, Torney D, Cobb H B, Johnson J 1985 The changing role of endodontics and orthodontics in the management of traumatically intruded permanent incisors. Pediatric Dentistry 7: 104–110

Stewart D J 1963 Stabilising appliances for traumatised incisors. British Dental Journal 115: 416–418

Zachrisson B J, Jacobsen I 1975 Long-term prognosis of 66 permanent anterior teeth with root fracture. Scandinavian Journal of Dental Research 83: 345–354

RECOMMENDED READING

Andreasen J O, Andreasen F M 1994 Textbook and color atlas of traumatic injuries to the teeth, 3rd edn. Munksgaard, Copenhagen

29 Intermediate and final treatment of traumatized permanent anterior teeth

29.1 RESTORATION OF THE CROWN

29.1.1 Teeth with fractures not involving the pulp

A fractured tooth may have been restored with composite resin as part of immediate treatment (Ch. 28), in which case this restoration is retained semi-permanently until such time as it is no longer satisfactory, usually for aesthetic reasons. If, on the other hand, immediate treatment involved only the placing of a protective bandage of composite resin (p. 210), the crown should be restored within a few weeks to prevent drifting of the tooth labially (if the fracture shortened the length of the crown and released it from control of the lower lip) or tilting of adjacent teeth over it (if there is incisor crowding).

The material most commonly used to restore a fractured incisor is composite resin. Satisfactory results have been obtained, but the main problem is gradual discoloration of the composite resin; these restorations are therefore only acceptable at present as semi-permanent restorations. In attempts to overcome the problem of discoloration, manufacturers have produced resins containing fillers of different types and particle size; the most satisfactory for the restoration of fractured incisors appear at present to be the 'hybrid' types, which contain a mixture of 'macro'- and 'micro'-sized particles.

Ideally, enamel extending about 3–4 mm from the fractured edge around the tooth is utilized to retain the restoration. Before proceeding it must be decided either to apply composite resin directly to these surfaces or to reduce the thickness of enamel first. If no enamel reduction is done (the approach often preferred, especially for children), it is inevitable that the restored crown will be thicker labio-palatally than the natural crown (and its contralateral tooth), but, despite this, the appearance is usually acceptable. If, however, it is decided to reduce enamel thickness, this may be limited to the labial surface or may be extended around the tooth to the palatal surface (palatal reduction is essential if addition of composite to the palatal surface would interfere with occlusion).

If it is decided not to reduce enamel thickness, the only mechanical preparation that is recommended is to bevel the enamel at the labial edge of the fractured surface (Fig. 29.1), to increase the thickness of composite material at this point.

If it is decided to reduce enamel thickness, enamel should be removed to a depth of about 0.5 mm, extending 3–4 mm from the edge of the fracture if possible (Fig. 29.2a). With oblique fractures there may be less supragingival enamel available beyond the gingival edge of the fracture, and the preparation can therefore only be carried to or just beyond this point (Fig. 29.2b).

The preparation may be finished at or just short of the incisal edge of the tooth if only labial enamel is

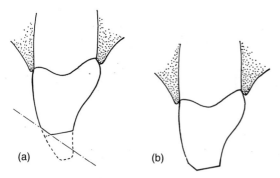

(a)   (b)

Fig. 29.1

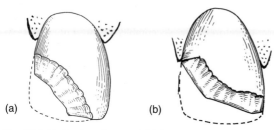

(a)   (b)

Fig. 29.2 Reduction of enamel thickness.

being reduced (Fig. 29.3a), but should be carried over the incisal edge to the palatal surface if the palatal surface is also being reduced (Fig. 29.3b).

Because of the limitations of composite resin restorations, a porcelain veneer or jacket crown is usually the ultimate restoration for a fractured incisor. Jacket crown restoration should be delayed until the child is at least 18 years of age, by which time pulp horns will have receded and tooth reduction can be done safely.

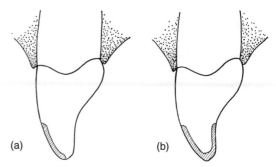

(a)   (b)

Fig. 29.3 Preparation finished (a) just short of the incisal edge; (b) on the palatal surface.

Technique: composite resin crown restoration

Procedure	Method	Rationale	Notes
1. Clean the tooth surface	Use a slurry of pumice in water or an oil-free prophylaxis paste to clean all surfaces of the crown. Ensure that dentine on the fracture surface is covered with calcium hydroxide. If composite was used previously to provide pulp protection (Ch. 28), stone and then pumice to produce a 'fresh' composite surface.	New composite will bond to old composite if the latter has a clean, uncontaminated surface.	This cleaning procedure is unnecessary if a fresh enamel surface has been exposed by reducing its thickness (see text).
2. Prepare a crown form	Select a cellulose acetate crown form matching the tooth size and shape.	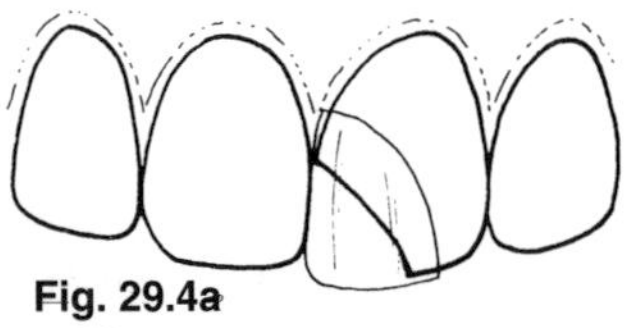	An alternative technique, not using a crown form, is to apply the composite directly to the tooth. Unless the fracture is very small, this technique is only feasible if a light-sensitive composite is used; the material is applied in increments, polymerizing each before adding the next.

Fig. 29.4a

| | Cut the crown form so that its margin lies about 4 mm from the fractured edge of the tooth (Fig. 29.4a). If labial enamel thickness was reduced, the margin of the crown form should lie over the periphery of the tooth preparation. With a probe, punch a small hole through the crown form at the incisal corner. | The crown form is cut so that its margin lies at the desired periphery of the restoration. About 4 mm from the fractured edge provides sufficient area for adequate bonding.

Small holes incisally allow the escape of air incorporated into the composite during mixing or when filling the crown form. | When the fracture is oblique, less than 4 mm will be available mesially or distally. This deficiency must be compensated by allowing more coverage elsewhere. |

Technique: composite resin crown restoration *(contd)*

Procedure	Method	Rationale	Notes
		when the crown form is placed on the tooth, thus preventing the formation of voids in the restoration.	
3. Isolate the tooth	Isolate the tooth, ideally with rubber dam but otherwise with cotton wool rolls and saliva ejector.	For successful bonding of composite resin to enamel to occur, it is essential that the tooth is kept isolated from saliva.	
4. Etch the enamel	As described on page 210, but extend the area of etching beyond the planned periphery of the composite restoration, i.e. at least 5 mm from the fractured edge if possible (Fig. 29.4b).	Etching must be extended beyond the planned periphery of the restoration, to ensure that the margin of the restoration is firmly bonded to etched enamel.	Any etched enamel not subsequently covered by composite quickly becomes remineralized.
5. Wash and dry the enamel surface	See page 210.		

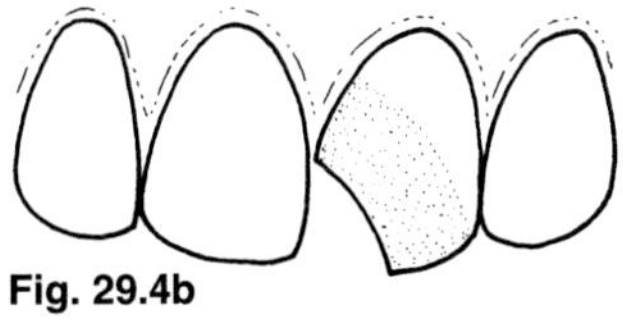

Fig. 29.4b

6. Apply unfilled resin	Apply unfilled resin to the etched enamel using a small brush or absorbent pad.		
7. Apply filled resin (i.e. composite 'paste') in the crown form	Fill the crown form with composite paste of the appropriate colour, place it on the tooth and vibrate it gently by hand into its previously determined position (Fig. 29.4c).	Vibrating the crown form into position encourages any entrapped air to escape through the holes made in the incisal corners.	

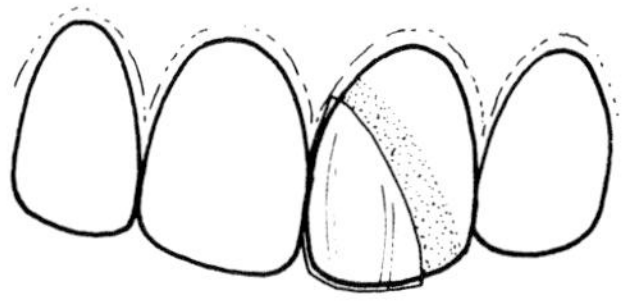

Fig. 29.4c

8. Remove excess composite	If using a light-sensitive material, support the crown form in position with a finger and, with a probe or other hand instrument, remove excess material that extruded from the crown form. Then polymerize the composite by applying an appropriate light source to labial and palatal surfaces in turn. If using an autopolymerizing resin, less time is available for removing excess; the material polymerizes within a few minutes.		
9. Trim and finish the restoration	When the composite has polymerized, remove the crown form by splitting it palatally with a probe or excavator and lifting it off. If possible, limit finishing procedures to the margin of the restoration, but if the whole restoration is too bulky, it must be reduced. Use diamond or tungsten carbide finishing burs in a high-speed handpiece, or abrasive discs in a slow-speed handpiece. For final polishing, use a tungsten carbide finishing bur, or the finest abrasive discs, or composite polishing paste.	No known method of polishing a composite restoration leaves its surface as smooth as that which polymerizes against a crown form or matrix strip.	However closely the crown form fitted initially, it inevitably becomes distorted to some extent when it is filled with composite and pressed into position on the tooth. It is therefore always necessary to trim the margin of the restoration.

29.1.2 Teeth with fractures involving the pulp

Retention of the composite crown restoration described above is dependent on its bond to etched enamel. When fractures involve the pulp, less natural crown remains, and the available enamel may be inadequate to retain the relatively large restoration that is required. If at least half of the crown remains and the tooth has received endodontic treatment, satisfactory retention can be obtained by utilizing part of the pulp chamber; a retentive cavity is prepared palatally into which composite resin is packed at the time of making the restoration.

If less than half of the crown remains, restoration with a post crown may be the most obvious solution, but this is not feasible for an immature tooth with a wide open root apex. In such a case, further measures are required to retain a crown for a few years until further closure of the root apex occurs. Pins and a dentine adhesive may be used to aid retention. Self-shearing pins are available which are inserted into dentine with a slow-speed handpiece and shear off at the depth of previously prepared hole (Fig. 29.5). A dentine adhesive is used instead of the unfilled resin.

If less than half of the crown remains but the tooth has a fully developed root, there are no special difficulties in restoring the tooth with a conventional post crown (Fig. 29.6). However, for an active child prone to accidents or involved in contact sports, it may be preferable to use a short cast or preformed post (Fig. 29.7), to reduce the risk of root fracture should further trauma occur. In either case, it is prudent to provide a mouthprotector for a patient who engages in contact sports.

A summary of intermediate and final treatments for crown restoration is given in Table 29.1.

29.1.3 Teeth with reattached crown fragment

The fractured tooth may have been restored initially by reattaching the fractured crown fragment (page 212). The durability of such a restoration is uncertain and its appearance may deteriorate as a result of discoloration of the composite resin bonding the fragment to the tooth. To overcome these problems a porcelain veneer may be fitted to cover the entire labial surface (page 146); this strengthens the attachment and improves the appearance.

29.2 PULP VITALITY TESTS

Root canal therapy does not usually form part of the immediate treatment of fractured teeth, except when a tooth with a fully developed root is fractured through the pulp. However, the pulp of any traumatized tooth may die, either quickly (within a few weeks) or slowly (during the next year or two). Therefore, regular assessment of pulp vitality is essential for at least 2 years after trauma, and root canal therapy is required if the pulp dies.

Tests of pulp vitality are, in fact tests of the sensitivity of pulpal nerves to thermal or electrical stimuli. Although pulp sensitivity is associated with pulp vitality, this not invariably the case. Thus, although a normal response to stimulation usually indicates that the pulp is healthy, and a reduced or negative response usually indicates that the pulp is partially or totally necrotic, it is possible for trauma to injure the pulpal nerves but not the blood vessels. In such a case the pulp would be healthy because it has a normal blood supply, but would not respond to stimuli (Bhaskar & Rappaport 1973). This would occur following the immediate replantation of an immature tooth; the pulp would revascularise but the nerve supply would not be re-established for at least 1 month.

Conversely, sensitivity to stimulation does not necessarily indicate that the pulp is vital. If the stimulus is transmitted through the tooth to periodontal rather than to pulpal nerves, a false positive response would be given. It has been estimated that a healthy pulp responds to an electrical stimulus of 150 μA from a monopolar pulp tester, and that stimuli

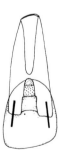

Fig. 29.5

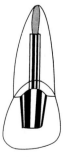

Fig. 29.6

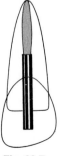

Fig. 29.7

Table 29.1 Summary of intermediate and final treatments for crown restoration.

Type of fracture	Root development	Immediate treatment previously performed	Intermediate treatment	Final treatment (after age 18)
Class II (through dentine)	open apex closed apex }	pulp protection	composite resin restoration (acid-etch retention)	porcelain veneer or jacket crown (or composite resin restoration)
Class III (through pulp) At least ½ crown remaining:	open apex	— pulpotomy	composite resin restoration (acid-etch retention + extra retention in pulp chamber)	porcelain veneer or jacket crown (or composite resin restoration)
	closed apex	— pulpotomy or pulpectomy and root filling		
Less than ½ crown remaining:	open apex	pulpotomy	composite resin restoration (acid-etch retention + extra retention in pulp chamber, from pins and from dentine adhesive)	root canal treatment, reduction of crown to gingival level and preparation for post and core (cast or preformed), porcelain crown
Less than ½ crown remaining:	closed apex	pulpectomy and root filling	1. short post projecting through fractured crown, composite resin restoration	removal of short post, reduction of crown to gingival level, preparation for conventional post and core, porcelain crown
			or	
			2. reduction of crown to gingival level and preparation for post and core, porcelain crown	if the margin of the crown has become supragingival and unaesthetic—cutting of porcelain crown from post, re-establishment of margin, new porcelain crown

greater than 200 μA may excite periodontal nerves (Matthews & Searle 1974).

Thus, pulp testing cannot provide definitive information about pulp vitality; it should be regarded only as an aid in diagnosis (Chambers 1982), to be considered in conjunction with clinical signs (for example tooth discoloration and the presence of a sinus), symptoms, sensitivity to percussion and radiographic evidence.

Thermal or electrical test may be used to assess pulp vitality. Thermal tests are of two kinds: the application of heat (usually heated gutta-percha) or of cold (usually frozen ethyl chloride on a cotton wool pledget). Electrical pulp tests are performed with instruments that are especially designed for the purpose, but which have different electrical characteristics (Drummer et al 1986). One of the newer instruments (Analytic Technology) has the advantage that the intensity of the stimulus can be increased very gradually, so that patients feel a warm, gentle tingling rather than the sudden jolting sensation sometimes experienced with other instruments (Cooley & Lubow 1984); a disadvantage of this instrument, however, is its relatively high cost.

The effect of wearing surgical gloves on electrical pulp testing has been investigated. With the dentist wearing gloves, the Pelton and Crane Vitalometer operates satisfactorily, although readings are higher when gloves are not worn (King & King 1977, Holan 1993), but the Analytic Technology instrument does not function. This problem, however, can be overcome by using a simple device supplied by the manufacturer or by asking the patient to grasp the metal handle of the pulp tester's probe with thumb and a finger (Anderson & Pantera 1988, Kolbinson & Teplitsky 1988).

Electrical tests provide the following important advantages over thermal tests:

1. It is easy to check the reliability of the response. If the patient responds at widely different points on successive tests, the reliability of the response is in doubt. Thermal tests do not allow such a check to be made.

2. Changes in the sensitivity of a tooth may be assessed by comparison with neighbouring teeth. If two or more teeth respond at similar points in one test and then, some time later, one tooth responds at a different point, that tooth would come under some suspicion thereafter. Comparisons of the relative sensitivity of different teeth are not possible with thermal tests.

Technique: electric pulp testing

Procedure	Method	Rationale	Notes
1. Prepare the patient and the equipment	Explain the purpose of the test in simple terms, e.g. "to check if the tooth is well" (avoid "to check if the tooth is dead"). Ask for the child's help in carrying out the test. Explain that: a. the tester will be placed on the tooth (demonstrate this on a finger nail); b. nothing will be felt at first but that, as the test progresses, a "little tingle" or "twinge" may be felt in the tooth. Ask the child to "signal" by raising an arm if a "tingle" or "twinge" is felt.	Cooperation is essential if meaningful information is to be obtained from the test; good patient management is therefore imperative. Encouraging active participation rather than expecting passive acceptance is good practice. Explaining the type of sensation to be expected prevents the child being surprised and upset by it.	
2. Perform the test	If the vitality of a particular tooth is in doubt, test that tooth first.	If a sound tooth is tested first and, despite careful preparation, the child dislikes the sensation, false positive responses may be given subsequently when a non-vital tooth is tested. If the first tooth tested is non-vital, the child will not respond and important information will have been obtained.	Occasionally a response may be obtained when testing a non-vital tooth, probably through stimulation of the periodontal nerves.
	Place the electrode tip on the middle of the labial surface, away from the gingival margin (Fig 29.8).	Contacting the gingival margin would provoke a false positive response.	

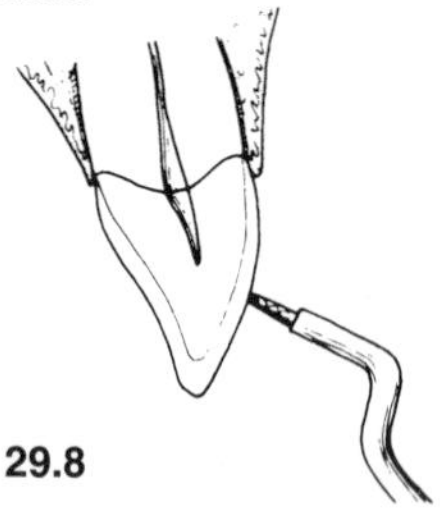

Fig. 29.8

| | Increase the current slowly. If and when the child signals by raising an arm, immediately remove the electrode from the tooth and note the reading on the dial. Repeat the test on the same tooth. If a similar reading is obtained, the result can be accepted with confidence. If a very different reading is obtained, the reliability of the child's response must be doubted. Repeat the procedure but place the electrode near, but not in contact with, the tooth. If the child again signals, the responses are clearly meaningless. Explain to the child once again the nature of the sensation to be expected. | Increasing the current quickly might result in the point of first stimulation being exceeded, causing unnecessary discomfort. | The ability to check the patient's response in this way is an advantage of electrical tests over thermal tests. Response may also be checked by use of the tester with the current switched off. |

Technique: electric pulp testing *(contd)*

Procedure	Method	Rationale	Notes
	Having established that the child is responding reliably, proceed to test neighbouring teeth. If no response is elicited from the first tooth tested, repeat the test two or three times to confirm. Then proceed to test neighbouring teeth.	In cases of trauma, several teeth may have been injured, even though they are not fractured and appear undamaged. If no response is elicited from one tooth but a positive response from neighbouring teeth, strong evidence will have been obtained that the first has a necrotic pulp.	It has been shown that teeth traumatized but not fractured are more liable to become non-vital than teeth fractured through enamel or dentine (Rock et al 1974).

29.3 PULPECTOMY

All traumatized teeth should be reviewed for at least 2 years, noting signs and symptoms, testing sensitivity to percussion, testing pulp vitality and taking radiographs. Pulpectomy is required if the pulp dies or if root resorption is diagnosed radiologically.

29.3.1 Mature teeth

Traumatized teeth that are not loosened or, if loosened, suffer little or no displacement, may be monitored as outlined above. In these cases, the risk of root resorption is minimal and the reason for endodontic treatment is almost always pulp death. For mature teeth conventional pulpectomy and root canal filling techniques can be used.

In contrast, endodontic treatment should be carried out within 2–4 weeks for teeth that are intruded or avulsed; not only is it almost certain that pulp death will occur but also that pulp death will be followed by external root resorption within this short period of time. After removing the pulp, and cleaning and washing the root canal, the canal should be filled with calcium hydroxide, which can inhibit root resorption. A radiograph should be taken every 3–6 months; if it is noted that root resorption is still progressing or that the calcium hydroxide is becoming resorbed at the root apex, it should be washed out and replaced. This treatment may need to be repeated several times, and completion of endodontic treatment by obturation of the canal should be delayed until external root resorption appears to have been controlled. Internal root resorption is less common, but should be treated similarly with calcium hydroxide.

29.3.2 Root-fractured teeth

The repair which takes place at the site of a root fracture is adversely affected by death of the pulp.

Since effective repair of the root fracture is crucial to the long-term survival of teeth with middle $\frac{1}{3}$ and cervical $\frac{1}{3}$ root fractures (p. 214), pulpectomy must be carried out promptly if pulp death occurs; this emphasizes the importance of regular monitoring of pulp vitality of root-fractured teeth (and, indeed, of any traumatized teeth). Pulp inflammation and necrosis of a root-fractured tooth is usually confined to the coronal fragment, pulp in the apical fragment remaining vital. Therefore, endodontic treatment may initially be restricted to the coronal fragment. Again, use of calcium hydroxide for several months as a root canal dressing is recommended.

If, following initial endodontic treatment, further signs or symptoms indicates that the pulp in the apical root fragment has died, further treatment is required. For apical $\frac{1}{3}$ fractures this treatment is simple: the apical fragment is surgically removed, and the tooth remains firm because sufficient length of root remains to provide adequate periodontal support. For middle $\frac{1}{3}$ and cervical $\frac{1}{3}$ root fractures, however, treatment is more complicated because the coronal fragment is not long enough to provide adequate periodontal support. Stability of the tooth must be achieved by splinting the two fragments together; this can be achieved by insertion of a post following root canal therapy. However, access to the canal in the apical fragment may be difficult if some hard tissue repair of the fractures has occurred, and the prognosis following this treatment is uncertain because necrotic remnants may remain between the two fragments. The alternative treatment is to extract the two fragments and to provide a prosthetic replacement: either a single-tooth partial denture, or a bridge (usually an etch-retained bridge for a child).

29.3.3 Immature teeth

Root canal treatment of non-vital immature teeth is complicated by the shape of the root canal. The walls of the root apex may be divergent ('blunderbuss'-

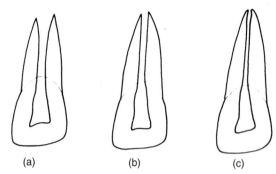

(a)   (b)   (c)

Fig. 29.9 The root apex at different stages of root development: (a) divergent walls, (b) parallel-sided walls, (c) convergent walls.

shaped), parallel-shaped or convergent (Fig. 29.9), depending on the extent of root development. When the walls are divergent it is impossible to achieve a good apical seal with a conventional root filling; when the walls are parallel-sided or convergent, it is not impossible but still difficult. In these cases calcium hydroxide is used not only to control root resorption if necessary but also to induce closure of the root apex (Cvek et al 1976); the technique is described on pages 231–233. Calcium hydroxide stimulates the deposition of a calcific barrier across the root apex or, in some cases, continued root development (Heithersay 1970). Whether a calcific barrier is formed or root development continues, the treatment with calcium hydroxide makes it easier later to achieve the fundamental objective of root canal therapy: the complete obturation and sealing of the root apex. The technique has been found to be highly successful (Mackie et al 1988, Cvek 1993).

The timing of final root canal filling is decided on the basis of clinical and radiographic assessment of apical barrier formation, continued root development, or arrest of root resorption. Usually, final treatment is carried out about 1 year after the initial treatment with calcium hydroxide.

If the root canal converges towards the apex, filling is uncomplicated and may be achieved with a large gutta-percha point, or by condensation of several gutta-percha points. However, if the canal is parallel-sided or divergent, it is more difficult to fill adequately. A calcific deposit at the root apex helps, but this cannot be expected to be a complete and impervious barrier. These wide canals may be filled by many gutta-percha points. Alternatively, a gutta-percha 'plug' may first be made by warming several points over a flame and rolling them together either with the fingers or between glass slabs. When a 'plug' of the

estimated diameter of the canal has been made, it is placed in the tooth to the known length of the canal, and a mark is made on it with a hot instrument at the level of the incisal edge of the tooth (a radiograph may be taken to check its position). When the 'plug' is a satisfactory fit, it is coated with a proprietary root canal sealing cement and placed into position (a little of the cement may first be introduced into the canal with a rotary filling instrument or reamer, placing the cement at the apex and on the walls of the canal). Further small gutta-percha points should be inserted if possible and condensed. The gutta-percha is then cut at the base of the pulp chamber (using fine scissors or a heated dental instrument) and the palatal cavity is sealed.

The pulp of a replanted immature tooth may survive if the tooth has a wide open root apex (e.g. in a 7–9-year-old child), especially if, after avulsion, the tooth was kept under ideal conditions and replanted within about 2 hours. The tooth should be radiographed about 3 weeks after replantation and at 3–4 week intervals afterwards. Thermal or electric pulp testing is not useful during this early stage, and the need for endodontic treatment is determined from clinical signs and symptoms or from the radiological diagnosis of external root resorption. Pulpectomy and root filling with calcium hydroxide should be carried out at the first sign of root resorption. In immature teeth that remain vital after replantation, a response to pulp testing may be elicited after 1–2 months.

Intruded immature teeth that are being extruded orthodontically or allowed to re-erupt (p. 216) should likewise be treated by pulpectomy and root filling with calcium hydroxide at the first radiological sign of root resorption.

29.4 PARTIAL PULPECTOMY

Sometimes an immature tooth is assessed as being dead but, on proceeding with pulpectomy, vital pulp tissue is encountered at some point in the root canal. The alternative courses of action (after achieving local analgesia) are either to proceed with pulpectomy or to resect the pulp at the level of the vital tissue. The latter approach allows vital apical tissue to remain, in the hope that further root development will occur; this constitutes a partial pulpectomy, and is especially desirable when the walls of the root apex are divergent or parallel. The root of canal up to the vital tissue is filled with calcium hydroxide paste. If subsequent radiographs show no further root development, suggesting death of the apical pulp, full pulpectomy can be performed, as described above.

Technique: pulpectomy of an immature tooth

Procedure	Method	Rationale	Notes
1. Prepare instruments and materials	Ideally, use a pre-packed sterile tray containing all the necessary instruments and materials.		
2. Prepare the site of operation	Place rubber dam (unless there is good reason for not doing so).	Rubber dam ensures good isolation from saliva and eliminates the risk of the patient, particularly if supine, swallowing or inhaling a reamer or other instrument if it should accidentally be dropped into the mouth.	If rubber dam is not used, isolation must be obtained with cotton wool rolls and saliva ejector, and the patient must be protected by using a 'parachute harness' attached to reamers and files.
3. Gain access to the pulp chamber	Use a diamond or tungsten carbide bur at high speed to outline the access cavity in the palatal surface of the tooth (Fig. 29.10a). Prepare this cavity in dentine but do not extend into the pulp. Make the cavity large enough to permit good access to the pulp chamber, and extend it over the region of the pulp horns (Fig. 29.10b). Dry the area, and then wipe the tooth, adjacent teeth and rubber dam with a cotton wool pledget soaked in hibitane solution (1:1000) or other antiseptic. Using a sterile round bur (size 4–6) deepen the access cavity until pulp is exposed. Either with the same bur or with a similar sized fissure bur, remove the entire roof of the pulp chamber (Fig. 29.10c).	Good access is essential for successful root canal therapy. All instrumentation from this stage must be under sterile conditions; although the necrotic pulp is infected, introduction of further infection should be avoided.	
4. Eliminate the cervical construction of the root canal	With a flame-shaped or tapered fissure bur in a slow-speed handpiece, open out the constricted area to the diameter of the canal immediately apical to it (Fig. 29.10d).	Removal of the cervical construction is necessary to ensure access to all of the radicular pulp.	

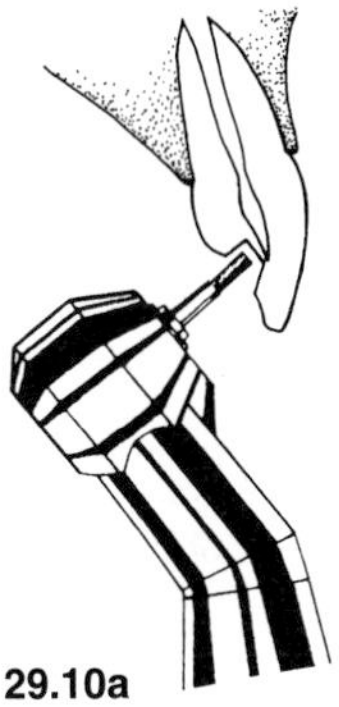

Fig. 29.10a

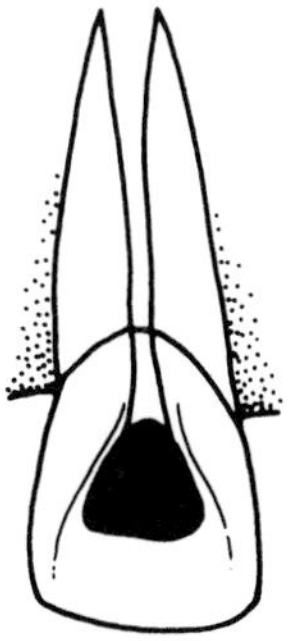

Fig. 29.10b 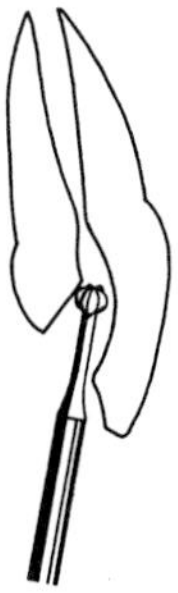   **Fig. 29.10c**

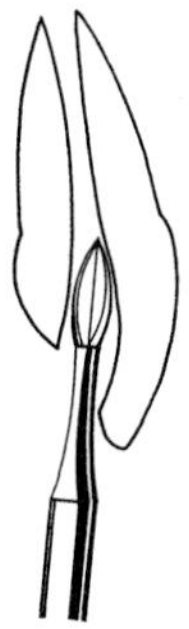

Fig. 29.10d

Technique: pulpectomy of an immature tooth *(contd)*

Procedure	Method	Rationale	Notes
5. Determine the length of the root canal	Place a reamer to the estimated length of the canal (judged from a pre-operative radiograph); support it in position with soft wax or warm gutta-percha, and obtain a periapical radiograph.	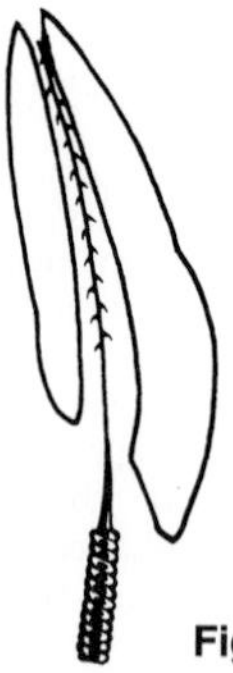	If vital tissue is encountered before reaching the root apex, partial pulpectomy may be performed (p. 230).
6. Extirpate the necrotic pulp	Use barbed broaches and/or reamers to extirpate the necrotic pulp tissue (Fig. 29.10e). Before inserting a broach or reamer into the canal, mark it in some way so that the distance from the mark to its tip is 1–2 mm less than the estimated length of the tooth. Insert each instrument until the mark is level with the incisal edge of the tooth.	The periapical tissues must not be traumatized.	Various methods may be used to mark the working length of root canal instruments.
7. File the walls of the root canal	Use files to cleanse the walls of the root canal, again to 1–2 mm of the root apex (Fig. 29.10f). Work carefully and methodically around the canal.	The use of files is essential because the root canal is not circular in cross-section. 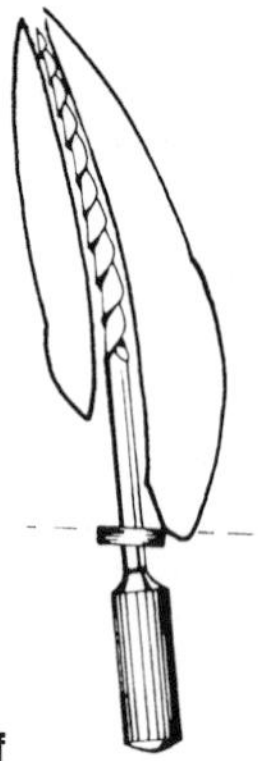	Meticulous mechanical cleansing of the root canal is crucial to the success of the treatment. 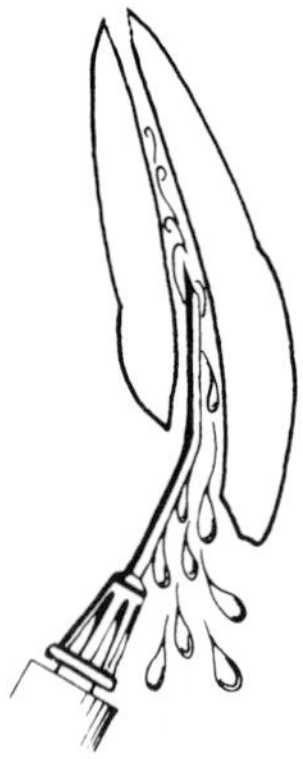
8. Wash the canal	Use a syringe containing sterile water or saline (Fig. 29.10g). Place the needle of the syringe at least half way up the canal; while syringing, hold the nozzle of a high-volume aspirator close to the palatal cavity in the tooth.	Simultaneous syringing and aspirating removes necrotic tissue from the canal.	The canal should be syringed several times during the filing procedure. 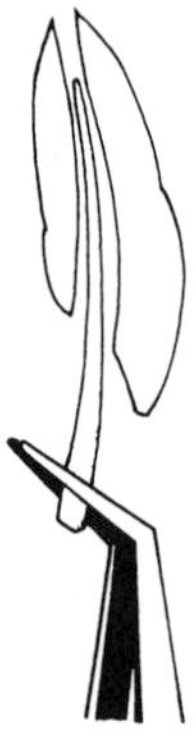
9. Dry the canal	Use absorbent paper points to dry the canal (Fig. 28.10h).		Large-diameter paper points are available, which are useful when drying wide root canals.

Fig. 29.10e

Fig. 29.10f

Fig. 29.10g

Fig. 29.10h

Technique: pulpectomy of an immature tooth *(contd)*

Procedure	Method	Rationale	Notes
10. Fill the canal with calcium hydroxide paste	Use a rotary filling instrument in a slow-speed handpiece (Fig. 29.10i). Mark it as above so that its tip will reach to 1–2 mm short of the root apex.	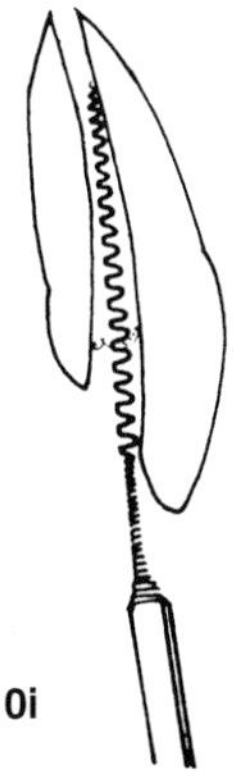	An alternative method is to use a proprietary material supplied in a cartridge that is loaded into a special syringe, so that the calcium hydroxide can be injected into the canal.
	Prepare a stiff mix of calcium hydroxide powder and sterile water, or use a proprietary material. Pick up some paste along the length of the rotary filler; do not pick up too much.	If a large bulk of paste is picked up, it is difficult to carry it beyond the entrance of the root canal.	A non-setting type of calcium hydroxide paste should be used so that it can easily be washed out of the canal when required.
	With the handpiece stationary, insert the filler into the canal and place it in light contact with the canal wall. Run the handpiece at slow speed in the forward direction while withdrawing the filler slowly from the canal; aim to deposit paste in the canal, not to spin it up. Repeat the procedure as often as is necessary to fill the canal completely.	Inserting the filler with the handpiece stationary avoids the risk of the filler jamming and fracturing.	Some types of rotary filler have a flexible connection between spiral and shank; this design greatly reduces the risk of fracture.
		If paste is spun up the canal it may pass into the periapical tissues.	Although calcium hydroxide introduced periapically becomes absorbed, the aim in this technique is to keep it within the root canal.
11. Seal the cavity	See 'vital pulpotomy' (Ch. 28).		

Fig. 29.10i

FOLLOW-UP

Check after 1 month, and then at 3- or 6-month intervals.

Radiograph 6-monthly to check for evidence of calcific barrier formation or continued root development. After 6 months, the calcium hydroxide may be washed out with sterile water or saline, and the presence of an apical barrier tested gently with a reamer or gutta-percha point. The canal may then either be refilled with calcium hydroxide for a further 6 months or filled with gutta-percha as described on page 230.

29.5 RETROGRADE ROOT CANAL FILLING

The recommended method of treating an immature, non-vital tooth is by pulpectomy and temporary root filling with calcium hydroxide, as described above. However, the alternative approach is retrograde root filling, which involves surgery to expose the root apex followed by sealing of the apex, usually with amalgam. The rest of the canal should previously have been filled with a dental cement (e.g. zinc oxide-eugenol), either at the time of operation (using a quick-setting material) or on the previous treatment visit; the amalgam can then be packed down on to the cement, and the whole of the canal is effectively obturated.

The principal disadvantage of this approach is that it is much more unpleasant for the child than the conservative approach described previously. Since conservative endodontic treatment is usually effective, there seems to be no justification for preferring the surgical approach. However, when periapical infection persists despite repeated attempts to control it by conservative methods, surgery may be the only solution if the tooth is to be saved; retrograde root filling is then accompanied by curettage of the infected periapical bone.

29.6 BLEACHING OF DISCOLOURED PULPLESS TEETH

Teeth that have received root canal treatment often become discoloured as a result of either haemolysis following diffusion of blood into dentinal tubules during pulpectomy, or decomposition of pulp tissue that was not removed from the pulp chamber. Haemorrhage during pulpectomy of a vital pulp is inevitable, but every effort should be made to wash blood from the root canal and pulp chamber. Incomplete removal of pulp usually results from making inadequate access to the pulp chamber.

There are several treatment alternatives for a discoloured root-filled tooth: bleaching the crown, covering the labial surface with a composite or porcelain veneer (p. 145–146); or, as a last resort, cutting off the crown and making a porcelain jacket crown on a post and core.

In the past, bleaching techniques involved applying concentrated hydrogen peroxide solution (30% w/v)

on a cotton wool pledget into the pulp chamber and then activating it with heat or ultraviolet light for 20–30 minutes (Grossman 1978, Howell 1980). The technique now used most commonly (described below) involves sealing a paste of sodium perborate and hydrogen peroxide in the pulp chamber for 1 or more weeks (Nutting & Poe 1967); the application of heat or light is not necessary. No studies have been conducted to compare the effectiveness of these methods, but the latter is certainly less time-consuming.

The use of hydrogen peroxide has been implicated as a cause of external root resorption that has sometimes been noted following bleaching procedures (Cvek & Lindvall 1985). In order to avoid this, Holmstrup et al (1988) used only sodium perborate as the bleaching agent, and reported good results and no evidence of root resorption after 3 years. Their technique was similar to that described below, but the sodium perborate was placed in the pulp chamber using an amalgam carrier, and lightly condensed with a moist cotton wool pledget.

Technique: bleaching

1. Isolate the tooth with rubber dam.
2. Remove all filling materials from the pulp chamber. Remove also about 2 or 3 mm of root canal filling to expose dentine in the cervical region of the tooth (at least on the labial side).
3. Inspect the periphery of the palatal cavity. If it does not allow excellent access to all parts of the pulp chamber, extend the cavity.
4. Clean the wall of the pulp chamber with a large round bur, removing any obvious stains.
5. Check that the root canal is well sealed. If in doubt, apply a small amount of quick-setting cement.
6. Swab the walls of the pulp chamber with a cotton wool pledget soaked in chloroform; this dissolves fatty substances produced during pulp decomposition, which would interfere with the penetration of hydrogen peroxide solution.
7. Dehydrate the dentine by swabbing with 100% ethyl alcohol, and dry thoroughly with compressed air; this aids the penetration of hydrogen peroxide solution.
8. Mix 1–2 drops of hydrogen peroxide solution and powdered sodium perborate to make a thick paste. Bocasan (Oral B Laboratories) is a convenient source of sodium perborate. Hydrogen peroxide solution must be handled with care because it is extremely irritant.
9. Fill the pulp chamber with paste. Alternatively, to facilitate removal, the paste may be incorporated into a cotton wool pledget.
10. Seal the pulp chamber with a quick-setting zinc oxide cement.
11. Assess in about 1 week. If necessary, repeat the treatment; it is desirable to overbleach slightly because some darkening usually follows.
12. When the bleaching treatment is completed, fill the palatal cavity with composite resin.

REFERENCES

Anderson R W, Pantera E A 1988 Influence of the barrier technique on electric pulp testing. Journal of Endodontic 14: 179–180

Bhaskar S N, Rappaport H M 1973 Dental vitality tests and pulp status. Journal of the American Dental Association 86: 409–411

Chambers I G 1982 The role and methods of pulp testing in oral diagnosis: a review. International Endodontic Journal 15: 1–5

Cooley R L, Lubow R M 1984 Evaluation of a digital pulp tester. Oral Surgery, Oral Medicine and Oral Pathology 58: 437–442

Cvek M 1993 Prognosis of luxated non-vital maxillary incisors treated with calcium hydroxide and filled with gutta-percha. Endodontics and Dental Traumatology 8: 45–55

Cvek M, Hollender I, Nord C E 1976 Treatment of non-vital permanent incisors with calcium hydroxide VI: a clinical, microbiological and radiological evaluation of treatment in one sitting of teeth with mature or immature roots.

Cvek M, Lindvall A-M 1985 External root resorption following bleaching of pulpless teeth with hydrogen peroxide. Endodontics and Dental Traumatology 1: 56–60

Drummer P M H, Tanner M, McCarthy J P 1986 A laboratory study of four electric pulp testers. International Endodontic Journal 19: 161–171

Grossman L I 1978 Endodontic practice, 9th edn. Lea & Febiger, Philadelphia, ch 18

Heithersay G S 1970 Study of root formation in incompletely developed pulpless teeth. Oral Surgery, Oral Medicine and Oral Pathology 29: 620–630

Holan G 1993 Influence of wearing latex gloves on electric pulp tester readings in children. International Journal of Paediatric Dentistry 3: 199–204

Holmstrup G, Palm A M, Lambjerg-Hansen H 1988 Bleaching of discoloured root-filled teeth. Endodontics and Dental Traumatology 4: 197–201

Howell R A 1980 Bleaching discoloured root-filled teeth. British Dental Journal 148: 159–162

King D R, King A C 1977 Use of the vitalometer with rubber gloves. Journal of the Canadian Dental Association 43: 182, 186

Kolbinson D A, Teplitsky P E 1988 Electric pulp testing with examination gloves. Oral Surgery testing with examination gloves. Oral Surgery, Oral Medicine and Oral Pathology 65: 122–126

Mackie I C, Bentley E M, Worthington H 1988 The closure of open spices in non-vital immature incisor teeth. British Dental Journal 165: 169–173

Matthews B, Searle B N 1974 Some observations on pulp testers. British Dental Journal 173: 307–312

Nutting E B, Poe G S 1967 Chemical Bleaching of discoloured endodontically treated teeth. Dental Clinics of North America (Nov) 655–662

Rock W P, Gordon P H, Friend L A, Grundy M C 1974 The relationship between trauma and pulp death in incisor teeth. British Dental Journal 136: 236–239

RECOMMENDED READING

Andreasen J O, Andreasen F M 1994 Textbook and color atlas of traumatic injuries to the teeth, 3rd edn. Munksgaard, Copenhagen

30 Trauma to primary teeth

The 1973 survey of child dental health in England and Wales reported that 8% of 5-year-old children showed signs of having suffered trauma to primary incisors (Todd 1975); the second and third national surveys in 1983 and 1993 did not include an examination for injuries to primary teeth. The most common results of trauma are loosening of the teeth (with or without displacement), intrusion and avulsion; crown or root fractures are rare (Ravn 1968).

30.1 LOOSENED (SUBLUXATED) OR DISPLACED (LUXATED) PRIMARY TEETH

Loosening of primary incisors (especially maxillary incisors) is a common injury of toddlers unsteady on their feet. Splinting of loosened teeth is difficult if not impossible in such young children, but fortunately periodontal reattachment usually occurs rapidly without splinting. If the tooth is displaced labially or palatally (and is not so loose as to require extraction) it should be repositioned by gentle finger pressure. Parents should be advised to provide a soft diet and to discourage the child from disturbing the tooth.

Intrusion and avulsion are more severe forms of displacement. An intruded primary tooth requires no immediate treatment because it usually re-erupts within a few weeks and attains its original position within 6 months (Ravn 1976). It is necessary to reassure the parents, to advise them to keep the area clean by gentle swabbing with warm antiseptic solution, and to inform them (while attempting not to alarm them) of the possibility that the permanent successor may have been damaged and that the primary tooth may require further treatment (see below). Appointments should be arranged at monthly intervals to assess re-eruption and pulp vitality of the primary tooth. Radiography to investigate possible damage that might affect the eruption of the permanent successor may be delayed until the child is about 7 years of age.

Although it is possible to replant an avulsed primary tooth (Mueller & Whitsett 1978) this is rarely done because of inadequate patient cooperation and the difficulty of splinting satisfactorily.

30.2 CROWN OR ROOT FRACTURES

In the rare cases of crown fracture, ideal treatment involving pulp protection or pulp treatment (as described for permanent teeth) may not be feasible because of inadequate cooperation from the child. Teeth with fractures not involving pulp may survive without treatment and may therefore be kept under supervision, but those fractured through pulp must be extracted if the appropriate pulp treatment cannot be performed.

The usual treatment for the very rare cases of root fracture is extraction, but teeth with apical- or middle-third root fractures may be kept under observation.

Loss of a primary incisor is distressing for the child and parents, but not as socially unacceptable as is the absence of a permanent incisor. A prosthetic replacement is therefore not usually demanded, nor is space maintenance necessary because loss of a primary incisor does not usually result in drifting of adjacent teeth into the space.

30.3 DAMAGE TO PERMANENT SUCCESSORS

A serious aspect of trauma to primary teeth is the damage that may be caused to the developing permanent successor, by either direct trauma associated with intrusion; labial displacement or avulsion of a primary tooth; or infection spreading from a non-vital primary tooth.

The most common forms of damage are hypoplasia and hypomineralization (Andreasen & Ravn 1971, von Arx 1993) which become apparent when the permanent tooth erupts. Since maxillary permanent incisors develop palatal to the roots of the primary incisors, it is the labial surfaces of the permanent teeth that are primarily affected. Mineralization of the crowns of permanent incisors begins 3–4 months after birth and is complete by about 4–5 years, and the position of the band or area of hypoplasia/hypomineralization on the labial surface reflects the age of the child when the trauma occurred. In general the more severe the injury and the younger the child the greater the chance that hypoplasia rather than hypomineralization will be the predominant form of damage.

Less common forms of damage are dilaceration (p. 152), odontome-like malformations, and arrested root development of the permanent successor, which may be detected by radiography when the child is about 7 years of age. There is no advantage in obtaining this information earlier.

The most severe types of injury to primary teeth are avulsion and intrusion. Damage to permanent successors is caused in almost all cases if avulsion occurs when the child is less than 2 years old, in about 80% of cases if it occurs between the ages of 2 and 4 years, and in only about 18% of cases when the child is over 5 years old (Ravn 1975). Intrusion of a primary tooth occurs mainly in children under 4 years of age and causes damage to permanent successors in 54% of cases (Ravn 1976).

30.4 NON-VITAL PRIMARY INCISORS

If a traumatized primary tooth subsequently dies, associated periapical infection may cause hypomineralization or hypoplasia of the developing permanent tooth crown; therefore traumatized teeth must be monitored closely. Unfortunately pulp testing may not give reliable results with a young child and radiographs are often unhelpful because of superimposition of the developing permanent tooth over the root of the primary tooth. The assessment of pulp death therefore depends largely on symptoms of pain and on clinical signs. The appearance of a sinus on the gingiva buccal to the root of the primary tooth is a certain sign of pulp death. The development of a blue-grey discoloration of the crown of the primary tooth suggests but does not invariably indicate pulp death, and a yellow discoloration is a sign of pulp calcification but not necessarily of pulp death. Many discoloured primary incisors remain symptomless and exfoliate normally (Jacobsen & Sangnes 1978). On the other hand, it is probable that the majority of such teeth have necrotic or chronically inflamed pulps (Soxman et al 1984), which may give rise to periapical infection, which in turn may affect the developing permanent successor; this risk is greatest in a child under the age of 4 years, when the crown of the permanent tooth is still developing.

Treatment

If discoloration of the tooth is the only sign suggesting pulp death, but there is no sinus in the labial sulcus or other signs or symptoms, it is reasonable to carry out no treatment, but to review the teeth regularly and inform the parents that treatment will be required if more definite signs of infection appear. If signs or symptoms indicate the presence of infection, the tooth must either be extracted or receive endodontic treatment. For young children, some compromise of ideal endodontic technique is usually necessary and justifiable.

1. Having made an adequate access cavity in the palatal surface, a small straight-shanked excavator may be used to remove pulp from the pulp chamber and root canal. Ideally this should be followed by mechanical cleansing of the canal with an endodontic file.
2. The length of the canal may have to be estimated roughly from a pre-operative radiograph; it may not be practicable to take another radiograph with an instrument in place in the canal to determine root length exactly.
3. Having sealed a cotton wool pledget soaked with disinfectant solution (e.g. formocresol, beechwood creosote or camphorated parachlorophenol) in the pulp chamber for 1–2 weeks, a resorbable material (e.g. zinc oxide-eugenol or iodoform should be used to fill the root canal).

The child's compliance is, of course, required, but this technique is simple enough to avoid causing distress. Local analgesia is not required and the operative procedures are quick and simple. A parent's support is often helpful, as illustrated in Fig. 1.1 on page 7. If the treatment succeeds the child will have been spared the more distressing experience of extraction under local or general anaesthesia. If it fails, however, there is a risk that associated periapical infection might damage the developing permanent successors.

REFERENCES

Andreasen J O, Ravn J J 1971 The effect of traumatic injuries to primary teeth or their permanent successors. II: a clinical and radiographic follow-up study of 213 teeth. Scandinavian Journal of Dental Research 79: 284–294

Jacobsen I, Sangnes G 1978 Traumatized primary anterior teeth: prognosis related to calcific reactions in the pulp cavity. Acta Odontologica Scandinavica 36: 199–204

Mueller B H, Whitsett B D 1978 Management of an avulsed deciduous incisor: report of case. Oral Surgery, Oral Medicine and Oral Pathology 46: 442–446

Ravn J J 1968 Sequelae of acute mechanical traumata in the primary dentition. Journal of Dentistry for Children 35: 281–289

Ravn J J 1975 Developmental disturbances in permanent teeth after exarticulation of their primary predecessors. Scandinavian Journal of Dental Research 83: 137–141

Ravn J J 1976 Development disturbances in permanent teeth after intrusion of their primary predecessors. Scandinavian Journal of Dental Research 84: 131–134

Soxman J A, Nazif M M, Bouquot J 1984 Pulpal pathology in relation to discoloration of primary anterior teeth. Journal of Dentistry for Children 51: 282–284

Todd J E 1975 Children's dental health in England and Wales 1973. Her Majesty's Stationery Office, London, p 44

von Arx T 1993 Developmental disturbances of permanent teeth following trauma to the primary dentition. Australian Dental Journal 38: 1–10

31 Non-accidental injuries to children

In 1995, child-protection registers in England recorded 12 900 children in categories of non-accidental injury involving physical abuse (Department of Health 1995). Most cases of non-accidental injury (NAI) do not come to the attention of a dentist, but 65% of injuries involve the face or head (Becker et al 1978), and dentists are therefore in a position to assist others in the detection and management of NAI. A particularly distressing feature is the frequency of repeated attacks, with injuries tending to become more serious, and this emphasizes the importance of early diagnosis. Many dentists are unaware of their legal and social responsibilities with respect to child abuse, and are reluctant to report suspected cases.

31.1 CLINICAL SIGNS

1. *Facial bruising*, especially if bilateral. Bruises of different colours indicate injuries that have been inflicted on more than one occasion. Fingertip-sized bruises may be found over bony prominences such as the forehead, zygoma and mandible. Blows around the eyes may produce orbital haematomas ('black eyes'). Bruised or swollen lips, or abrasions at the corners of the mouth, are suggestive of blows from a fist.
2. *Severe head injuries.* Superficial scalp bruising may indicate more serious underlying damage. Intracranial bleeding may produce a subdural haematoma, which causes headache, drowsiness and vomiting. Injuries to the scalp must be investigated by radiography to exclude the possibility of skull fracture.
3. *Burns.* Facial burns caused by hot solid objects are common, but cigarette burns are more common on the limbs and trunk. The typical circular outline of a cigarette burn is easily recognized. A recent burn will be a raw weeping wound; this is later covered by a scab, and further healing produces a depressed and puckered scar.
4. *Bite marks.* These are found most commonly on the limbs, but are sometimes found on the face. Careful study of the marks will usually reveal whether they were inflicted by a child or an adult (Sims et al 1973).
5. *Laceration of labial mucosa*, especially of the upper lip, often involving tearing of the labial frenum, may be caused by aggressive bottle feeding or by forcing a spoon into the child's mouth.
6. *Fractured or displaced teeth*, often associated with alveolar fracture, if the history of the injury is unconvincing.

31.2 DIAGNOSIS

If clinical signs suggest the possibility of NAI, it is most important to obtain a detailed history from the parent or guardian and later, if possible, to question the child separately. Parents must not be challenged directly but questioned gently and tactfully to avoid antagonizing them. It may be difficult not to appear critical but it must be borne in mind that the parents may themselves be in great need of care and attention. Most parents who injure their children are poor and socially deprived, and may also have been unloved and abused during childhood (Sims 1985).

Suspicion of NAI is increased if there is a discrepancy between the history given by the parents and the clinical signs; if there has been delay in bringing the child for treatment; if replies to questions are inadequate or evasive; if there is evidence that injuries have been suffered on more than one occasion; and if the child is dirty and appears generally neglected.

31.3 MANAGEMENT

Health authorities have established guidelines for dealing with suspected cases of NAI. The recommended procedures include the following:

1. Perform emergency treatment of dental and soft tissue injuries, and prescribe antibiotic and antitetanus toxoid if necessary.
2. a. *If there is only a suspicion of NAI:* contact the family's doctor or a hospital paediatrician immediately by telephone, and arrange for the child to have a full medical examination. Explain the need for this examination to the parents in a careful and tactful manner, to avoid arousing their suspicion that child abuse is suspected.

   Check later that the parents took the child for examination. If they did not, suspicion of NAI would be strengthened and the local social services department should be informed immediately. The local administrative dental or medical officer would help, if required, in contacting the appropriate agency and in giving general advice. Every health authority maintains a child abuse register; telephone to enquire whether the child is on the register.

   b. *If there is strong evidence of NAI:* arrange for the child to be admitted immediately to a hospital. Ideally, arrange for an ambulance to take the child and the parents to the hospital. Alternatively, escort them personally or arrange for a colleague to do so. Hospital personnel will then be responsible for notifying the social services department.

   Admission to hospital is necessary to ensure the safety of the child while medical and social investigations are undertaken. When investigations and enquiries are complete, a case conference is convened for doctors, social workers, health visitors, and any other professional workers involved in the case, such as the dentist. It is therefore most important that the dentist keeps a detailed record of the child's injuries and of the history given by the parents. A decision is made either to return the child home and give the parents the support they need, or to place the child under local authority care.

Child abuse is most distressing and its causes are complex. Management of suspected cases requires tact and understanding by all professional staff, including the dentist. The most difficult cases to deal with are those in which there is only a suspicion of NAI, when investigation may be hampered by the scepticism of professional colleagues. However, it is better to risk being rebuffed and proved wrong than to risk exposing the child to further suffering.

REFERENCES

Becker D B, Needleman H L, Kotelchuck M 1978 Child abuse and dentistry: orofacial trauma and its recognition by dentists. Journal of the American Dental Association 97: 24–28

Department of Health 1995 Children and young people on child-protection registers: England. Government Statistical Service, London

Sims A P T 1985 Non-accidental injury in the child presenting as a suspected fracture of the zygomatic arch. British Dental Journal 158: 282–293

Sims B G, Grant J H, Cameron J M 1973 Bite marks in the battered baby syndrome. Medicine, Science and the Law 13: 207–210

RECOMMENDED READING

MacIntyre D R, Jones D M, Pinckney R C N 1986 The role of the dental practitioner in the management of non-accidental injury to children. British Dental Journal 161: 108–110

McDonald R E, Badger G R, Needleman H L 1988 Child abuse and neglect. Pediatric Dentistry 8 (special issue 1): 66–121

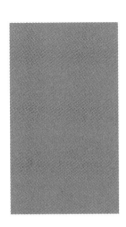

Appendix 1: Bur numbering system

In this book the UK bur numbering system is used when referring to burs. The equivalent numbers by the international and USA systems are given below:

	0.60	0.80	0.90	1.00	1.20	1.40	1.60	1.80	2.10	2.30	2.50	2.70	2.90	3.10
	Maximum diameter of bur head (mm)													
ISO*	006	008	009	010	012	014	016	018	021	023	025	027	029	031
United Kingdom														
Round	$\frac{1}{2}$	1		2	3	4	5	6	7	8	9	10	11	12
Inverted cone	$\frac{1}{2}$	1		2	3	4	5	6	7	8	9	10		
Flat fissure														
(plain & cross cut)		$\frac{1}{2}$	1	2	3	4	5	6	7	8	9	10	11	12
Tapered fissure (plain cut)				2	3		5							
Tapered fissure (cross cut)				700	701		702		703					
USA														
Round	$\frac{1}{2}$	1		2	3	4	5	6	7	8	9	10		
Inverted cone	$33\frac{1}{2}$	34	$34\frac{1}{2}$	35	36	37	38	39	40	41	42	43		
Flat fissure (plain cut)		55	56	57	58	59	60	61						
Flat fissure (cross cut)	$555\frac{1}{2}$	556		557	558	559	560	561	562	563				
Tapered fissure (plain cut)		168	169	170	171		172		173					
Tapered fissure (cross cut)		669		700	701		702		703					

*International Organisation for Standardisation

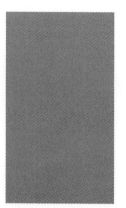

Appendix 2: Antibiotic prophylaxis of infective endocarditis before tooth extraction, scaling or periodontal surgery

Approved by the Endocarditis Working Party of the British Society for Antimicrobial Chemotherapy and by the Dental Formulary Subcommittee, 1995.

LOCAL OR NO ANAESTHESIA

Allergic to penicillin or
received penicillin more than
once in previous month?

NO	YES

amoxycillin
3 g orally 1 hr pre-op.
Child < 10 years: $\frac{1}{2}$ adult dose
< 5 years: $\frac{1}{4}$ adult dose

clindamycin
600 mg orally 1 hr pre-op.
Child < 10 years: $\frac{1}{2}$ adult dose
< 5 years: $\frac{1}{4}$ adult dose

GENERAL ANAESTHESIA
(Refer patient to a hospital dental department)

Special risk*?

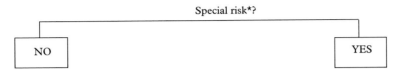

| NO | YES |

NO branch:

NOT allergic to penicillin
or received penicillin more
than once in previous month

amoxycillin
1 g in 2.5 ml 1% lignocaine
intramuscularly or intravenously at induction
+ 500 mg orally 6 hr later
Child < 10 yr: $\frac{1}{2}$ adult dose
< 5 yr: $\frac{1}{4}$ adult dose

or

amoxycillin
3 g orally 4 hr pre-op.
+ 3 g orally as soon as possible post-op.
Child < 10 yr: $\frac{1}{2}$ adult dose
< 5 yr: $\frac{1}{4}$ adult dose

YES branch:

Allergic to penicillin or
received penicillin more than
once in previous moth?

| NO | YES |

YES → NO:

amoxycillin
1 g in 2.5 ml 1% lignocaine
intramuscularly or intravenously
+ gentamicin
120 mg intramuscularly or
intravenously at induction
+ amoxycillin
500 mg orally 6 hr later
Child < 10 yr: amoxycillin $\frac{1}{2}$ adult dose
gentamicin 2 mg/kg
< 5 yr: amoxycillin $\frac{1}{4}$ adult dose
gentamicin 2 mg/kg

YES → YES:

vancomycin
1 g intravenously over
at least 100 min,
followed by
gentamicin
120 g intravenously
at induction
or 15 min pre-op.
Child < 10 yr:
vancomycin 20 mg/kg,
gentamicin 2 mg/kg

or

teicoplanin 400 mg
+ gentamicin 120 mg
intravenously at induction
or 15 min pre-op.
Child < 14 yr: teicoplanin
6 mg/kg, gentamicin 2 mg/kg

or

clindamycin
300 mg intravenously over at
least 10 min at induction or
15 min pre-op.
followed by
clindamycin
15 mg orally or intravenously
6 hr later
Child < 10 yr: $\frac{1}{2}$ adult dose
< 5 yr: $\frac{1}{4}$ adult dose

* Special risk – previous endocarditis, prosthetic heart valve

Index